Diagnostic Endometrial Pathology

SECOND EDITION

Diagnostic Endometrial Pathology

SECOND EDITION

T. Yee Khong, MD, FRCPath, FRCPA
Department of Anatomical Pathology
Women's and Children's Hospital, North Adelaide, Australia
and
Clinical Professor, University of Adelaide, Australia

Annie N. Y. Cheung, MBBS, MD, PhD, FRCPath, FHKAM(Path)
Laurence LT Hou Professor in Anatomical Molecular Pathology
Clinical Professor of Pathology, The University of Hong Kong
Hong Kong, China

Wenxin Zheng, MD, FCAP
Mark and Jane Gibson Distinguished Professor in Cancer Research
Professor of Pathology, Obstetrics and Gynecology
University of Texas Southwestern Medical Center, Dallas, Texas, USA

With contributions from

Richard Wing-Cheuk Wong, FRCPA
Department of Clinical Pathology, Pamela Youde Nethersole Eastern Hospital
The University of Hong Kong, Hong Kong, China
(Chapters 7 and 10)

Hao Chen, MD, PhD
Department of Pathology, University of Texas Southwestern Medical Center
Dallas, Texas, USA
(Chapters 8 and 9)

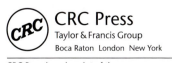

CRC Press is an imprint of the
Taylor & Francis Group, an **informa** business

CRC Press
Taylor & Francis Group
6000 Broken Sound Parkway NW, Suite 300
Boca Raton, FL 33487-2742

© 2019 by Taylor & Francis Group, LLC
CRC Press is an imprint of Taylor & Francis Group, an Informa business

No claim to original U.S. Government works

Printed on acid-free paper

Printed and bound in India by Replika Press Pvt. Ltd.

International Standard Book Number-13: 978-1-138-62641-6 (Hardback)

This book contains information obtained from authentic and highly regarded sources. While all reasonable efforts have been made to publish reliable data and information, neither the author[s] nor the publisher can accept any legal responsibility or liability for any errors or omissions that may be made. The publishers wish to make clear that any views or opinions expressed in this book by individual editors, authors or contributors are personal to them and do not necessarily reflect the views/opinions of the publishers. The information or guidance contained in this book is intended for use by medical, scientific or health-care professionals and is provided strictly as a supplement to the medical or other professional's own judgement, their knowledge of the patient's medical history, relevant manufacturer's instructions and the appropriate best practice guidelines. Because of the rapid advances in medical science, any information or advice on dosages, procedures or diagnoses should be independently verified. The reader is strongly urged to consult the relevant national drug formulary and the drug companies' and device or material manufacturers' printed instructions, and their websites, before administering or utilizing any of the drugs, devices or materials mentioned in this book. This book does not indicate whether a particular treatment is appropriate or suitable for a particular individual. Ultimately it is the sole responsibility of the medical professional to make his or her own professional judgements, so as to advise and treat patients appropriately. The authors and publishers have also attempted to trace the copyright holders of all material reproduced in this publication and apologize to copyright holders if permission to publish in this form has not been obtained. If any copyright material has not been acknowledged please write and let us know so we may rectify in any future reprint.

Except as permitted under U.S. Copyright Law, no part of this book may be reprinted, reproduced, transmitted, or utilized in any form by any electronic, mechanical, or other means, now known or hereafter invented, including photocopying, microfilming, and recording, or in any information storage or retrieval system, without written permission from the publishers.

For permission to photocopy or use material electronically from this work, please access www.copyright.com (http://www.copyright.com/) or contact the Copyright Clearance Center, Inc. (CCC), 222 Rosewood Drive, Danvers, MA 01923, 978-750-8400. CCC is a not-for-profit organization that provides licenses and registration for a variety of users. For organizations that have been granted a photocopy license by the CCC, a separate system of payment has been arranged.

Trademark Notice: Product or corporate names may be trademarks or registered trademarks, and are used only for identification and explanation without intent to infringe.

Library of Congress Cataloging-in-Publication Data

Names: Khong, T. Yee, author. | Cheung, Annie N. Y. author. | Zheng, Wenxin, author. | Wong, Richard Wing-Cheuk, contributor. | Chen, Hao, M.D., contributor.
Title: Diagnostic endometrial pathology / T. Yee Khong, Annie N.Y. Cheung, Wenxin Zheng ; with contributions from Richard Wing-Cheuk Wong, Hao Chen.
Other titles: Handbook of endometrial pathology
Description: 2e. | Boca Raton : CRC Press, 2018. | Preceded by Handbook of endometrial pathology / T. Yee Khong, Sezgin M. Ismail. 2005. | Includes bibliographical references and index.
Identifiers: LCCN 2018026101| ISBN 9781138626416 (hardback : alk. paper) | ISBN 9781315228686 (e-book)
Subjects: | MESH: Endometrium--pathology | Uterine Diseases--diagnosis | Diagnosis, Differential
Classification: LCC RG316 | NLM WP 400 | DDC 618.1/4--dc23
LC record available at https://lccn.loc.gov/2018026101

Visit the Taylor & Francis Web site at
http://www.taylorandfrancis.com

and the CRC Press Web site at
http://www.crcpress.com

Contents

Preface		vii
Preface to the first edition		ix
Acknowledgments		xi
Authors		xiii
1	Sampling the endometrium	1
2	The normal endometrium	7
3	Pregnancy	21
4	Endometrial inflammation	35
5	Functional abnormal uterine bleeding	43
6	Iatrogenic disease	47
7	Benign tumors and tumor-like conditions, including metaplasia	65
8	Endometrial premalignant lesions	91
9	Endometrial malignant lesions	113
10	Gestational trophoblastic disease	147
Index		175

Preface

The aim and scope of this book are similar to those of the first iteration, which was published as *Handbook of Endometrial Pathology*. This edition remains a working bench book, and we have retitled the book to emphasize the diagnostic aspects. To this end, we have incorporated the numerous advances in gynecological practice and in our knowledge of endometrial pathology.

T. Yee Khong
Adelaide, Australia

Annie N. Y. Cheung
Hong Kong, China

Wenxin Zheng
Dallas, Texas

Preface to the first edition

The endometrium is one of the most commonly examined tissues in anatomic pathology. In the past two decades, the literature on endometrial pathology has expanded exponentially. There have been many advances in our understanding of endometrial disease, and gynecological practice has changed enormously. Some of the literature is not as clear as it ought to be. Some of the concepts still in circulation are outdated or simply not clinically practical.

We have therefore written a bench book that, we believe, distils the literature in an accessible manner while retaining a practical histopathological outlook. For those lesions that cause much diagnostic difficulty, we have tried to emphasise not only the differential diagnosis but also the route to the diagnosis proper. We have also stressed the clinical correlates of the pathology to make this a clinically useful book. To this end, we have omitted some of the recent developments that remain of unproven utility.

We are both practicing pathologists in busy departments, and we think our experience complements each other's. The book is aimed at trainees and practicing histopathologists. Gynecologists should also benefit from it, as they would gain an understanding of how and why pathologists report the endometrium the way they do.

T. Yee Khong
Sez Ismail

Acknowledgments

We thank our colleagues for their support during the writing of this book. We acknowledge Sez Ismail for the use of some of the photomicrographs from the first edition.

We thank Miranda Bromage, editor (medicine), and the production team at CRC Press for their work and professionalism.

T. Yee Khong
Annie N. Y. Cheung
Wenxin Zheng

Authors

Professor T. Yee Khong: Dr Khong is a Clinical Professor in the Department of Pathology and Department of Obstetrics and Gynaecology, University of Adelaide, and is a Senior Consultant at SA Pathology in Women's and Children's Hospital, Adelaide. He graduated MBChB from University of Sheffield Medical School and MSc in Immunology from University of London. He gained his MD with a recommendation from the University of Sheffield. He did his pathology training at the Royal Free Hospital and St George's Hospital in London and at the John Radcliffe Hospital in Oxford, UK. Among his awards were the Edgar Research Fellowship, awarded by the Royal College of Obstetricians and Gynaecologists, and the American Cancer Society Eleanor Roosevelt International Cancer Research Fellowship, awarded by the International Union Against Cancer (UICC).

Professor Annie N. Y. Cheung: Professor Cheung is the Laurence L. T. Hou Professor of Anatomical Molecular Pathology and Clinical Professor in the Department of Pathology, University of Hong Kong (HKU). She is the key pathologist for gynaecological histopathology and cytology at Queen Mary Hospital, Director of the HKU Cervical Cytology Laboratory and the University Pathology Laboratory (Molecular Pathology) as well as the Chief of Service of Pathology, HKU-Shenzhen Hospital.

Professor Cheung was an HKU MBBS graduate and continued her studies at HKU for her MD and PhD. She received her postgraduate gynaecological pathology training at the University of Manchester, UK, Massachusetts General Hospital, Harvard Medical School and The Armed Forces Institute of Pathology, USA. Professor Cheung's research focuses on ovarian, endometrial and cervical cancers as well as gestational trophoblastic disease, aiming at investigating diagnostic and prognostic markers as well as molecular targets for better therapy.

Professor Cheung is currently a Standing Member of the Editorial Board of *WHO Classification of Tumours, 5th Edition*. She is also Advisor to the Executive Board of the Asian Oceania Research on Genital Infections and Neoplasia and immediate ex-president of the Hong Kong College of Pathologists. Professor Cheung has been President of the Hong Kong Society for Colposcopy and Cervical Pathology as well as a Council Member of the International Federation for Cervical Pathology and Colposcopy and a Council Member at Large of the International Society of Gynecological Pathologists.

Professor Wenxin Zheng: Dr Wenxin Zheng, tenured Professor of Pathology and tenured Professor of Obstetrics and Gynecology, University of Texas Southwestern Medical Center, is also the Mark and Jane Gibson Distinguished Professor in Cancer Research. Dr Zheng graduated from Shanghai Medical College, Fudan University. He completed his pathology residency training at Cornell University New York Hospital, his research fellowship at Columbia University (New York), and his gynecologic pathology fellowship at Brown University Women and Infants' Hospital (Rhode Island).

Dr Zheng has published more than 180 peer-reviewed articles in many prestigious scientific journals. His main scientific contributions include: (1) Defining and naming the precancerous lesion of endometrial serous carcinoma; (2) leading the research of endometrial serous carcinogenesis; (3) identifying the tubal origin of low-grade ovarian serous carcinoma; (4) defining the 'initial endometriosis' as the earliest recognizable endometriosis in the ovary; and (5) developing a 'one-stop cervical care' clinic for cervical cancer early detection and prevention.

Dr Zheng is a physician-scientist, who is an internationally well-recognized gynaecologic pathologist and consultant. Within the field of gynaecologic pathology, Dr Zheng served as the leading Editor-in-Chief for the book *Gynecologic and Obstetrics Pathology* both in Mandarin (Science Press, Beijing) and in English (Springer, Germany), which is one of the major gynecologic pathology textbooks in the field of gynecologic pathology.

Sampling the endometrium

Indications for sampling the endometrium	1	Tissue artifacts	3
Sampling of the endometrium	1	References	4
When is the endometrial tissue sufficient?	3		

INDICATIONS FOR SAMPLING THE ENDOMETRIUM

Among the many indications for sampling the endometrium, abnormal uterine bleeding is the commonest (Table 1.1). When used in conjunction with other techniques, histological examination of an endometrial sample may help to exclude significant endometrial pathology such as endometritis, hyperplasia or carcinoma. Age over 45 years as a cut-off has previously been a guideline for sampling the endometrium in order to detect atypical hyperplasia and cancer in premenopausal women with abnormal uterine bleeding. This may no longer be appropriate as obesity, resulting in relative unopposed estrogen, increases the risk of atypical hyperplasia or carcinoma and the cut-off may place women at risk of delayed or missed diagnosis.[1-3]

Transvaginal ultrasonography and hysteroscopy are increasingly being used in conjunction with endometrial biopsy for the evaluation of women with abnormal uterine bleeding. Transvaginal ultrasonography with assessment of endometrial thickness may determine which women would benefit from an endometrial biopsy; thresholds for endometrial thickness in relation to risk of endometrial hyperplasia and cancer appear to differ between symptomatic and asymptomatic women.[4,5] Under certain circumstances, hysteroscopy may help identify pathological lesions missed by blind endometrial biopsy and enable a directed biopsy of abnormal areas. Both transvaginal ultrasonography and hysteroscopy used together with endometrial biopsy can reassure the patient or physician that a negative biopsy is the result of an atrophic mucosa.

Table 1.1 Indications for sampling the endometrium

Premenopausal abnormal uterine bleeding
Postmenopausal bleeding
Screening
Infertility
Abnormal pregnancy

Endometrial sampling is carried out periodically in order to rule out malignancy and premalignant changes in the endometrium of asymptomatic women receiving postmenopausal hormone replacement or tamoxifen for breast cancer. Women at high risk of developing endometrial cancer, such as those with Lynch syndrome, may benefit from screening, although there is a lack of consensus as to optimal screening technique, and whether endometrial sampling should be included, frequency and age at which to commence screening.[6] Women with polycystic ovary syndrome are also monitored because of an increased risk of endometrial hyperplasia and cancer. The finding that asymptomatic, morbidly obese patients have a high prevalence of occult hyperplasia, associated with a relatively high hormone receptor expression, suggests that those women would also benefit from screening.[7]

Histological evaluation of endometrial biopsy is also carried out in the investigation of infertility.

Endometrial sampling, in addition to clinical history, examination and other tests, may be necessary for the detection of an intrauterine pregnancy when the diagnosis of an ectopic pregnancy is in doubt.[8]

SAMPLING OF THE ENDOMETRIUM

DILATATION AND CURETTAGE

The introduction of antiseptics allowed the procedure of cervical dilatation and endometrial curettage to become widespread. It is used also for the treatment of early pregnancy loss and for investigation of abnormal uterine bleeding.

Between 77% and 94% of such procedures have been reported to yield specimens deemed adequate for histological interpretation.[9] At a time when it was the practice to perform curettage prior to hysterectomy for ruling out unsuspected endometrial cancer, in 16% of 50 consecutive pre-hysterectomy curettage specimens, less than one-fourth of the cavity had been curetted, and in 60%, less than half

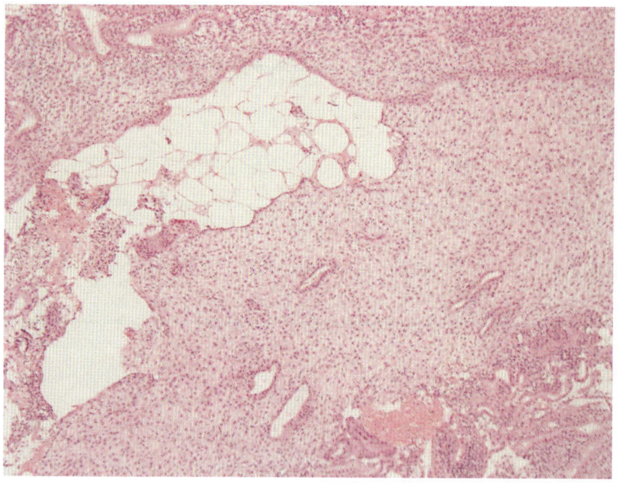

Figure 1.1 Adipose tissue admixed amongst endometrium may be derived from a uterine lipoleiomyoma, lipoma, adenolipoleiomyoma or liposarcoma but as these are rare, more critically, may indicate uterine perforation.

of the uterine cavity was sampled. However, recent appraisals support a high sensitivity of the method to detecting endometrial cancer in premenopausal and postmenopausal women.[10,11] Lesions that were missed most often were endometrial polyps, pedunculated submucous leiomyomas, endocervical polyps and placental polyps.

Dilatation and curettage necessitates hospital admission and involves an anesthetic risk. There is potential for infection and, especially in women who have not had children, trauma. Trauma can result in an incompetent cervix from excessive dilatation, uterine perforation and hemorrhage (Figure 1.1). As a result, it has largely been replaced by hysteroscopy and by office sampling methods.

OUTPATIENT SAMPLING BY ENDOMETRIAL ASPIRATE

Monitoring of the endometrium nowadays is often performed as an outpatient or office procedure with endometrial aspirate sampling.

Most instruments available for sampling the endometrium in an outpatient setting use a suction mechanism to sample the endometrial lining; these include the Vabra aspirator and Pipelle. Others, such as the Tao brush, rely on mechanical removal of the endometrium. The rates of perforation, infection and hemorrhage with an aspiration sampling technique are lower when compared with curettage.

One of the most commonly used devices is the Pipelle sampler and its variants. The Pipelle device is known to sample 4.2% of the endometrial surface area and, as expected with the low percentage, the sampling is distributed over a small fraction of the uterine surfaces. Pipelle biopsies provide limited diagnostic accuracy in cases with focal pathologies. The Tao brush is said to provide fewer insufficient specimens than the Pipelle method. Tissues obtained using the Tao brush have been interpreted by conventional histology, as well as by cytology, using either smear examination or liquid-based techniques.

Hysteroscopic-directed sampling may also be performed in the outpatient setting without general anesthetic or as a procedure in the hospital under local or general anesthetic. Hysteroscopy permits direct visualisation of the endometrium.

Comparison of these outpatient sampling methods with each other and with dilatation and curettage in terms of diagnostic accuracy is difficult. The more complete the first procedure for obtaining samples of endometrium, the less likely a second procedure is to produce tissue that will lead to the same diagnosis. Thus, the first procedure artificially reduces the diagnostic accuracy of the second. Furthermore, there are diagnostic limitations of the curettage biopsy itself. Comparison of the different sampling techniques is dependent also on the diagnostic outcome being interrogated: samples may be considered inadequate to reliably exclude hyperplasia but may be sufficient to exclude malignancy.

Endometrial tumors localized to a polyp or to a small area of endometrium may go undetected using outpatient endometrial-biopsy methods. As with a specimen obtained using a formal dilatation and curettage, polyps themselves may go undetected using these sampling techniques. In women with known endometrial carcinoma who were subjected to a Pipelle endometrial biopsy pre-hysterectomy, well-differentiated, low-volume and minimally invasive tumors, i.e. most early tumors, were likely to be misinterpreted. This may be due to sampling errors as well as to interpretative difficulties associated with smaller biopsies and would appear to preclude its use as a screening tool. Outpatient sampling of endometrial tumors is reliable in diagnosing endometrial cancer when an adequate specimen is obtained. A positive test result

> **SUMMARY BOX 1.1: Sampling the endometrium**
>
> Dilatation and curettage
>
> - Hospital admission procedure; has risk of infection and trauma
> - High sensitivity to detect endometrial cancer in premenopausal and postmenopausal women
> - May miss lesions such as polyps and pedunculated submucous leiomyomas
>
> Suction/aspiration sampling
>
> - Outpatient sampling; minimises trauma or infection risk
> - Smaller volume of tissue sampled than dilatation and curettage
> - Focal and small lesions may be missed, while early carcinomas may be misinterpreted
> - More useful when disease is identified; a negative result does not rule out pathology

is more accurate for ruling in disease than a negative test result is for ruling it out.

The histological subtyping and grading of endometrial carcinoma, particularly the endometrioid subtype, can be discrepant between pre-hysterectomy specimens, whether obtained by formal cervical dilatation and curettage or by outpatient endometrial sampling, and hysterectomy specimens.[12] Thus, treatment protocols based solely on pre-hysterectomy endometrial histology may result in inappropriate management (Summary Box 1.1).

WHEN IS THE ENDOMETRIAL TISSUE SUFFICIENT?

There are no agreed published criteria for an insufficient endometrial biopsy sample. The reported rate of insufficient samples range from 2% to 76%.[13] The quality of the specimen can be assessed on the quantity of the intact endometrium present and the lack of tissue fragmentation. These two factors mean that an adequate specimen is defined as one that is of sufficient size to determine the gland-to-stroma ratio and to demonstrate endometrial morphological features. Dimensions and numbers of intact strips of tissue have been used variably.[14,15]

Inadequate specimens more often arise in an outpatient office setting, such as using the aspiration Pipelle device. It is likely that this reflects the increasing use of these procedures in perimenopausal and postmenopausal women. Such specimens often contain blood and mucus with disaggregated fragments of surface or glandular epithelium with a variable quantity of stroma attached (Figure 1.2). The scanty material that is obtained with these methods should not be dismissed as being inadequate for histological diagnosis. Mitotic figures, even if only one is present, will confirm proliferative phase endometrium while secretory vacuoles will confirm secretory phase endometrium.

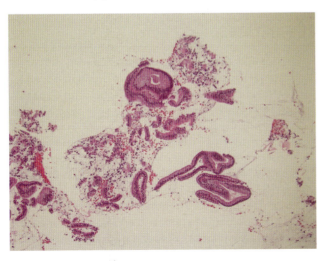

Figure 1.2 Inadequate endometrial Pipelle specimen with insufficient material to assess gland-stroma ratio or endometrial morphological features.

Some authors advocate the reporting of the tissue components that are present, including those that are non-endometrial in origin, and leave the decision of whether any follow-up is needed or not to the gynecologist.[16] The specimen received can be classified as being no tissue identified, tissue insufficient for diagnosis, no endometrium identified and endometrial tissue insufficient for diagnosis.

TISSUE ARTIFACTS

Several artifacts can ensue from procuring or processing of the specimen, but awareness of their possibility usually ensures that diagnostic errors are unlikely (Table 1.2).

Table 1.2 Tissue artifacts

Clots or blood obscuring pathological detail • Can be overcome using a lysis buffer/ethanol solution before applying conventional fixation techniques
Insufflation procedure during hysteroscopy or suction evacuations introducing air into tissue • Vacuolated spaces in blood or tissue mimicking fat vacuoles – pseudolipomatosis (Figure 1.3)[17] • Artifact should not to be mistaken for adipose tissue and erroneous overdiagnosis of uterine perforation
Impressions from biopsy bags for processing resulting in tic-tac-toe, serrated contour or elongated oval space artifacts • Reportedly present in as much as 60% of endometrial specimens • Focal and does not interfere with the diagnosis
Biopsy trauma compressing glands • Intussusception of the glands to produce a gland-within-gland appearance • Described as a telescoping effect • Complicated glandular pattern can lead to an initial impression of complex hyperplasia (Figures 1.4 and 1.5). Each glandular structure is, however, surrounded by a rim of normal glandular epithelium, thereby discounting the diagnosis of hyperplasia.
Traumatic disruption or fragmentation of the stroma • May result in glands appearing more crowded than normal or may be separated by clear space or blood • Careful examination will rule out an erroneous diagnosis of hyperplasia (Figure 1.6).
Poor or delayed fixation of specimen • Commonly encountered with hysterectomy specimens • Retraction of the stroma from the glands, leaving a halo-like space around the glands (Figure 1.7) • Does not normally create any diagnostic problems • Injecting formalin through the external cervical os into the endometrial cavity, or bivalving the specimen prior to immersion in formalin is effective in reducing the endometrial autolysis in hysterectomy specimens.

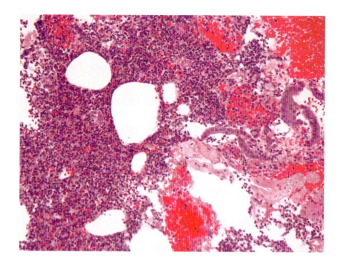

Figure 1.3 Pseudolipomatosis: Irregular clear vacuoles devoid of nuclei are seen within the inflamed tissue.

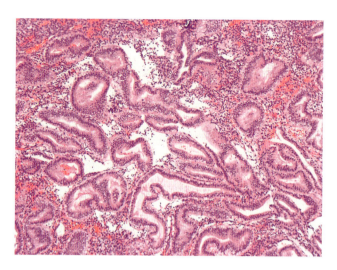

Figure 1.6 Artifactual crowding of glands resulting from artifactual stromal fragmentation.

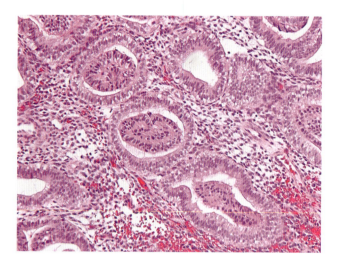

Figure 1.4 Telescoping effect of glands may simulate cribriform structures, where tumor cells grow within glandular lumina.

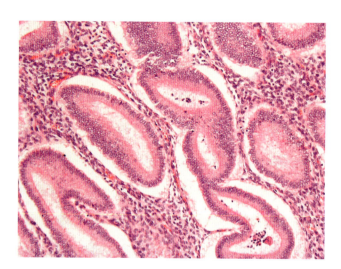

Figure 1.7 Retraction of stroma around glands to create an artifactual halo effect.

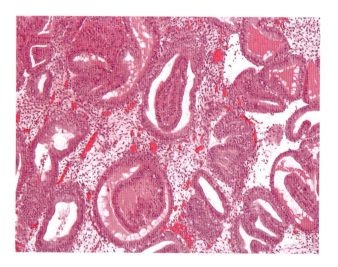

Figure 1.5 Gland-within-gland artifact may simulate glandular crowding.

REFERENCES

1. Wise MR, Jordan V, Lagas A et al. Obesity and endometrial hyperplasia and cancer in premenopausal women: A systematic review. *Am J Obstet Gynecol* 2016;214:689 e1–689 e17.
2. Wise MR, Gill P, Lensen S, Thompson JM, Farquhar CM. Body mass index trumps age in decision for endometrial biopsy: Cohort study of symptomatic premenopausal women. *Am J Obstet Gynecol* 2016;215:598 e1–598 e8.
3. Aune D, Navarro Rosenblatt DA, Chan DS et al. Anthropometric factors and endometrial cancer risk: A systematic review and dose-response meta-analysis of prospective studies. *Ann Oncol* 2015;26: 1635–48.
4. Aston B, Weaver E. Risks and benefits of hysteroscopy and endometrial sampling as a standard procedure

for assessing serendipitous findings of endometrial thickening in postmenopausal women. *Aust N Z J Obstet Gynaecol* 2014;54:597–9.
5. Louie M, Canavan TP, Mansuria S. Threshold for endometrial sampling among postmenopausal patients without vaginal bleeding. *Int J Gynaecol Obstet* 2016;132:314–7.
6. Downes MR, Allo G, McCluggage WG et al. Review of findings in prophylactic gynaecological specimens in Lynch syndrome with literature review and recommendations for grossing. *Histopathology* 2014;65:228–39.
7. Argenta P, Svendsen C, Elishaev E et al. Hormone receptor expression patterns in the endometrium of asymptomatic morbidly obese women before and after bariatric surgery. *Gynecol Oncol* 2014;133:78–82.
8. Batig AL, Elliott D, Rumjahn H et al. Pipelle endometrial sampling in the evaluation of abnormal first trimester pregnancies. *Mil Med* 2014;179:1030–5.
9. Grimes DA. Diagnostic dilation and curettage: A reappraisal. *Am J Obstet Gynecol* 1982;142:1–6.
10. Barut A, Barut F, Arikan I et al. Comparison of the histopathological diagnoses of preoperative dilatation and curettage and hysterectomy specimens. *J Obstet Gynaecol Res* 2012;38:16–22.
11. Moradan S, Ghorbani R, Lotfi A. Agreement of histopathological findings of uterine curettage and hysterectomy specimens in women with abnormal uterine bleeding. *Saudi Med J* 2017;38:497–502.
12. Batista TP, Cavalcanti CL, Tejo AA, Bezerra AL. Accuracy of preoperative endometrial sampling diagnosis for predicting the final pathology grading in uterine endometrioid carcinoma. *Eur J Surg Oncol* 2016;42:1367–71.
13. van Hanegem N, Prins MM, Bongers MY et al. The accuracy of endometrial sampling in women with postmenopausal bleeding: A systematic review and meta-analysis. *Eur J Obstet Gynecol Reprod Biol* 2016;197:147–55.
14. Kandil D, Yang X, Stockl T, Liu Y. Clinical outcomes of patients with insufficient sample from endometrial biopsy or curettage. *Int J Gynecol Pathol* 2014;33:500–6.
15. Sakhdari A, Moghaddam PA, Liu Y. Endometrial samples from postmenopausal women: A proposal for adequacy criteria. *Int J Gynecol Pathol* 2016;35:525–30.
16. Anderson MC, Robboy SJ, Russell P, Morse A. The normal endometrium. In: Robboy SJ, Anderson MC, Russell P (eds) *Pathology of the Female Reproductive Tract*. London: Churchill Livingstone, 2002;241–65.
17. Unger ZM, Gonzalez JL, Hanissian PD, Schned AR. Pseudolipomatosis in hysteroscopically resected tissues from the gynecologic tract: Pathologic description and frequency. *Am J Surg Pathol* 2009;33:1187–90.

2

The normal endometrium

General considerations	7	Postmenopausal endometrium	17
Composition of the endometrium	9	Dating the endometrium	18
The menstrual cycle	11	References	19

GENERAL CONSIDERATIONS

The endometrium forms the mucosal lining of the myometrium between the interstitial segments of the fallopian tubes in the uterine cornua on either side of the fundus and the isthmical portion above the cervix. It is a complex tissue composed of surface epithelium, glands, stromal and inflammatory cells and blood vessels.

Prior to the onset of menarche, the endometrial cavity is lined by cuboidal epithelium with clefts dipping into spindly stroma (Figure 2.1). With the onset of puberty, estrogenic influences initiate endometrial proliferation to commence the cyclical changes (Figure 2.2). In the early phase of menarche, ovulation is not regular and anovulatory bleeding is frequent. When regular ovulatory cycles are established, the endometrium undergoes regular cyclical changes in response to the recurrent hormonal changes and, except during lactation and pregnancy, true menstruation is experienced. After menopause, the endometrium reverts to forming a mucous membrane for the myometrium.

The endometrial response to cyclical hormonal changes is crucial to implantation and development of the fertilized ovum. The menstrual cycle commences on the first day of bleeding and ends just before the next menstrual period; this cycle lasts for approximately 28 days, although the length of this cycle can vary from one woman to another and between cycles in the same woman. The menstrual cycle is divided into three phases: follicular, ovulatory and luteal. Follicles in the ovary are stimulated under the influence of follicle-stimulating hormone (FSH), and there is a rise in plasma estrogen level. This rise in estrogen level leads to an inhibitory feedback for production of FSH and a positive feedback for the production of luteinizing hormone (LH). Just prior to ovulation, there is a rapid upsurge of the plasma gonadotropins, LH and FSH, which results in follicular rupture and ovulation. Following conversion of the ruptured follicle to a corpus luteum, the previously very low levels of plasma progesterone rises rapidly. After ovulation, there is a rapid decline in the plasma LH and

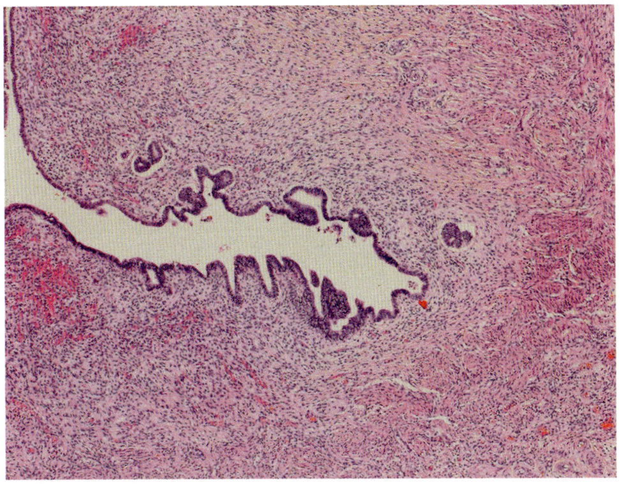

Figure 2.1 Endometrium in a three-year-old showing simple endometrial pattern with surface epithelium and clefts dipping into spindly stroma.

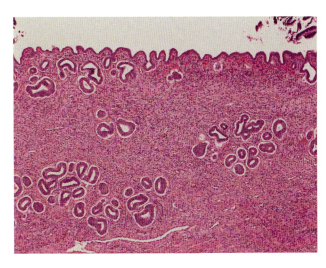

Figure 2.2 Endometrium in a ten-year-old showing beginnings of glandular development.

FSH levels while the plasma progesterone levels remain high for about 10 days. Estrogen levels decline for a few days after ovulation but there is a midluteal phase rise. If conception does not occur, both plasma estrogen and progesterone levels decline rapidly during the last week of the cycle, associated with regression of the corpus luteum. Plasma FSH and LH levels also fall in the last week of the cycle but rise again before menstruation commences in preparation for the next cycle.

The morphology of the endometrium is dependent on its anatomical location within the uterus. In the isthmus, there is a transition between endocervical and endometrial mucosa. Here, the endometrial glands are not responsive to hormonal stimulation and are poorly developed. In biopsy specimens, the clue to this setting is the stroma that becomes progressively more fibrous and less cellular the further it is from the body of the uterus. Isthmic glands are lined by ciliated epithelial cells (Figure 2.3). The endometrium is generally fairly uniform in appearance in the fundus and body and is conventionally divided into two components: the basal layer, adjacent to the myometrium, and the functional layer, superficial to the basal layer (Figure 2.4). There is no sharp line of

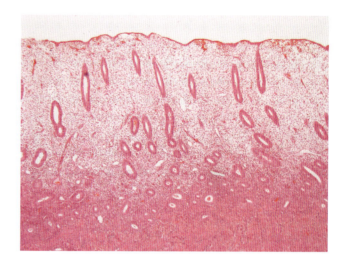

Figure 2.4 Endometrium in the body of the uterus showing superficial functional zone and deeper basal layer with slightly denser stroma. Note the absence of a clear demarcation between the two layers and between the basal layer and underlying myometrium.

demarcation either between the basal endometrium and the myometrium or between the functional and basal layers.

The basal layer, which forms the regenerative layer, does not normally respond to hormonal stimulation. The glands within it show no secretory activity, and there is minimal or no mitotic activity. The stroma is relatively more prominent as the volume of glands is smaller in comparison with the functional layer (Figure 2.5). The stromal cells are composed of largely spindled nuclei with scanty cytoplasm.

The more superficial functional layer is responsive to the hormonal changes of the ovulatory cycle. It is mitotically active in the proliferative phase and is shed during the menstrual period in the reproductive years (Figure 2.6). This layer is further subdivided into the stratum compactum and the stratum spongiosum. This subdivision is more

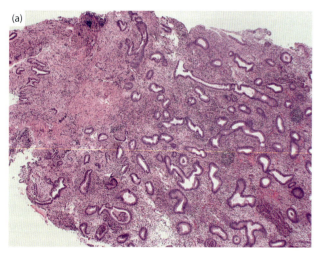

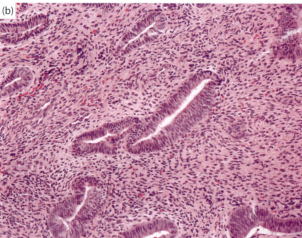

Figure 2.3 Endometrium in the lower segment showing (a) disordered arrangement of glands and (a, b) fibrous stroma.

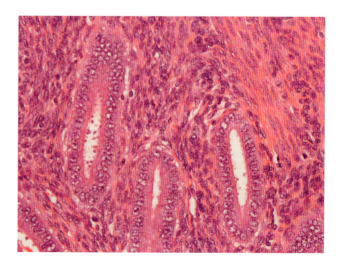

Figure 2.5 Basal layer of proliferative-phase endometrium showing absence of mitotic activity and dense stroma.

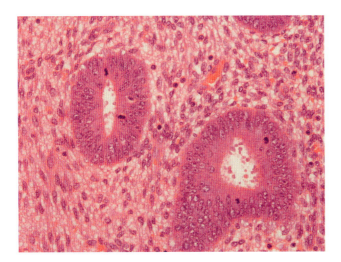

Figure 2.6 Functional layer of proliferative-phase endometrium showing glandular mitotic activity and looser stroma.

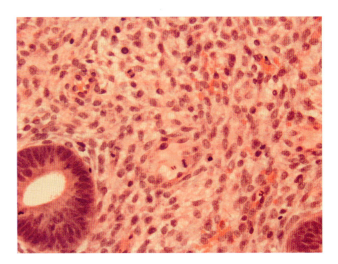

Figure 2.7 Stromal cells in early proliferative phase with oval nuclei and inconspicuous cytoplasm. Mitotic activity is readily seen within stromal cells.

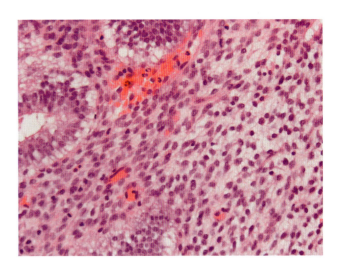

Figure 2.8 Stromal cells in early secretory phase showing spindle-shaped and slightly vesicular nuclei.

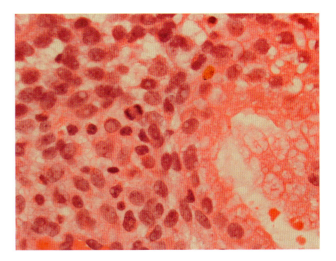

Figure 2.9 Stromal mitosis in late secretory-phase endometrium.

apparent during the late secretory phase when the stroma in the spongiosum layer is more edematous.

COMPOSITION OF THE ENDOMETRIUM

ENDOMETRIAL GLANDS

The glandular epithelium is in continuity with the surface epithelium, but the latter shows less of the hormonally-induced cyclical variation. The morphology of the glandular epithelium varies with the stage of the menstrual cycle, which will be detailed in the later section.

STROMA

The stromal cells vary considerably throughout the endometrial cycle, especially during the last seven or so days of the normal cycle. During the proliferative phase, they resemble fibroblasts with oval hyperchromatic nuclei and inconspicuous cytoplasm (Figure 2.7). In the late proliferative phase and early secretory phase, the nuclei become slightly larger and, with organelle accumulation, the cytoplasm becomes more noticeable (Figure 2.8). In the second half of the secretory phase, the nuclei become vesicular and larger and there is swelling of the cytoplasm with increasing accumulation of glycogen. This pre-decidualization of the stromal cells commences around the spiral arteries and arterioles cuffing those vessels, as a forerunner of the Streeter's columns of spiral arteries cuffed by decidua in pregnancy (Figure 2.9). Stromal edema becomes prominent and delineates the middle of the endometrium into the spongy layer. Pre-decidualization continues into the upper layer of the endometrium to form a more or less compact zone of swollen stromal cells, the compact layer. The stromal cells in the basal and parabasal layers are less responsive to progesterone and remain largely unchanged from those seen in the proliferative phase.

By tradition, the nomenclature of progestogen-induced stromal changes is influenced by the setting in which they take place. The terms decidualization and decidua are generally confined to describing the changes seen during pregnancy. Generally, pre-decidua is used to describe the change seen in the stromal cells during the secretory phase of the menstrual cycle while pseudodecidua refers to those induced by exogenous progesterone therapy. The stromal changes induced by endogenous progesterone during the secretory phase or pregnancy and those induced by synthetic progesterone therapy are largely similar; they are more extensive and uniform in pregnancy.

INFLAMMATORY CELLS

The numbers and distribution of leucocytes vary during the menstrual cycle, but leucocytes constitute some 10%–25% of all endometrial cells. The majority of endometrial leucocytes are natural killer cells (CD56+ NK cells). Macrophages constitute about 30% of the leucocyte population. T lymphocytes are found mainly in the basal endometrium in lymphoid aggregates and throughout the endometrial stroma and epithelium; most of the T lymphocytes are CD8+ (Figure 2.10). Other inflammatory cells seen in small numbers within the endometrium are CD83+ dendritic cells, CD16+ NK cells and mast cells.[1] Neutrophils are seen in the endometrium during the menstrual phase. Plasma cells and eosinophils are rarely seen, and their presence in significant numbers raises the possibility of a chronic endometritis. In fetuses, neonates and children, the majority of endometrial inflammatory cells are macrophages and monocytes; CD56+ natural killer cells are only present postnatally and in relatively small numbers.

The uterine NK cells have now been shown to be bone marrow-derived and are known as endometrial granulocytes, large granulated lymphocytes or K cells (Körnchenzellen). These are small, rounded cells with indented nuclei and eosinophilic intracytoplasmic granules of varying size. These

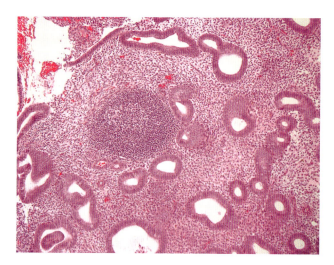

Figure 2.10 Lymphoid aggregate in the stroma of proliferative-phase endometrium.

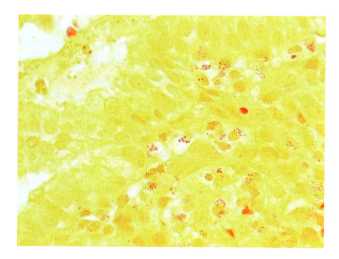

Figure 2.11 Prominent numbers of inflammatory cells, many of which contain phloxinophilic granules, near a gland. Phloxine-tartrazine stain.

granules, which are readily apparent using the phloxine-tartrazine stain, have led the unwary to mistake them for polymorphonuclear leucocytes (Figure 2.11). There is a marked increase in the number of these cells during early pregnancy such that they comprise as much as 70%–80% of all endometrial leucocytes. It has been suggested that they play a role in implantation and placentation either by acting as cytotoxic effector cells or by secretion of various cytokines.[2,3]

BLOOD SUPPLY

The uterine artery reaches the uterus at the level of the upper cervix where the ascending branch runs lateral to the uterus and a descending branch anastomoses with the vaginal artery. The ascending branch of the uterine artery anastomoses with branches of the ovarian artery at the lateral upper part of the uterus below the isthmic part of the fallopian tube. These paired uterine arteries that run lateral to the uterus, with anastomotic contributions from the ovarian arteries, supply the uterus predominantly. Branches from this utero-ovarian anastomosis penetrate the serosa and form a circular arcuate system in the outer myometrium. Arteries from the arcuate arterial system radiate into the inner myometrium. These radial arteries terminate, just proximal to the junction of the endometrium and myometrium as the basal arteries and the spiral arteries. The basal or straight arteries ramify in the innermost layers of the myometrium and terminate in the basal endometrium, which they supply. The spiral or coiled arteries, that are destined to become the uteroplacental arteries during pregnancy, traverse the endometrium in their course towards the uterine lumen. The spiral arteries give off anastomosing branches to the glands and stroma of the functional layer, and they terminate in a complex anastomotic network in the superficial layer of the endometrium (Figure 2.12). The venous drainage from the endometrium, in general, follows the arterial supply. The human endometrium also contains lymphatic vessels that are predominantly seen in the basal layer but sometimes also in the functional layer.

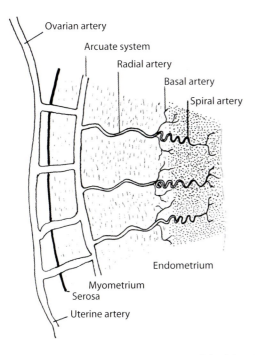

Figure 2.12 Diagrammatic representation of the blood supply to the uterus.

The spiral arteries and arterioles are hormonally responsive. Estrogen and progesterone receptors have been demonstrated in the smooth-muscle cells of these arteries, although there is some heterogeneity in distribution and quantity of these receptors.[4] Estrogen and progesterone receptors have been found also in the perivascular cells. It is unclear to what degree the actions of estrogen and progesterone on endometrial blood vessels are mediated directly or indirectly via paracrine or autocrine factors.

The spiral arteries grow by hyperplasia and hypertrophy throughout the menstrual cycle as the endometrium grows in thickness. In the late proliferative and secretory phases and in early pregnancy, their growth exceeds that of the endometrium so that their natural coiled configuration is exaggerated further. Various factors are implicated in the cyclical regeneration of spiral arteries, including vascular endothelial growth factor (VEGF), angiopoietin-1 and -2 and receptors such as Flt-1, Flk1/KDR and Tie-1 and -2. It is not clear how steroids affect the growth process and the paracrine signals involved.[5]

THE MENSTRUAL CYCLE

The salient features of the endometrium through the menstrual cycle is summarised (Table 2.1).

PROLIFERATIVE

The endometrium regenerates from the basal layer and that part of the functional layer that remains after menstruation.

The normal proliferative phase lasts about two weeks. However, the time taken for follicles to develop and to mature tends to vary between cycles and from one woman to the next so that it is impossible to date the proliferative phase with any degree of accuracy. As the daily morphologic changes are not sufficiently distinctive for accurate dating, it is not necessary to date the endometrium during the proliferative phase, although many pathologists split the phase into early, middle and late proliferative phases.

In the early stages, the glands have a low columnar epithelium and a straight, simple tubular arrangement (Figure 2.13). The elongated nucleus fills most of the cell and the nuclei are arranged at different levels, giving a pseudostratified appearance. Mitotic activity is seen in the glands and in the stroma (Figures 2.14 and 2.15). The stroma appears dense and the stromal cells, which change little throughout the proliferative phase, appear to contain little cytoplasm, giving an appearance of naked nuclei on hematoxylin-and-eosin staining (Figure 2.7).

In the mid-proliferative phase, the glands continue to elongate and stromal edema develops. Although the endometrium thickens during this period, the elongation of the glands outstrips the stromal edema and endometrial thickening resulting in tortuosity of the glands (Figure 2.16). Mitotic activity continues in the glands and stroma.

In the late proliferative phase, the stromal edema subsides, resulting in further tortuosity of the glands. Mitotic activity is maximal in the glands and stroma, corresponding to the maximal pre-ovulation peak of estrogen. The columnar epithelium is tall and becomes heaped to give a pseudostratified appearance (Figure 2.17). Accumulation of glycogen and glycoproteins occurs in the late proliferative phase before ovulation occurs, but this is evident by electron microscopy or histochemistry only. The glandular lumina may also become distended with glycogen and glycoproteins.

The endometrial spiral arteries are relatively inconspicuous during the proliferative phase, being identifiable as thin-walled blood vessels (Figure 2.18).

SECRETORY

The secretory phase is best divided into two stages. Glandular changes predominate in the first stage while stromal changes predominate in the second.

The exact day of ovulation can be determined only by daily plasma hormone measurements to pinpoint the peak of the LH surge. The day of ovulation cannot be established from endometrial histology as there is a lag phase of between 36 and 48 hours between ovulation and the appearance of progestogenic effects on the endometrium. During this period, sometimes termed the interval phase, there is little change in the morphology of the endometrium except for further distension and tortuosity of the glands. There is gradual loss of the pseudostratification in the epithelium while mitotic activity is still readily evident. Focal subnuclear vacuolation may be seen.

Subnuclear vacuolation occurs some 36–48 hours following ovulation (Figure 2.19). A clear vacuole made of glycogen and mucin is formed between the nucleus and the base

Table 2.1 Histological features of the endometrium through the menstrual cycle

	Glands	Stroma	Vessels
Proliferative – early	Small straight glands mitoses	Dense spindle cell stroma; mitoses	Relatively inconspicuous spiral arteries with thin walls
Proliferative – mid	Slightly tortuous glands	Loose, edematous stroma with spindled cells	
Proliferative – late	Pseudostratified appearance; nuclei at various heights but most in basal half; smooth luminal surface; lumina sharp outline	Less edematous stroma	
Secretory POD 1	Mitotic; subnuclear vacuolation	No change	
POD 2	Tortuous		
POD 3			
POD 4	Less regular subnuclear vacuoles; secretory vacuoles on luminal side		
POD 5	Outline of glands irregular; widening diameter of glands; papillary infoldings – sawtooth; no longer pseudostratified; apical surface of rough and indistinct nuclei – round, vesicular and pale staining	Edema starts; therefore can distinguish basal from functional date 8 = max edema	
POD 6			
POD 7			
POD 8			
POD 9		Edema starts to regress	Spiral arteries appear more prominent
POD 10			Pre-decidual cuffing of spiral arteries
POD 11		Decidual change starts	
POD 12	Central–Sawtooth endometrium secretions ++ tall columnar epithelium Surface may have flat to cuboidal cells; some luminal breakdown	Solid stroma; no edema superficial still decidual change; granulated lymphocytes	
POD 13			
POD 14			
Menstrual	Glandular collapse; clumped epithelial glandular cells with secretory exhaustion	Crumbling stroma; compact balls of stromal cells; overlying epithelial cells	Thrombosed spiral arteries

Abbreviation: POD, postovulatory day.

of the cell. This subnuclear vacuolation may be patchy initially, and ovulation should be assumed to have taken place only when the majority of the endometrial glandular epithelial cells are vacuolated. Taking Day 0 as the day of ovulation, on postovulatory Day 2 (Day 16 of a 28 day 'normal' menstrual cycle), the pseudostratification will have smoothened out. The epithelial nucleus will have moved upwards to the mid-region of the columnar cells, apparently pushed up by the accumulation of secretory material beneath them. Mitotic activity continues in the glands and stroma but is much decreased (Figure 2.20).

As the plasma progesterone levels rise, secretory activity increases to such an extent that the nucleus occupies the upper half of each cell, and this feature is maximal at postovulatory Day 3–4 (Day 17–18) (Figure 2.21). As the secretory material of the subnuclear vacuole moves to the apex of the cell, the nucleus starts to assume a more basal position and there is supra- and subnuclear vacuolation (Figure 2.22). The glands are distended and mitotic activity in the glands comes to an end. There may still be occasional stromal mitoses (Figure 2.23).

By postovulatory Day 6–7 (Day 20–21), the nuclei are basal in position. The secretory material may protrude into the gland lumen with secretory blebs apparent and, as it is shed by the apocrine method, the epithelial surface assumes a more irregular border. Dilatation of the glands by luminal secretory material is prominent (Figure 2.24). The stroma starts becoming edematous.

If pregnancy does not ensue, the corpus luteum starts to involute and progesterone levels fall. Estrogen levels, which have fallen following ovulation, reach a second lower peak by postovulatory Day 7–8 (Day 21–22). These hormonal changes coincide with a change in emphasis of the endometrial morphology from the glands to the stroma. Thus, secretory activity declines after Day 22. The glands begin to involute, and there is inspissation or gradual disappearance of the luminal secretions; the glandular nuclei are now basal (Figure 2.25). Stromal edema is maximal by Day 22–23. The involuting glands collapse and show a saw-tooth appearance (Figure 2.26). As the stromal edema begins to subside by Day 23–24, the spiral arterioles become prominent. There is an increase in length of the arterioles and mitotic activity can be seen in them. Pre-decidual change of the stroma immediately around the spiral arterioles leads to a prominent cuffing appearance (Figure 2.27).

Thereafter, from Days 26–28, the stromal changes allow the endometrium to be divided into three separate zones, or strata. The stromal cells enlarge and accumulate a polygonal shape with small rounded nuclei; the cytoplasm accumulates glycogen and lipid and is conspicuous. The area adjacent to the endometrial surface forms the stratum compactum in which the decidualized stromal cells predominate and the glands are inconspicuous, either due to compression by the stroma or to a lack of secretions (Figure 2.28). The

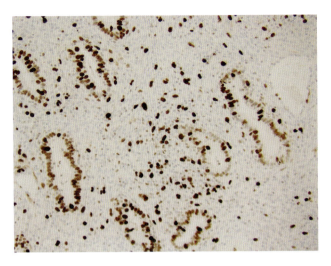

Figure 2.15 Proliferative-phase endometrium showing strong and diffuse immunolabeling of glandular and stromal cell nuclei with Ki-67; immunolabeling of occasional endothelial cells of endometrial capillaries.

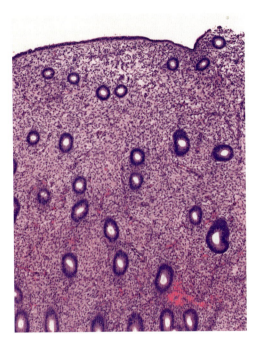

Figure 2.13 Early proliferative-phase endometrium showing glands with a straight, simple tubular arrangement.

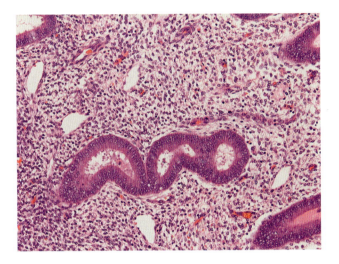

Figure 2.16 Mid proliferative-phase endometrium with tortuous glands. The spiral arteries are thin-walled.

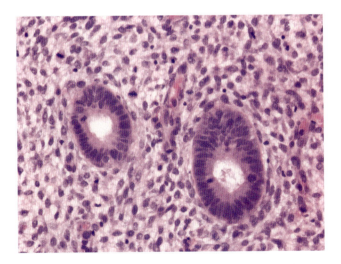

Figure 2.14 Early proliferative-phase endometrium showing low columnar epithelium with pseudostratified appearance of the elongated nuclei. There is mitotic activity in glands and stroma.

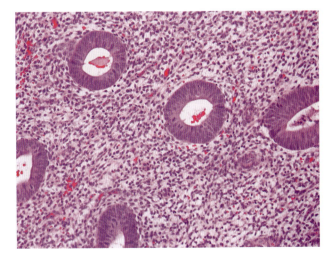

Figure 2.17 Late proliferative-phase endometrium with tall columnar epithelium and pseudostratification of nuclei.

14 The normal endometrium

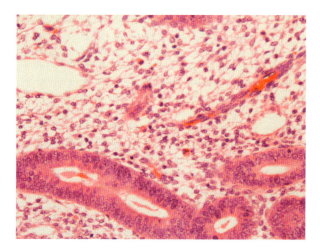

Figure 2.18 Inconspicuous spiral arteries in proliferative phase endometrium.

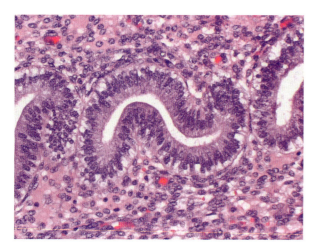

Figure 2.19 Secretory-phase endometrium, postovulatory Day 1, with the pseudostratified epithelium almost smoothed out and almost uniform subnuclear vacuolation. The nuclei are now located in the mid-region of the epithelium.

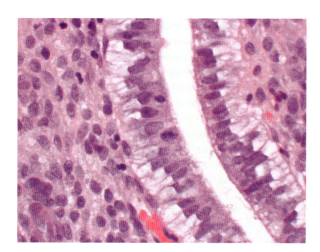

Figure 2.20 Secretory-phase endometrium (postovulatory Day 3) showing nucleus near to luminal border of the epithelial cells and residual mitosis.

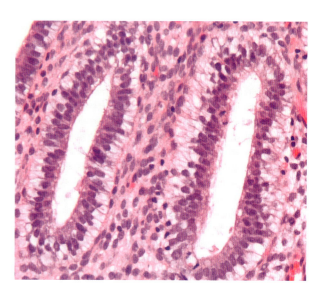

Figure 2.21 Secretory-phase endometrium (postovulatory Day 3–4) with maximal subnuclear vacuolation and nuclei pushed near to the luminal border.

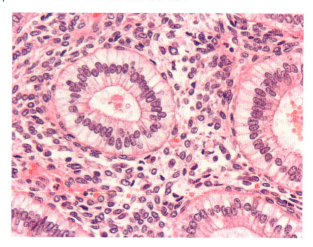

Figure 2.22 Secretory-phase endometrium (postovulatory Day 4–5) showing supranuclear and subnuclear vacuolation.

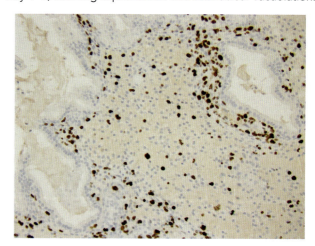

Figure 2.23 Secretory-phase endometrium showing absence of immunolabeling of glandular cells with Ki-67 with immunolabeling of stromal cells reduced from that seen in the pre-ovulatory endometrium.

The menstrual cycle / Secretory

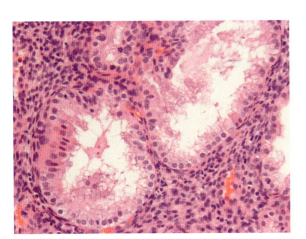

Figure 2.24 Secretory-phase endometrium (postovulatory Day 6–7) showing dilatation of glands and irregular border of epithelial surface with secretory blebs on the luminal aspect of the glandular cells.

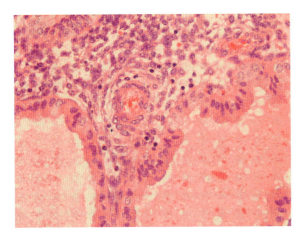

Figure 2.25 Secretory-phase endometrium (postovulatory Day 8) with basal nuclei and secretions in the lumen. Note the endometrial granulocytes around the spiral artery.

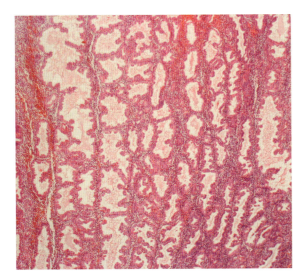

Figure 2.26 Secretory-phase endometrium with infolding of the glandular epithelium to give a saw-tooth appearance (postovulatory Day 8–9).

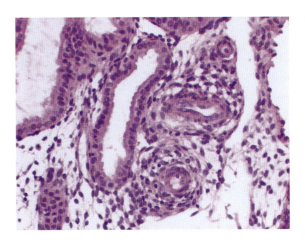

Figure 2.27 Prominent spiral arteries with predecidua cuffing in late secretory-phase endometrium.

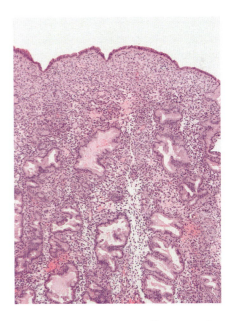

Figure 2.28 Stratum compactum adjacent to the endometrial surface in late secretory-phase endometrium showing decidualized stromal cells; there is a relative absence of glands and the stroma is more compact compared with the subjacent stratum spongiosum which contains tortuous glands separated by sparse stroma.

intermediate layer or stratum spongiosum shows tortuous dilated glands with a saw-toothed appearance and separated by scant stroma. The spiral arterioles, with their predecidual cuff, course through this layer. The basal layer or stratum basale adjacent to the myometrium contains the deep portions of the glands set in a stroma that shows little change throughout the menstrual cycle. The glands progressively become effete. Granulated lymphocytes infiltrate the stroma, particularly the compact layer, during Days 26 and 27, with the numbers being greater on Day 27 than 26 (Figure 2.29).

The endometrial granulated lymphocytes are present in the endometrium throughout the secretory phase, tending to aggregate around the glands and spiral arteries. These

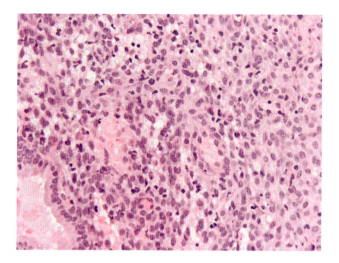

Figure 2.29 Granulated lymphocytes in the stratum compactum in the late secretory phase.

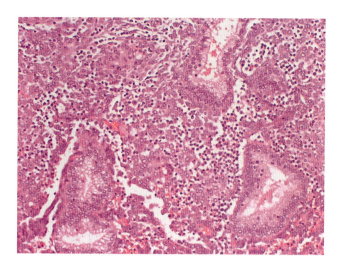

Figure 2.31 Menstrual-phase endometrium showing secretory exhaustion: dilated glands are disrupted and lined by flattened cells showing a frayed border.

lymphocytes proliferate between Day 21 and 27, but the stimulus for this proliferation is unclear.

MENSTRUAL PHASE

Much of the endometrial lining is shed at the end of each menstrual cycle if pregnancy has not occurred. Menstrual endometrium is characterised by disintegrating fragments of fully developed secretory endometrium (Figure 2.30). The glands show secretory exhaustion: there is disruption of the dilated glands that are lined by flattened cells showing a frayed border (Figure 2.31). Apoptosis is seen in the glandular epithelium. There is a marked infiltration of the stroma by endometrial granulated lymphocytes and leucocytes (Figure 2.32). The coiling of the spiral arteries is accentuated due to collapse and the stroma is markedly condensed (Figure 2.33). The stromal condensation reflects a sharp shrinkage in endometrial thickness because of fluid loss secondary to the fall in progesterone and estrogen levels.

Commensurate with this, there is also a further reduction in the already sluggish blood flow because of the increase in coiling of the arteries. After a time, red blood cells pass through the damaged walls of the ischemic blood vessels. Small hematomas ensue (Figure 2.34). When the necrotic epithelium is shed, the blood is then shed directly into the uterine lumen. The shedding of the endometrium starts superficially and proceeds to the deeper layers. Shedding is along irregular lines of necrosis in the functional layer and rapid disintegration of the endometrium then takes place. The endometrium is usually shed in a piece-meal fashion but can be shed in larger fragments or even in the form of a uterine cast. There is now a heavy infiltration of the tissue by acute inflammatory cells.

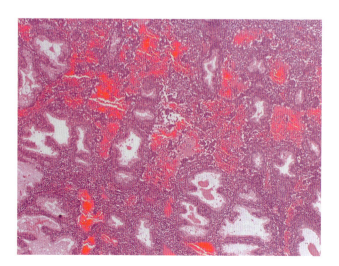

Figure 2.30 Menstrual-phase endometrium showing characteristic disintegrating fragments of fully developed secretory endometrium.

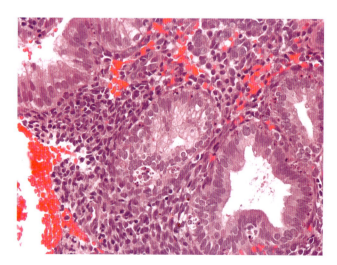

Figure 2.32 Early breakdown in menstrual-phase endometrium showing marked apoptosis of glandular epithelium, stromal condensation and infiltration of the stroma by endometrial granulocytes.

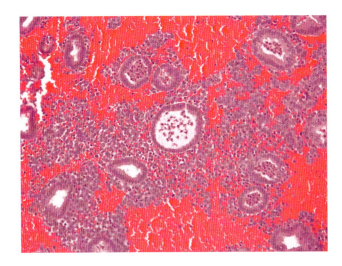

Figure 2.33 Menstrual-phase endometrium with breakdown of the stroma with marked stromal infiltration by granulocytes and leucocytes and interstitial hemorrhage; neutrophils are seen in the glandular lumina.

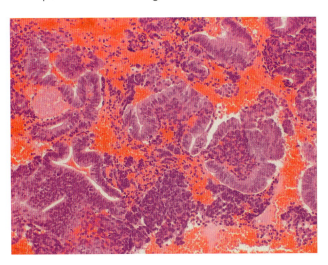

Figure 2.34 Menstrual-phase endometrium showing degenerate glands and condensed stroma.

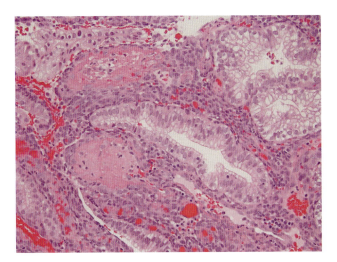

Figure 2.35 Menstrual-phase endometrium with fibrin thrombi within spiral arteriole.

Hemostasis is secured by the formation of fibrin and platelet plugs (Figure 2.35). Regeneration starts well before cessation of obvious menstrual flow and is largely complete by the time that occurs. Menstruation usually lasts for four days, although it can vary from three to five days. Regeneration begins in the remnants of glands in the basal layer and in those parts of the functional layer that are not shed in the menstrual process.

POSTMENOPAUSAL ENDOMETRIUM

The end of the reproductive phase is characterised by falling sex hormones as a result of involution of the ovaries. Anovulatory cycles become more frequent and menstruation increasingly becomes irregular. There is a gradual reduction in size of the uterus: the endometrium becomes

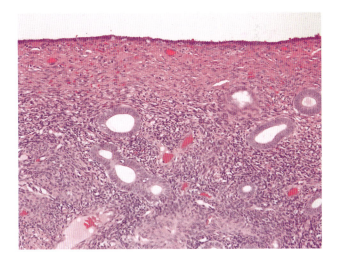

Figure 2.36 Hysterectomy specimen of postmenopausal endometrium showing thinning of endometrium, small numbers of glands and dense stroma.

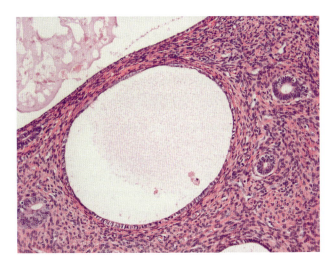

Figure 2.37 Postmenopausal endometrium with cystically dilated glands lined by cuboidal epithelium.

thinner and the glands are reduced in numbers and are lined by a cuboidal or low columnar epithelium and the stroma is rather dense (Figure 2.36). The endometrium is no longer differentiated into functional and basal layers. Occasionally, the glands become cystically dilated, being lined by a cuboidal or flattened epithelium (Figure 2.37). There is usually an associated fibrous stroma with diminished cellularity. Benign cystic polyps may frequently coexist with this atrophic postmenopausal endometrium.

DATING THE ENDOMETRIUM

There are several essential principles for dating the endometrium (Table 2.2).

Noyes and his colleagues established criteria for the histological dating of the endometrium.[6] This method is imprecise, however.[7]

A theoretical contribution to the imprecision is that endometrial dating is discontinuous and arbitrary in that it is measured in days whereas the biological event of endometrial cycling is presumably continuous. The actual time difference between the day the biopsy was obtained and the biological date as predicated by the onset of the next menses may be one day more or less, and this can introduce an error of one day in about 15% of the biopsies.[8]

At any stage of the cycle, there are regional variations in the histological date of the endometrium. The endometrium responds differently to the cyclical hormonal changes depending on its anatomical location within the uterus. The basal endometrium responds to estrogen by proliferating while the functional zone is responsive to progesterone. The superficial portion of the endometrium responds to both estrogen and progesterone. Furthermore, the most reactive part of the endometrium is in the body and fundus, whereas the lower segment and isthmic endometrium are poorly responsive. These differences, however, contribute only minimally to the imprecision, and there is little basis for advocating sampling from specific locations within the fundal portion of the uterus for purposes of dating the endometrium.

Table 2.2 Principles for dating the endometrium

Biopsy is dated by the most advanced area.
Dating should be performed on endometrium from the functional layer; the basal endometrium does not respond to the hormonal changes to the same degree.
The lower segment should not be dated; this area is relatively less responsive to hormonal changes.
Abnormal endometrium should not be dated.
Polyps or endometria showing hyperplasia or endometritis should not be dated.
Inactive or atrophic endometrium cannot be dated.

Intra-observer variation can be greater than two days in about 10% of observations, without any consistency in the direction of the discrepancy, while inter-observer discordance is even greater.[9]

The duration of the follicular phase can vary substantially between cycles and between women, rendering the ascertainment of the date of ovulation based on the date of the last menstrual period somewhat inaccurate. Dating of the endometrial biopsy generally assumes a 14-day luteal phase in women, but the duration of the luteal phase can also vary significantly. Only a small percentage of women ovulate 14 days before the onset of menses, even for women with regular 28-day cycles. Time from ovulation to the next menses can range from 7 to 19 days (Day 10 to Day 22 of the menstrual cycle). Thus, the variability in the duration of the luteal phase adds further to the difficulty in ascertaining the date of ovulation based on the usual cycle length and duration of the menstrual period.

DATING THE ENDOMETRIUM AND INFERTILITY

The most common application of dating the endometrium had been determining the presence of luteal phase defects in the investigation of the infertile woman. Uterine receptivity is defined as the state during the period of endometrial maturation when the uterus is receptive to blastocyst attachment and implantation. Outside this time, called the 'window of implantation or receptivity', the uterus is thought to be resistant to attachment by the blastocyst. The endometrial preparedness is coordinated by the ovarian hormones,[10] and deficient production of the hormones or a failure of the endometrium to respond is thought by some to be a cause of recurrent spontaneous miscarriage and infertility. This condition, referred to as luteal phase defect, is defined as endometrial histology that is inconsistent with the chronological date of the menstrual cycle based on the woman's next menses, with the benchmark to establish the diagnosis of luteal phase defect being that the biopsy must be out-of-phase in two consecutive menstrual cycles. The usefulness of histological dating of the endometrium in investigating infertility or recurrent miscarriage is now disputed. As indicated in the section 'Dating the epithelium', histological dating of the endometrium lacks accuracy. More cogently, it does not guide clinical management of the infertile woman as out-of-phase biopsies are seen just as frequently in fertile as in infertile women.[11,12]

Molecular mediators involved in the development of the endometrium, such as growth factors, cytokines, chemokines, lipids and adhesion molecules, have been proposed as alternative non-histological markers for distinguishing receptive from non-receptive endometrium, but none have proven to be clinically useful at this stage.[13]

These, and other candidate molecules need to be assessed critically for reproducibility and relation to pregnancy outcome. It is possible that the presence or absence of these markers may be an epiphenomenon of abnormal endometrial development during the particular cycle of study. Furthermore, it is unclear whether aberrant expression of any of these molecules is a primary cause of reproduction failure or whether some underlying endometrial pathology has a deleterious effect on embryo implantation and causes the aberrant molecule expression.

While the emphasis has moved away from histological dating of the endometrium in the routine evaluation of the infertile couple, the endometrial biopsy is still necessary for excluding other morphologic causes such as tuberculous endometritis and also to provide tissue for transcriptomic molecular analysis.[14]

REFERENCES

1. Berbic M, Ng CH, Fraser IS. Inflammation and endometrial bleeding. *Climacteric* 2014;17(Suppl 2):47–53.
2. Small HY, Cornelius DC, Guzik TJ, Delles C. Natural killer cells in placentation and cancer: Implications for hypertension during pregnancy. *Placenta* 2017;56:59–64.
3. Wallace AE, Fraser R, Cartwright JE. Extravillous trophoblast and decidual natural killer cells: A remodelling partnership. *Hum Reprod Update* 2012;18:458–71.
4. Perrot-Applanat M, Groyer-Picard MT, Garcia E, Lorenzo F, Milgrom E. Immunocytochemical demonstration of estrogen and progesterone receptors in muscle cells of uterine arteries in rabbits and humans. *Endocrinology* 1988;123:1511–9.
5. Girling JE, Rogers PA. Recent advances in endometrial angiogenesis research. *Angiogenesis* 2005;8:89–99.
6. Noyes RW, Hertig AT, Rock J. Dating the endometrial biopsy. *Fertil Steril* 1950;1:3–25.
7. Noyes RW, Haman JO. Accuracy of endometrial dating: Correlation of endometrial dating with basal body temperature and menses. *Fertil Steril* 1953;4:504–17.
8. Gibson M, Badger GJ, Byrn F et al. Error in histologic dating of secretory endometrium: Variance component analysis. *Fertil Steril* 1991;56:242–7.
9. Duggan MA, Brashert P, Ostor A et al. The accuracy and interobserver reproducibility of endometrial dating. *Pathology* 2001;33:292–7.
10. Paulson RJ. Hormonal induction of endometrial receptivity. *Fertil Steril* 2011;96:530–5.
11. Coutifaris C, Myers ER, Guzick DS et al. Histological dating of timed endometrial biopsy tissue is not related to fertility status. *Fertil Steril* 2004;82:1264–72.
12. Kazer RR. Endometrial biopsy should be abandoned as a routine component of the infertility evaluation. *Fertil Steril* 2004;82:1297–8.
13. Thouas GA, Dominguez F, Green MP et al. Soluble ligands and their receptors in human embryo development and implantation. *Endocr Rev* 2015;36:92–130.
14. Katzorke N, Vilella F, Ruiz M, Krüssel JS, Simón C. Diagnosis of endometrial-factor infertility: Current approaches and new avenues for research. *Geburtshilfe Frauenheilkd* 2016;76:699–703.

3

Pregnancy

Placentation	21	Postpartum hemorrhage	30
Abortion	24	Pregnancy following therapy	32
Abnormal pregnancy	27	References	33

Fertilization of the ovum normally takes place in the ampullary segment of the fallopian tube about 24 hours after ovulation. There is then an interval of about six days before the blastocyst, having developed from the zygote through the morula stage in its passage through the fallopian tube, embeds in the endometrium. Thus, at about seven days post ovulation, or at about 21 days of a normal 28-day cycle, the blastocyst implants interstitially within the stroma between the glands of the endometrium. At this time the glands are at the peak of their secretory activity, but the stroma has not shown pre-decidualization yet.

Gonadotrophin production by the primitive trophoblast of the blastocyst begins possibly before, but at the latest at the time of, implantation of the blastocyst. Thus, the corpus luteum comes under the influence of the luteotrophic hormones and does not involute as it would do in the absence of a conceptus. Further development of the corpus luteum results in higher levels of plasma progesterone, which sustain the endometrium and lead to the formation of a true decidua.

The word 'decidua' was first used to describe that part of the uterine tissue shed on parturition, that is the gestational endometrium. The term is now restricted to the transformed stromal part of the gestational endometrium and to similar mesenchymal tissue elsewhere in the genital tract and, occasionally, outside it, during pregnancy. The pre-pregnancy changes that occur during the luteal phase should be called decidua or predecidua (Figure 3.1). Decidualization is associated with a marked increase in uterine natural killer cells. The changes produced in the endometrium by prolonged administration of progestins can be termed pseudodecidua.

PLACENTATION

Soon after implantation, the cytotrophoblastic shell is formed around the developing conceptus, and streamers of these cytotrophoblastic cells permeate the decidua basalis.

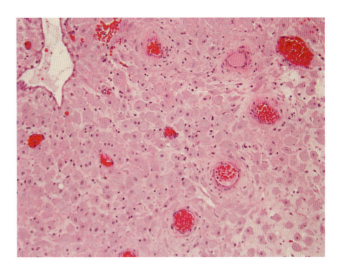

Figure 3.1 Decidua vera at six weeks gestation with spiral arteries and gland.

By the 20th postovulatory day, the decidua is overrun by this extravillous trophoblast that is also termed as nonvillous migratory trophoblast (Figure 3.2). Large numbers of uterine natural killer and myelomonocytic cells and smaller numbers of T cells accumulate, particularly around infiltrating trophoblast cells.[1]

There are two subsets of extravillous trophoblast: one subset, termed the interstitial trophoblast, infiltrates the interstitium of the decidua while the other, termed the endovascular trophoblast, infiltrates the spiral arteries (Figure 3.3). This population of interstitial and endovascular trophoblast, sometimes also called intermediate trophoblast, is a mixture of mononuclear cytotrophoblast, multinuclear syncytiotrophoblast and cells that are truly intermediate in form.

One of the prime functions of the proliferating cytotrophoblast is to open up the decidual terminations of the spiral arteries. By the 12th day (conceptual age) of pregnancy, there is a system of well-developed lacunae in the trophoblastic syncytium of the implanted embryo. The lacunae

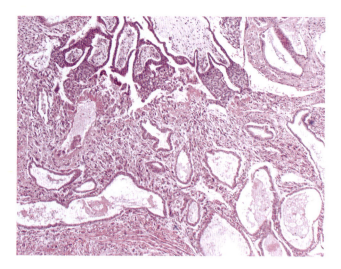

Figure 3.2 Implantation site and nine weeks gestation showing anchoring villi and overrunning of the decidua by interstitial trophoblast. The spiral artery already shows transformation into the uteroplacental artery with intraluminal endovascular trophoblast present. Note the abundant secretions within the glands.

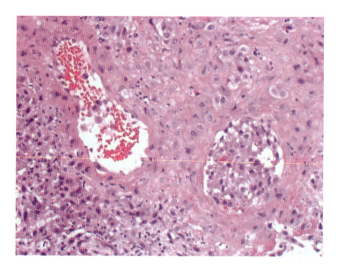

Figure 3.3 Interstitial trophoblast infiltrating the interstitium of the decidua and surrounding two spiral arteries. Endovascular trophoblast is present within the lumina of both spiral arteries and has formed a plug in the artery on the right. Some endovascular trophoblastic cells are seen embedded within the fibrinoid matrix of the uteroplacental arterial wall.

communicate with several sinusoids that have arisen from endometrial venules and capillaries. The first maternal vessels to be 'tapped' by the lacunae are slightly dilated venules or capillaries in the decidua. With further extension of the invading syncytium and more dilatation of blood vessels, the blood supply of the lacunae comes from venous sinusoids. Several spiral arteries are present in the vicinity of the implantation site but with no connections between them, and the lacunar spaces are found in conceptuses at the presomite embryo stage. Since there are no direct arterial connections into the intervillous space at this stage, flow into lacunar spaces is by a 'controlled seepage' from the veins. With increase in the extent and depth of trophoblastic invasion, it would seem that the maternal vessels are eroded progressively back to the level of arterioles and venules, thus permitting a through circulation. Prior to the full establishment of circulation, nutrition to the developing conceptus is histiotrophic, being derived from secretions from the endometrial glands.[2]

Prior to the arrival of the endovascular trophoblast, the spiral arteries become dilated and there is swelling and loosening of the media and endothelium. It is thought that this change is effected by the uterine natural killer cells.[3] From the period when the spiral arteries can definitely be seen to communicate with the intervillous space, the endovascular cytotrophoblast is seen within their lumina. These endovascular trophoblastic plugs restrict the flow of red blood cells into the developing placenta and the relative hypoxemia protects the conceptus from oxidative damage from free radicals. The endovascular trophoblastic cells replace the endothelium and cause much damage to the vessel wall such that the muscular and elastic tissues within the arterial walls are replaced by fibrinoid material. Eventually, the endovascular trophoblastic plugs disappear as the cells are embedded within this fibrinoid material (Figures 3.3 and 3.4); this permits a true uteroplacental circulation, and the oxygen level in the intervillous space rises considerably at the end of the first trimester. This also corresponds to the approximate time when the conceptus switches from histiotrophic to hematotrophic nutrition.

The uterine natural killer cells may regulate trophoblastic invasion into maternal tissue: maternally inherited variable killer immunoglobulin-like receptors (KIR) expressed by uterine natural killer cells bind to polymorphic fetal human leukocyte antigen-C molecules displayed by the extravillous trophoblast. It is unclear, however, how this translates into different functions of uterine natural killer

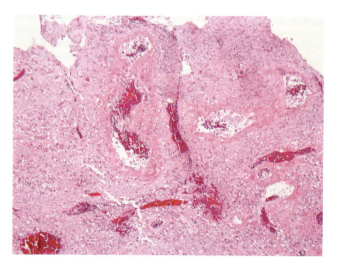

Figure 3.4 Distended spiral arteries, some with intraluminal endovascular trophoblast, with fibrinoid material already replacing the walls amidst plentiful interstitial trophoblast within the decidua.

cells to permit controlled invasion during placentation so the arteries are effectively transformed by the trophoblast and yet prevent undue penetration of the uterus.[4] The relative roles and interactions of other decidual leukocytes (macrophages, dendritic cells, effector T cells and Tregs) are also unclear at this stage.[5]

As the primitive anchoring villi are developing, fibrinoid material called Rohr's striae and Nitabuch's layer can be seen deposited between the villi and the decidua (Figure 3.5). Another feature that is not appreciated generally is the degree of necrosis within the decidua basalis and margin of the decidua vera (Figure 3.6).

The morphological transformation of the spiral arteries from muscular vaso-reactive arteries into compliant distensible arteries provides an increasing blood supply to the growing placenta and conceptus. Thus, these changes have been termed 'physiological vascular changes'. Detailed studies of

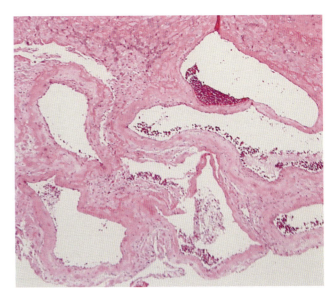

Figure 3.7 Uteroplacental artery showing distended lumina and fibrinoid matrix replacing the muscular and elastic tissues within the wall.

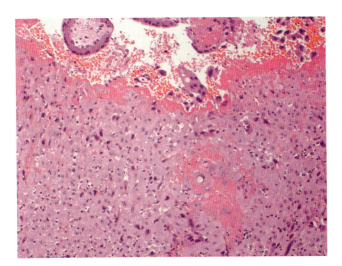

Figure 3.5 Fibrinous material called Rohr's striae and Nitabuch's layer seen deposited between the developing anchoring villi and the decidua.

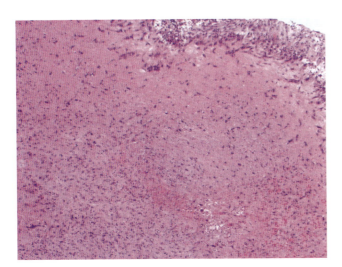

Figure 3.6 Focal necrosis of the decidua without significant inflammation present.

hysterectomy specimens with precise known menstrual dates have shown that endovascular migration and transformation of the spiral arteries take place in two topographical and temporal phases. The first stage, between approximately 6 and 12 weeks of gestation, is limited generally to the intradecidual portions of the spiral arteries and, after a relatively quiescent period, a renewed migratory phase takes place between approximately 16 and 22 weeks of gestation, transforming the myometrial portions of the spiral arteries.[6,7] These spiral arteries dilate further with the expansion in the woman's blood volume as pregnancy progresses and become true utero-placental arteries (Figures 3.7 and 3.8).

The spiral arteries in the decidua vera do not undergo these physiological changes as the extravillous trophoblast migrates only into the decidua basalis from the cytotrophoblastic shell and anchoring villi. Indeed, the decidua vera is distinguished from the basalis by the absence of the extravillous trophoblast, physiological changes or fibrinoid deposition (Summary Box 3.1 and Figure 3.9).

SUMMARY BOX 3.1: Normal placentation

Priming of the endometrium

- Decidualization – histiotrophic nutrition
- Increase in uterine natural killer cell numbers

Remodeling of spiral arteries

- Infiltration of decidua and spiral arteries by extravillous trophoblast
- Replacement of musculo-elastic media by fibrinoid
- Expansion in caliber of spiral arteries, now utero-placental arteries – hematotrophic nutrition

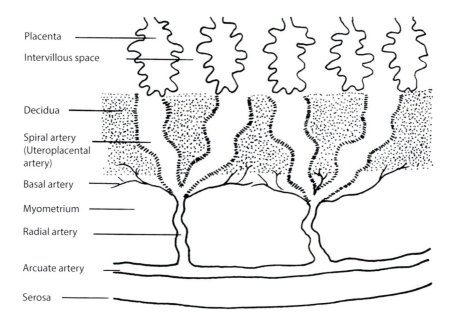

Figure 3.8 Diagrammatic representation of normal blood supply to the placenta. The hatched lines in the intramyometrial and intradecidual segments of the spiral arteries indicate physiological vascular changes, which extend from the origins from the radial arteries to the openings in the intervillous space. (Reproduced with permission from Khong TY, Liddell HS, Robertson WB. *Br J Obstet Gynaecol* 1987;94:649–55.)

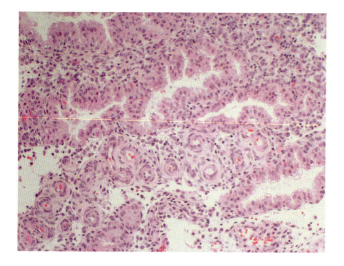

Figure 3.9 Decidua vera in early pregnancy with endometrial glands, 'unconverted' spiral arteries and a sprinkling of K cells.

ABORTION

The medical profession divides the term abortion into two categories: induced and spontaneous. The lay public, however, tends to equate the term abortion with one which is induced, therapeutically, self or criminal, whereas the term miscarriage to them means spontaneous abortion. Spontaneous abortion is usually defined as the involuntary loss of a conceptus before the fetus has attained viability. This seemingly simple definition can be challenging: firstly, the gestational age at which the fetus attains viability is subject to biological variants, such as improved medical care of extremely premature or extremely low-birth-weight infants, and, secondly, the legal criteria on viability of the fetus vary between jurisdictions.

TISSUE FROM INDUCED ABORTIONS

A prudent policy is to identify any gestational tissue obtained from induced or voluntary terminations of pregnancy to verify an intrauterine pregnancy and successful termination.

The relative proportions of pregnancy tissue, *viz* decidua, placenta and embryo/fetus, vary depending on the gestational age. Decidual tissue predominates during the first 4–6 weeks of pregnancy and placental tissue during the 7–16 weeks of pregnancy, while fetal tissue predominates thereafter. Various methods of correlating weight or volume of the conceptual products with complete removal of the gestation have been described, but these are not flawless. Gross examination alone can be unreliable also and is clearly dependent on the experience of the observer and lacks permanent documentation of an intrauterine pregnancy.

Universal histological examination of ostensibly normal tissue from induced abortions is difficult to justify because of the large numbers. The theoretical possibility that an occasional abnormal conceptus, such as a molar pregnancy, may be missed does not seem to be a reasonable justification for routine examination because of the low prevalence of molar pregnancy in the population and the frequency that a molar pregnancy will progress to persistent gestational trophoblastic disease. If, however, villi or fetal parts cannot be identified grossly with certainty in a specimen or when scanty material is obtained at termination of pregnancy, then it should be sent for histological examination to confirm successful termination. A cautionary note is that fibrillary tissues that look like villi under the dissecting microscope may sometimes be friable decidua only on histological examination.

Little is known about the outcome for an eutopic pregnancy following a procedure for terminating the pregnancy if all tissue examined identifies no products of conception histologically. Failed terminations of pregnancy occur in about 1 in 300 surgical procedures.[8] The failure rate of medical terminations depends on the gestational age at which they are performed: it ranges from 0.5% to 1% in the early first trimester[9] to 10% in the second trimester.[10] Curettage specimens obtained following a failed medical termination show increased inflammation as evidenced by increased numbers of T and B lymphocytes on immunohistology and increased extent of necrosis.[11] Few women who have opted for the termination in the first instance change their minds prior to a repeat procedure and decide instead to continue with their pregnancy. Ultrasound and hCG assays can confirm rapidly continuation of the pregnancy, following which a repeat procedure can be performed when the gestation is more mature and products are more likely to be obtained.

TISSUE FROM SPONTANEOUS ABORTIONS

With miscarriage (spontaneous abortion), the conceptus is often expelled in its entirety at the beginning. Women may be managed expectantly, dependent upon symptoms and amount of blood lost, or be managed actively, where the uterine cavity is evacuated formally under anesthesia as it is not possible often to decide whether the abortion has been complete or incomplete.

The amount and nature of the material depends upon the gestation, the method of management of the miscarriage and the timing of the abortal tissue in relation to the abortion or fetal demise. The material may include a complete gestational sac with or without a dead fetus and curettings from the uterus. The examination of the fetus and the gestational sac is out of the scope of this monograph. Instead, attention will be concentrated on the histology of the curettage specimens commonly received in the laboratory.

In the majority of cases, there is little difficulty in confirming the diagnosis of an abortion or retained products of conception. Typically, there is a mixture of decidua, placental villi and blood clot. Finding fetal somatic tissue makes confirmation of products of conception easier. The decidua may show varying degrees of necrosis and inflammation. Decidua basalis and decidua vera and parietalis may be included.

In many early miscarriages, the failure of embryonic development, together with deficient placental growth, results in the majority of the products of conception consisting of decidua only.[12] In the absence of chorionic villi, an intrauterine pregnancy can be diagnosed from changes in the decidua. It will be recalled that the extravillous trophoblast infiltrates the decidua basalis in the formation of the placental bed. The extravillous trophoblast may be difficult to identify using conventional staining with hematoxylin and eosin, but multiclefting and grooving of hyperchromatic nuclei facilitate differentiation of the extravillous trophoblast from decidual cells (Figure 3.10). Immunohistochemistry using anti-human placental lactogen or anti-keratin antibodies can help in the identification of the extravillous trophoblast. Two other features of pregnancy are the vascular changes in the spiral arteries and deposition of fibrinoid matrix in the developing Rohr's and Nitabuch's striae. It has been claimed that these are so specific that, when present, intrauterine pregnancy can be ruled in. The stromal fibrinoid matrix changes can be highlighted by the use of reticulin staining which shows a distinct increase in reticulin staining around the decidual and trophoblast cells and also accentuation around stromal vessels, glands and myometrial cells (Figure 3.11).[13]

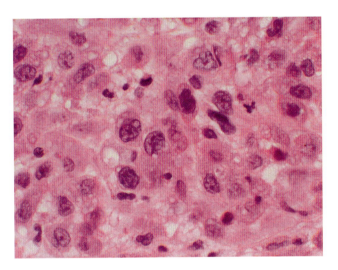

Figure 3.10 Multiclefting and grooving of hyperchromatic nuclei facilitate differentiation of extravillous trophoblast from decidual cells.

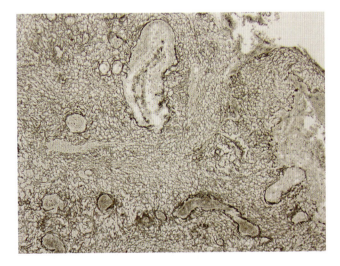

Figure 3.11 Reticulin stain around decidual and trophoblast cells and also accentuation around uteroplacental vessels and glands (same field as Figure 3.4).

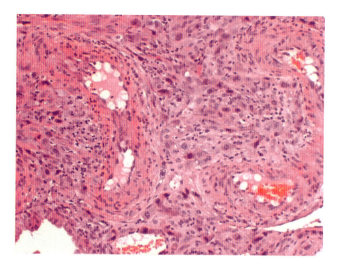

Figure 3.12 Spiral arteries in the decidua showing absence of vascular changes despite the presence of plentiful interstitial trophoblast in this miscarriage.

Undue emphasis is given to the finding of chorionic villi in uterine curettings, but the presence of villi, per se, does not indicate necessarily an intrauterine pregnancy: it is possible that they are derived from a tubal pregnancy that has aborted spontaneously into the uterine cavity. The only absolute confirmation of an intrauterine pregnancy is the finding of implantation-site changes in the intrauterine decidua.

Features of the chorionic villi or decidua to predict if the miscarriage is chromosomally normal are neither specific nor sensitive enough to be of use clinically. Abnormal placentation may be an etiological factor in miscarriage. In many cases of miscarriages, whether sporadic or recurrent, there is reduced trophoblastic infiltration into the decidua and into the spiral arteries, with consequent limited or absent physiological vascular changes (Figure 3.12).[14] Trophoblastic proliferation within the villous columns and the outer shell is reduced.

The endometrial histology subsequent to a miscarriage is seldom examined unless there is persistent bleeding. In the first two menstrual cycles after miscarriage, curettage findings include proliferative endometrium, proliferative glands with decidualized stroma, endometritis and luteal insufficiency.

TISSUE FROM PREGNANCIES OF UNKNOWN LOCATION AND ECTOPIC PREGNANCY

The endometrium responds to the hormonal influences of pregnancy regardless of whether nidation of the blastocyst has occurred in the uterine cavity or not. A true decidua is formed with the appropriate changes within the stroma and glands. In the absence of an intrauterine conceptus, the secondary changes in the gestational endometrium are not seen. Thus, there is no trophoblastic infiltration, fibrinoid matrix deposition or vascular reaction.

Curettage material obtained from women with ectopic pregnancy can be quite varied: decidual reaction, secretory endometrium and proliferative endometrium can be encountered.[15] When the embryo or fetus in an ectopic pregnancy dies, as it usually does early on, the decidua may be sloughed off as a cast, in which case it will be found to be a relatively bland specimen devoid of necrosis and inflammatory reaction. More commonly, there is gradual breakup of the decidua. The decidua will show a variable degree of necrosis and cellular infiltration admixed with blood clots or a picture of irregular shedding because of the slow involution of the corpus luteum. If the interval between the embryonic or fetal loss and curettage is long, the original decidua may have disappeared altogether to be replaced by proliferative endometrium and, because the first few cycles may be anovulatory, it is not uncommon to find the characteristic mildly hyperplastic endometrium of the anovulatory cycle. If there are still viable portions of the original decidualized endometrium in the curettings, then the Arias-Stella phenomenon may be identifiable.

The diagnosis of an extrauterine pregnancy is facilitated by transvaginal ultrasound, laparoscopy and hormonal assays. Nevertheless, the pathologist often is presented with uterine curettings in situations in which the location of the pregnancy is uncertain. The pathologist's task is to rule in an intrauterine gestation. The presence of chorionic villi, trophoblast or implantation site will rule in an intrauterine gestation, but the pathologist cannot exclude an ectopic pregnancy because there may be a concurrent ectopic pregnancy. The prevalence of heterotopic pregnancy is approximately 0.9:1000 in patients conceiving with assisted reproductive technologies[16] and estimated to be as high as 1:2600 in all pregnancies.[17]

Curettage material may be devoid of villi or the implantation site despite coming from an intrauterine pregnancy and can then be misinterpreted as coming from a case of ectopic pregnancy, particularly when there is only decidua with Arias-Stella changes. The sensitivity of an endometrial suction curette in detecting products of conception in most women with an intrauterine gestation during the first trimester when sonographic visualisation has not been attained is only moderate, which means that routine use of the endometrial biopsy in the algorithms for the diagnosis and treatment of ectopic pregnancy should be approached with caution.

The finding of bland non-necrotic or partly necrotic decidua with the Arias-Stella changes and little inflammatory response is strongly suggestive of an ectopic pregnancy, and the pathologist may suggest further clinical evaluation but cannot diagnose an ectopic pregnancy (Figure 3.13). Indeed, identical Arias-Stella changes may, on occasion, occur outside the endometrium or in nonpregnant women. Arias-Stella changes can be seen in endometria of peri- or postmenopausal nonpregnant women who have received exogenous hormones, particularly progestational agents (Summary Box 3.2).

Abnormal pregnancy 27

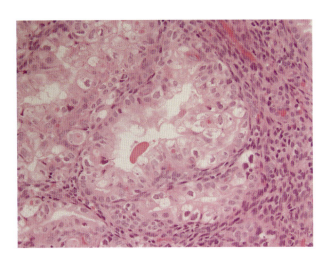

Figure 3.13 Endometrial glands with Arias-Stella phenomenon. The glands are hypersecretory with vacuolated cytoplasm and there is nuclear pleomorphism.

SUMMARY BOX 3.2: Approach to histopathology of early pregnancy

Tissue from induced abortion

- May be difficult to examine all cases because of numbers of cases
- Gross examination, including under dissecting microscope, may confirm villous tissue
- Not all fibrillary tissues are placental villi
- May require histological confirmation of pregnancy, including examining all tissue

Tissue from miscarriage

- The finding of fibrinoid tissues may be sufficient to confirm recent pregnancy
- Less imperative to examine all tissue to absolutely confirm pregnancy products

Tissue from pregnancy of unknown location

- May require histological confirmation of pregnancy, including examining all tissue
- Histological confirmation of pregnancy does not, however, exclude an heterotopic pregnancy

ABNORMAL PREGNANCY

In complicated pregnancies, the physiological vascular adaptive changes do not occur to the same extent or depth. The resulting compromise in blood supply to the placenta and conceptus can result in early pregnancy loss, intrauterine growth restriction, preeclampsia and intrauterine death. While the morphological features of abnormal placentation have been well documented, the molecular mechanisms leading to it are as yet unclear.[18]

In pregnancies that are destined to be complicated by preeclampsia or by small-for-gestational-date infants, the temporally and spatially related extravillous trophoblast migration during early pregnancy is impaired. Endovascular trophoblast migration and conversion of the spiral arteries into uteroplacental arteries fail to occur. This could affect part of one circumference of a vessel or be confined to part of the length of the spiral arteries, affecting only the intramyometrial segments only, or be more extensive and affect the entire length from their opening into the intervillous space through the intradecidual segments to their origin from the radial arteries in the superficial myometrium (Figures 3.14 to 3.16). Some or all of the spiral arteries in the decidua basalis and subjacent myometrium may exhibit this deficit of placentation. Since unconverted arteries retain high resistance and low capacitance properties, blood flow through these arteries is compromised.

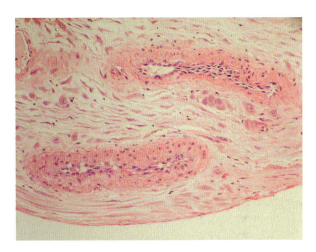

Figure 3.14 Absent vascular changes in intradecidual spiral artery in preeclampsia. Interstitial trophoblast can be seen adjacent to the wall of the upper artery.

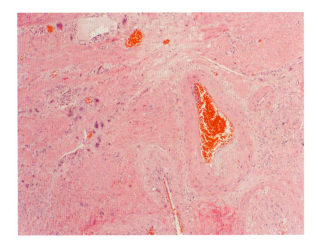

Figure 3.15 Absence of physiological changes with retention of muscular and elastic tissue within intramyometrial segment of spiral artery in preeclampsia. Adjacent basal artery shows no physiological changes.

28 Pregnancy

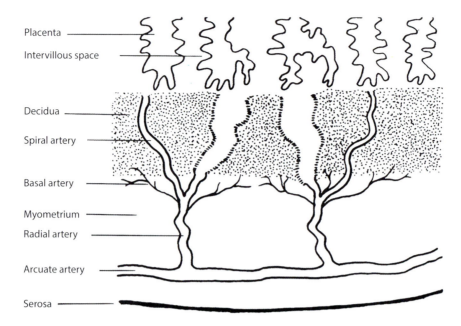

Figure 3.16 Diagrammatic representation of blood supply to the placenta in intrauterine growth restriction and in preeclampsia. The hatched lines in some intradecidual segments of the spiral arteries indicate physiological vascular changes, which are absent in other intradecidual or in the intramyometrial segments. (Reproduced with permission from Khong TY, Liddell HS, Robertson WB. *Br J Obstet Gynaecol* 1987;94:649–55.)

In women with essential hypertension, vessels that fail to display the physiological changes may manifest intimal or medial hyperplasia as a consequence of long-standing hypertension (Figure 3.17).

To emphasise the disordered migration of extravillous trophoblast in these pregnancy complications, endovascular trophoblast may be seen within the lumen in the spiral or uteroplacental arteries in the third trimester, when they would not normally be expected to be present then (Figure 3.18). This has been thought to reflect a teleological attempt to effect the physiological changes to ensure an adequate blood supply in the face of a compromised blood supply.[19] The density of the interstitial trophoblast is reduced in preeclampsia, recapitulating the defect in miscarriage.

Arteries in the decidua and superficial myometrium that have not undergone physiological changes may develop a lesion that, because of its resemblance to atheroma, has been designated as acute atherosis. The lesion is characterised by fibrinoid necrosis of the vessel wall, accompanied by a perivascular lymphocytic infiltrate and lipid-laden macrophages (Figures 3.19 and 3.20). Acute atherosis may be seen in basal arteries as well as arteries in the decidua parietalis.

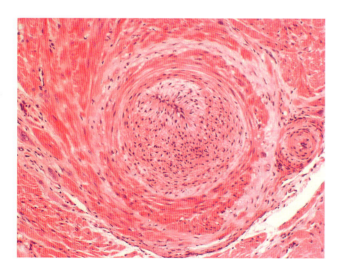

Figure 3.17 Medial hyperplasia and absence of vascular changes in long-standing hypertension superimposed on preeclampsia.

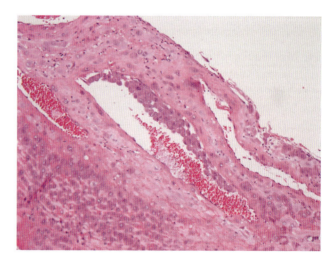

Figure 3.18 Intraluminal endovascular trophoblast in the spiral artery showing physiological changes in late third trimester in preeclampsia; some elastic tissue is present within the intima and media on the left side of the artery.

Abnormal pregnancy 29

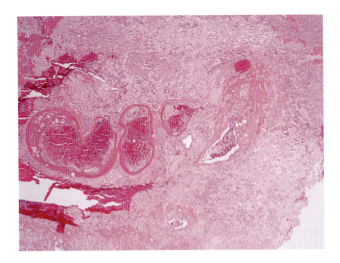

Figure 3.19 Acute atherosis: vessel showing mainly fibrinoid necrosis.

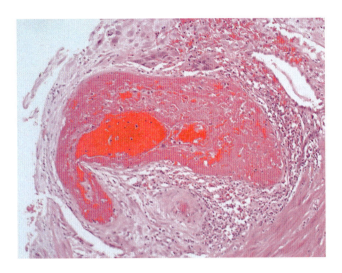

Figure 3.21 Acute atherosis: thrombosis within vessel showing mainly fibrinoid necrosis with a moderate perivascular lymphocytic infiltrate.

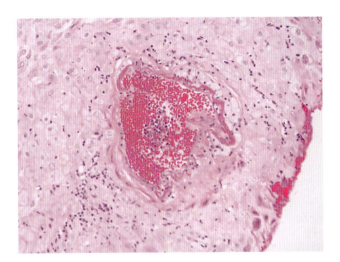

Figure 3.20 Acute atherosis: vessel showing fibrinoid necrosis, lipid-laden macrophages and scanty perivascular lymphocytic infiltrate.

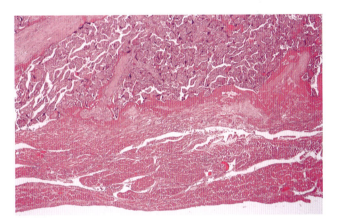

Figure 3.22 Placenta accreta in second trimester showing early pregnancy placental villi embedding directly onto myometrium.

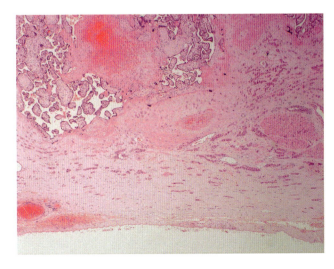

Figure 3.23 Placenta increta with placental villi almost reaching the serosa.

The similarity of acute atherosis to similar lesions seen in allograft rejection has prompted some authors to suggest that this is a histological marker for aberrant maternal-fetal immunological interaction. Acute atherosis is important because of its effect on reducing the caliber of the spiral arterial lumen, which is already compromised by the lack of physiological changes, as well as being associated with vascular thrombosis (Figure 3.21).

Another pregnancy disorder characterised by abnormal placentation is placenta accreta, the incidence of which has reached epidemic proportions.[20] There are three degrees of severity, but common to all three is placental villi embedding directly onto the myometrium without intervening decidua (Figure 3.22). In placenta accreta vera, placental villi attach directly to the myometrium, but the villi may invade or even penetrate the myometrium, conditions known as placenta increta and placenta percreta,

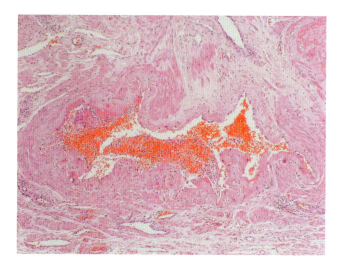

Figure 3.24 Placenta accreta: pregnancy-induced vascular changes extend to a radial artery deep in the myometrium.

respectively (Figure 3.23). Defective decidualization has been proposed as a pathogenetic mechanism but adequate decidual tissue is often found away from the placental site. There is often focal proliferation of cytotrophoblastic cells, accompanied by deeper penetration of the myometrium by extravillous trophoblast and pregnancy-induced vascular changes extending further into the radial arteries than in normal pregnancies (Figure 3.24). It is this last feature which accounts for the torrential bleeding that occurs when the placenta is removed manually in placenta accreta, as these larger vessels, devoid of the muscular and elastic tissue, are able to conduct more blood than the relatively smaller spiral arteries (Summary Box 3.3).

SUMMARY BOX 3.3: Abnormal placentation

Limited infiltration of interstitial trophoblast
Limited infiltration of endovascular trophoblast

- Seen in preeclampsia, intrauterine growth restriction, stillbirth, miscarriage
- Reduction in numbers and depth of spiral arteries with physiological changes
- Fibrinoid necrosis and acute atherosis of intrauterine arteries

Extensive infiltration of interstitial and endovascular trophoblast
Diminished decidualization

- Seen in placenta accreta with deep implantation of placental villi into myometrium
- Physiological changes seen deep in radial and arcuate arteries

POSTPARTUM HEMORRHAGE

Postpartum hemorrhage is estimated to occur in 6%–11% of births and is a leading cause of maternal morbidity and mortality worldwide. Postpartum hemorrhage is classified clinically into primary or secondary postpartum hemorrhage.

Primary postpartum hemorrhage is clearly defined as occurring within 24 hours of parturition and quantified as excessive blood loss. The excessive blood loss is defined variously as 500, 600 or 1000 mL, although it is acknowledged that quantification of the blood loss can be inaccurate. Uterine atony accounts for at least 80% of cases of primary postpartum hemorrhage, while placenta accreta is increasing as a cause.

Secondary postpartum hemorrhage, also termed late or delayed postpartum hemorrhage or bleeding, is less clearly defined. It refers to excessive hemorrhage that occurs after the first 24 hours postpartum until six weeks after the delivery. The upper limit is imposed because it is often difficult to determine whether bleeding after six weeks is related to the previous pregnancy, to subsequent menstruation or even to a spontaneous abortion of a new conception. However, there are reported cases where bleeding has either persisted for or commenced as late as six months after delivery. To overcome the imprecision of the definition, where the bleeding is merely a subjective impression of an increased amount, another definition is to include women who had bleeding excessive after hospital discharge enough to merit readmission or an operative procedure.

Generically, involution of the placental bed, subinvolution of the placental bed and retained placental fragments represent products of conception[21] (Table 3.1).

Involuted placental beds are characterised by the presence of ghost-like hyalinized residua of uteroplacental (spiral) arteries that are either collapsed or completely obliterated by thrombosis. Occasional hemosiderin-laden macrophages can be seen adjacent to these vascular outlines. Recanalisation of the lumina of regenerating vessels can be seen sometimes (Figure 3.25). In these women, the cause of postpartum hemorrhage remains unexplained by these findings, although dislodgment of thrombi is a possibility.

In contrast, the reason for bleeding in women with subinvolution, sometimes also known as noninvolution, of the placental bed is more obvious. The partly hyalinized uteroplacental arteries are widely distended or only partly

Table 3.1 Tissue types obtained from women presenting with secondary postpartum hemorrhage

Retained placental fragments
Involution of the placental bed
Subinvolution of the placental bed
Endometritis
Normal endometrium or decidua
Insufficient tissue for diagnosis

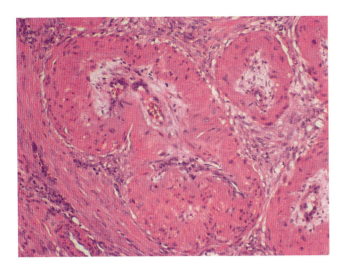

Figure 3.25 Involution of the placental bed: there is recanalisation of the arterial lumen while the residua of the fibrinoid matrix wall can still be seen.

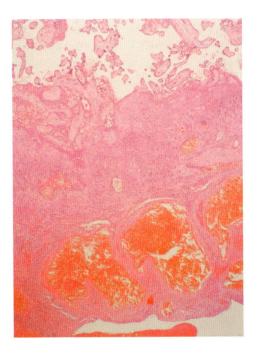

Figure 3.27 Retained placental fragment stenting open subinvoluted vessels in endometrium in postpartum hemorrhage.

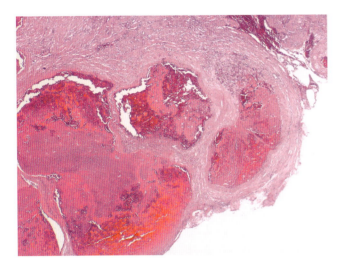

Figure 3.26 Partly hyalinized uteroplacental arteries that are only partly occluded by fresh thrombi with the artery on the right being occluded completely by thrombus.

occluded by fresh thrombi superimposed on organizing thrombi, thus allowing blood to percolate through them (Figure 3.26). Intraluminal endovascular trophoblast can be seen occasionally. Not infrequently, the curettage may have subinvoluted and involuted areas. Subinvolution of the placental bed can be a cause of bleeding following voluntary terminations of pregnancy, miscarriage and molar pregnancy in addition to following a third-trimester pregnancy.

Retained placental fragment is a better term than placental polyps as the former term is accurate and readily understood by both obstetrician and pathologist. A polyp implies the presence of a neoplastic lesion arising from a stalk with stroma and blood vessels; that is evidently not the case. Retained placental fragment is likely to be the largest cause of secondary postpartum bleeding.[22] The placental fragments may vary in viability, ranging from viable to necrotic fragments with dystrophic calcification. The accompanying inflammatory response is also variable and can be acute or chronic. Very often, subinvoluted vessels are seen either in adjacent or contiguous endometrial tissue. Bleeding is exacerbated by stenting of these maternal vessels by the placental fragments (Figure 3.27). It is appropriate, therefore, that the diagnosis of retained placental fragments takes precedence over subinvolution of the placental bed as the diagnosis in these women.

The frequency of infection as a cause of postpartum hemorrhage may be overstated. Bacterial cultures are not routinely performed to ascertain the prevalence of infection. The diagnostic criterion for endometritis, namely that of acute inflammation in excess of that normally seen following parturition, is nebulous and unhelpful as necrosis and inflammation are seen during the process of involution of the placental bed.

Quite commonly, the material obtained following curettage from women with postpartum hemorrhage is inadequate for diagnosis, or contains blood clots only. In others, decidua, if obtained shortly after delivery, or endometrium is found. In these cases, an anatomical cause for hemorrhage is not readily apparent.

An infrequent finding in abnormal uterine bleeding is the placental site nodule or plaque (see also Chapter 10). These are usually microscopic singular or multiple well-circumscribed plaques that are extensively hyalinized, giving an eosinophilic fluffy appearance (Figures 3.28 and 3.29). Rarely, they can be identified grossly. These nodules are generally paucicellular but persistent extravillous trophoblast is present within these nodules indicating their origin from a

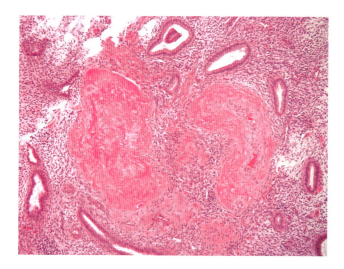

Figure 3.28 Placental site nodule: prior pregnancy was a miscarriage 48 days before curettage for abnormal uterine bleeding. The partly involuted uteroplacental arterial outline with effete trophoblastic cells can be seen in the right side of the hyalinized nodule.

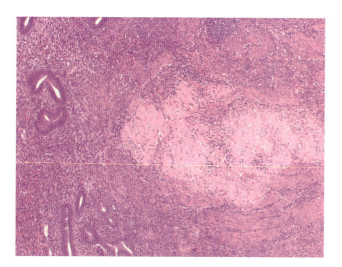

Figure 3.29 Placental site nodule at the endo-myometrial junction: prior pregnancy was two years before curettage. The hyalinized nodule has a more 'fluffy' acelllular appearance, and trophoblastic cells are no longer evident.

pregnancy that had occurred either knowingly up to several years previously or unbeknown to the woman.[23] Apart from this lack of immediate temporal relationship to pregnancy, they do not differ significantly from the nodules that are present in subinvolution of the placental bed.

Endometrial ossification is rare and while more likely to present as a cause of infertility, it can also present as postpartum hemorrhage or abnormal uterine bleeding. Retention of fetal bones following miscarriage or, more commonly, a voluntary termination of pregnancy is reported in most cases. In others, osseous metaplasia leads to endometrial ossification.

Endometrial implantation of fetal tissue following voluntary termination of pregnancy is well described. In addition to the fetal bones mentioned above, glial or adipose tissue have been described. Endometrial extramedullary hematopoiesis thought to be due to implanted fetal hematopoietic elements from the fetus or yolk sac has been described.

PREGNANCY FOLLOWING THERAPY

ENDOMETRIAL ABLATION

Endometrial ablation has become a well-established alternative to medical treatment or hysterectomy to treat abnormal uterine bleeding. The rationale is to replicate Asherman's syndrome so that there is little or no endometrium remaining. Placenta accreta is not an invariant accompaniment in pregnancies following endometrial resection.[24,25] Endometrial ablation, by necessity, will cause damage to the superficial portions of the endometrial vessels but will also likely cause scarring to the endometrial interstitium and the superficial myometrial layer, all of which are anatomically involved in the development of the maternal response to pregnancy. Thus, it is not surprising that case reports of subsequent pregnancies frequently describe fetal growth restriction and intrauterine fetal demise.[25]

PELVIC ARTERY EMBOLIZATION

Pelvic transcatheter artery embolization, involving successive introduction of a catheter into the bilateral femoral, internal iliac and finally uterine arteries to release embolization material, has been widely used for the management of postpartum hemorrhage. The endometrial ischemia resulting from the embolization leads to thinning of the endometrium. The incidence of placenta accreta, and further postpartum hemorrhage, is more frequent after pelvic artery embolization than in the general population.[26]

RADIOTHERAPY

The pregnancy outcome of women who had radiotherapy during their childhood for treatment of intraabdominal neoplasms is poorer than those whose treatment consisted of chemotherapy or surgery. Increased risk of miscarriages, preterm delivery and pregnancies with small-for-gestational-age infants have been reported, attributed to the effects of radiotherapy on the spiral arteries that render them unable to respond to the trophoblast invasion during the first half of pregnancy or to a reduction in uterine volume.[27]

CHEMOTHERAPY

A later effect of chemotherapy that has been described is partial placenta accreta. Partial placenta accreta has been described in pregnancies following chemotherapy for gestational trophoblastic neoplasms.

REFERENCES

1. Moffett A, Colucci F. Uterine NK cells: Active regulators at the maternal-fetal interface. *J Clin Invest* 2014; 124:1872–9.
2. Burton GJ, Watson AL, Hempstock J, Skepper JN, Jauniaux E. Uterine glands provide histiotrophic nutrition for the human fetus during the first trimester of pregnancy. *J Clin Endocrinol Metab* 2002;87:2954–9.
3. Robson A, Harris LK, Innes BA et al. Uterine natural killer cells initiate spiral artery remodeling in human pregnancy. *FASEB J* 2012;26:4876–85.
4. Moffett A, Chazara O, Colucci F. Maternal allorecognition of the fetus. *Fertil Steril* 2017;107:1269–72.
5. Small HY, Cornelius DC, Guzik TJ, Delles C. Natural killer cells in placentation and cancer: Implications for hypertension during pregnancy. *Placenta* 2017;56: 59–64.
6. Pijnenborg R, Dixon G, Robertson WB, Brosens I. Trophoblastic invasion of human decidua from 8 to 18 weeks of pregnancy. *Placenta* 1980;1:3–19.
7. Pijnenborg R, Bland JM, Robertson WB, Brosens I. Uteroplacental arterial changes related to interstitial trophoblast migration in early human pregnancy. *Placenta* 1983;4:397–413.
8. Heath V, Chadwick V, Cooke I, Manek S, MacKenzie IZ. Should tissue from pregnancy termination and uterine evacuation routinely be examined histologically? *Br J Obstet Gynaecol* 2000;107:727–30.
9. Cameron ST, Glasier A, Johnstone A, Dewart H, Campbell A. Can women determine the success of early medical termination of pregnancy themselves? *Contraception* 2015;91:6–11.
10. Pongsatha S, Tongsong T. How to manage unresponsiveness to misoprostol in failed second trimester pregnancy termination. *J Obstet Gynaecol Res* 2013;39:154–9.
11. Fuchs N, Maymon R, Ben-Ami I et al. Clinical, surgical, and histopathologic outcomes following failed medical abortion. *Int J Gynaecol Obstet* 2012;117:234–8.
12. Rushton DI. Examination of products of conception from previable human pregnancies. *J Clin Pathol* 1981;34:819–35.
13. Stewart CJ, Little L. Use of reticulin stain in the diagnosis of intra-uterine gestation. *Pathology* 2008;40: 365–71.
14. Khong TY, Liddell HS, Robertson WB. Defective haemochorial placentation as a cause of miscarriage: A preliminary study. *Br J Obstet Gynaecol* 1987;94: 649–55.
15. Lopez HB, Micheelsen U, Berendtsen H, Kock K. Ectopic pregnancy and its associated endometrial changes. *Gynecol Obstet Invest* 1994;38:104–6.
16. Perkins KM, Boulet SL, Kissin DM, Jamieson DJ. Risk of ectopic pregnancy associated with assisted reproductive technology in the United States, 2001–2011. *Obstet Gynecol* 2015;125:70–8.
17. Chan AJ, Day LB, Vairavanathan R. Tale of 2 pregnancies: Heterotopic pregnancy in a spontaneous cycle. *Can Fam Physician* 2016;62:565–7.
18. Brosens I, Khong TY. *Defective Spiral Artery Remodelling. Placental Bed Disorders*. Cambridge University Press. London, 2010.
19. Khong TY, De Wolf F, Robertson WB, Brosens I. Inadequate maternal vascular response to placentation in pregnancies complicated by pre-eclampsia and by small-for-gestational age infants. *Br J Obstet Gynaecol* 1986;93:1049–59.
20. Khong TY. The pathology of placenta accreta, a worldwide epidemic. *J Clin Pathol* 2008;61:1243–6.
21. Khong TY, Khong TK. Delayed postpartum hemorrhage: A morphologic study of causes and their relation to other pregnancy disorders. *Obstet Gynecol* 1993;82:17–22.
22. Dossou M, Debost-Legrand A, Dechelotte P, Lemery D, Vendittelli F. Severe secondary postpartum hemorrhage: A historical cohort. *Birth* 2015;42: 149–55.
23. Young RH, Kurman RJ, Scully RE. Placental site nodules and plaques. A clinicopathologic analysis of 20 cases. *Am J Surg Pathol* 1990;14:1001–9.
24. Bauer AM, Hackney DN, El-Nashar S, Sheyn D. Pregnancy outcomes after endometrial ablation in a multi-institutional cohort. *Am J Perinatol* 2018;35: 931–5.
25. Kohn JR, Shamshirsaz AA, Popek E et al. Pregnancy after endometrial ablation: A systematic review. *BJOG* 2018;125:43–53.
26. Soro MP, Denys A, de Rham M, Baud D. Short & long term adverse outcomes after arterial embolisation for the treatment of postpartum haemorrhage: A systematic review. *Eur Radiol* 2017;27:749–62.
27. Teh WT, Stern C, Chander S, Hickey M. The impact of uterine radiation on subsequent fertility and pregnancy outcomes. *Biomed Res Int* 2014;2014: 482968.

4

Endometrial inflammation

Normal endometrium	35	Morphological subtypes of endometritis	39
Endometritis	37	References	41
Nonspecific endometritis	37		

NORMAL ENDOMETRIUM

In order to arrive at a definition of clinically and morphologically significant endometrial inflammation it, is necessary to understand that the normal human endometrium contains a population of inflammatory cells and that these comprise some 10%–25% of all endometrial cells (see Chapter 2). Normal endometrial inflammatory cells are distributed between the basal layer, the functional layer stroma and within the endometrial epithelium. The predominant inflammatory cell type in normal endometrium comprises T lymphocytes with smaller numbers of macrophages, B lymphocytes and granulated lymphocytes (NK cells or stromal granulocytes). The relative composition of endometrial leucocytes undergoes cyclical alterations during the menstrual cycle.

The inflammatory cells within the basal layer are arranged into lymphoid aggregates (Figures 4.1 and 4.2)

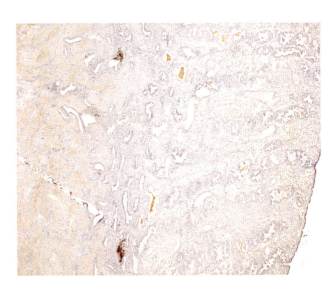

Figure 4.2 Low-power view of late secretory-phase endometrium: the basal lymphoid aggregates are highlighted by CD20 immunostaining for B cells.

composed of a central zone of B lymphocytes surrounded by CD8+CD4− T lymphocytes and an outermost zone of macrophages.[1] The lymphoid aggregates develop and increase in size during the proliferative phase (Figure 4.1) and are present during the secretory phase (Figure 4.2), but are absent in the immediate postmenstrual phase.

The stroma of the functional layer contains macrophages, CD56+ granulated lymphocytes as well as CD4+ and CD8+ T lymphocytes (Figures 4.3 through 4.5). The absolute number and relative proportion of different endometrial stromal leucocytes varies markedly throughout the menstrual cycle. The absolute number of T cells peaks in the early proliferative phase and decreases subsequently. The absolute number of CD56+ granulated lymphocytes, also referred to as NK cells or stromal granulocytes, increases sharply in the mid to late secretory phase and decreases following menstruation (Figures 4.6 and 4.7). Endometrial granulated lymphocytes tend to aggregate around the glands and spiral arteries. The number of macrophages remains constant throughout the cycle.

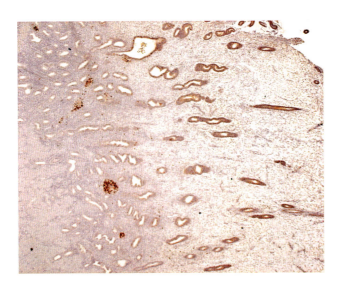

Figure 4.1 Low-power view of early proliferative-phase endometrium: the basal lymphoid aggregates are highlighted by CD20 (B cell) immunostaining.

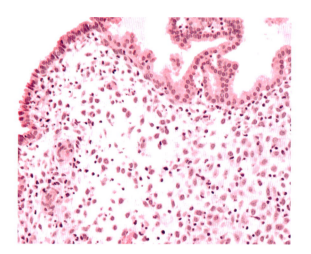

Figure 4.3 Late secretory-phase endometrium: contains numerous granulated lymphocytes seen in the stroma of the functional layer.

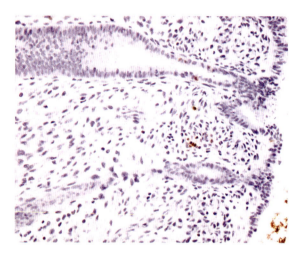

Figure 4.4 Early proliferative-phase endometrium: CD3 immunostaining showing T cells within glandular epithelium and stroma in the upper functional layer.

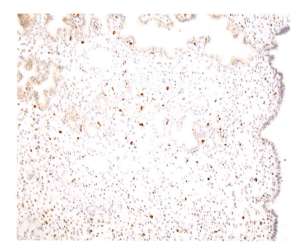

Figure 4.5 Late secretory-phase endometrium: CD68 immunostaining showing macrophages within the stroma and luminal epithelium within the upper functional layer.

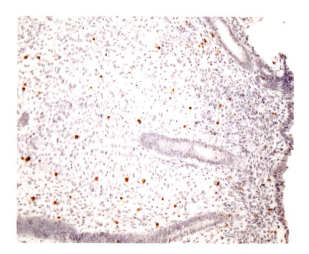

Figure 4.6 Early proliferative-phase endometrium: CD56 immunostaining showing granulated lymphocytes within the stroma.

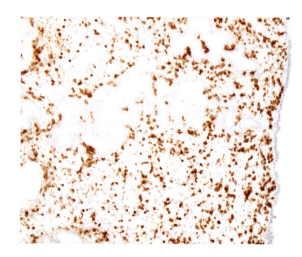

Figure 4.7 Late secretory-phase endometrium: CD56 immunostaining showing granulated lymphocytes within the stroma.

Intraepithelial lymphocytes are found in both the surface epithelium and the glandular epithelium. The type and number of intraepithelial lymphocytes also undergo cyclical variations. During the proliferative phase, most intraepithelial lymphocytes are predominantly CD8+ T lymphocytes, but the proportion of CD56+ granulated lymphocytes peaks in the secretory phase.[2]

Mast cells are found throughout the endometrium at all stages of the menstrual cycle, and the number of mast cells does not appear to vary with the phase of the menstrual cycle.[3] Eosinophils are found in groups within the functional zone during and immediately prior to menstruation, but are absent during the proliferative and secretory phase.[3] Neutrophils are found in very small numbers throughout the cycle but are seen in large numbers in areas of tissue breakdown during the menstrual phase.[4] Plasma cells are commonly seen in the endometrium of healthy women but not in significant numbers.[5]

Relatively little information is available about leucocytes in the postmenopausal endometrium. The total number of leucocytes is reduced compared with the cycling endometrium, but the relative proportion of different leucocyte types is similar to that found in the secretory endometrium.[6] Others have found a similar number of T cells as in cycling endometria and in the same compartments.[7]

ENDOMETRITIS

Endometritis is characterised by increased numbers and abnormal distribution of endometrial inflammatory cells, frequently accompanied by morphological abnormalities of endometrial glands and stroma. Depending on the pathological findings, endometritis is traditionally classified into nonspecific endometritis and other morphological subtypes (see Table 4.1). With few exceptions, this classification gives little or no indication of the cause of the inflammation.

NONSPECIFIC ENDOMETRITIS

PATHOLOGICAL FEATURES

On microscopic examination, these endometria show a variable appearance (Figures 4.8 through 4.12). There are an increased number of stromal lymphoid cells and prominent lymphoid aggregates within the functional layer. The stroma also contains numerous plasma cells and/or eosinophils; mast cells may also be present (Figure 4.9). In some cases, there are numerous neutrophils within the stroma and within the glandular lumina. There may be associated ulceration and epithelial regenerative changes. In premenopausal women with significant nonspecific endometritis, the glandular and stromal morphology may differ from the normal cyclical pattern, leading to problems

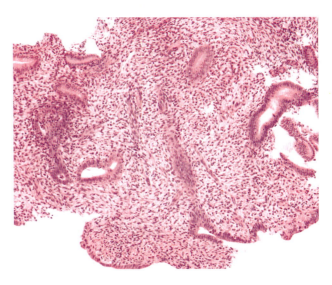

Figure 4.8 Nonspecific endometritis: postpartum chronic endometritis following a miscarriage.

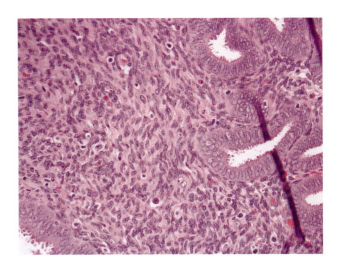

Figure 4.9 Nonspecific chronic endometritis showing stromal inflammatory infiltrate of plasma cells, mast cells and lymphocytes.

Table 4.1 Classification of endometritis

Type of endometritis	Causes
Nonspecific endometritis	Postpartum or post-abortion
	Polyps or neoplasms
	Instrumentation
	Intrauterine contraceptive devices
	Infections, e.g. gonococcal, mycoplasma or chlamydial
Other types	
Granulomatous endometritis	Post-TCRE, tuberculosis, histoplasmosis, sarcoidosis
Xanthogranulomatous endometritis	Related to necrosis, irradiation of tumors
Malakoplakia	Infections with Gram negative organisms
Viral endometritis	Herpesvirus or cytomegalovirus
Nodular histiocytic hyperplasia	Not known
Ligneous endometritis	Type-1 congenital plasminogen deficiency
Focal necrotising endometritis	Not known

Abbreviation: TCRE, transcervical resection of endometrium.

38 Endometrial inflammation

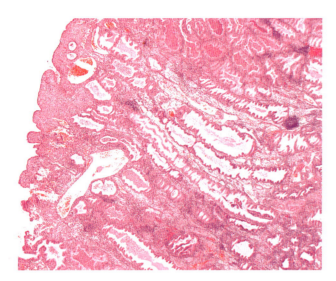

Figure 4.10 Low-power view of secretory endometrium with nonspecific endometritis. There are collections of neutrophils within endometrial glands (top) and dilated capillaries some traversing the endometrial glands transverse.

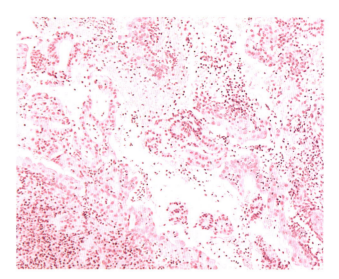

Figure 4.12 Nonspecific endometritis: marked distortion of glandular architecture with cribriform glands (bottom left); epithelial cells show reactive atypia.

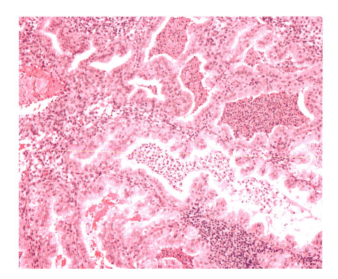

Figure 4.11 Nonspecific endometritis: neutrophils within the glands and chronic inflammatory cells within the stroma.

with endometrial dating. Florid acute endometritis may be associated with abnormalities of glandular architecture and cellular differentiation (Figure 4.12).

Where there is significant nonspecific endometritis, abnormalities should be discernible when scanning the endometrium at low power. The clinical significance of scanty stromal plasma cells or eosinophils that can only be identified after laborious high-power examination is doubtful, and a diagnosis of definite endometritis should not be made in these circumstances. This is corroborated by a contemporary study in which there was an underdiagnosis rate of 16% that was not clinically material, and only 3% who were diagnosed were treated with antibiotics.[8] To reiterate, plasma cells are commonly found in the normal human endometrium and may not represent upper genital tract inflammation.[5] A cautionary note is that the use of immunohistochemistry staining with CD138 to identify plasma cells will result in a significantly higher prevalence of chronic endometritis compared with the use of hematoxylin-and-eosin staining and morphological assessment alone.[9] Kiviat et al. found that the best indicator of upper female genital tract infection was the simultaneous demonstration of five or more neutrophils within surface epithelium per x400 field and one or more stromal plasma cell per x120 field.[10] The finding of eosinophils in an endometrial biopsy specimen should prompt a search for plasma cells for the diagnosis of chronic endometritis.[11]

ETIOLOGY

Endometritis is now rare in developed countries. During the reproductive period, it may be the reason for vaginal bleeding and infertility.

Nonspecific endometritis is most commonly seen in endometrial specimens sampled following delivery or an abortion (Figure 4.8). In these cases, there are often other histological features (such as chorionic villi, necrotic decidua, Arias-Stella change or implantation site) that indicate the presence of intrauterine gestation. Necrotic decidual fragments, where present, are infiltrated by neutrophils. Any endometrial fragments present may contain a stromal infiltrate of lymphoid cells and plasma cells. The stromal cells themselves often have a spindly appearance and mitotic activity. The inflammation in these post-pregnancy endometria is probably a normal component of endometrial repair and remodeling that must necessarily follow the end of gestation. Some cases of nonspecific postpartum endometritis may have an infective component, as prophylactic antibiotics appear to decrease the risk of endometritis.[12]

Chronic endometritis may be seen also in association with endometrial neoplasms and polyps with stromal lymphocytes and plasma cells in the background endometrium in these settings. This finding may represent a response either to mechanical factors or the presence within the endometrial cavity of necrotic tissue. Similarly, the presence of intrauterine devices may also elicit a chronic inflammatory response; progestin-containing devices often provoke an asymptomatic lymphoplasmacytic infiltration.

Nonspecific chronic endometritis can be a manifestation of infection with specific pathogens such as *Chlamydia trachomatis* and *Neisseria gonorrhoea*, the two commonest causes of pelvic inflammatory disease. In recent times, only a small percentage of patients had pelvic inflammatory disease (4%) in contrast to findings from past studies.[8] Severe plasma cell endometritis (defined as confluent stromal plasma cells, neutrophils within glandular epithelium and architectural disturbances making dating impossible) and stromal lymphoid aggregates are reportedly commoner in chlamydial than non-chlamydial endometritis.[13] However, these features are by no means specific and do not exclude non-chlamydial infection.

Similarly, mycobacterial infection in the endometrium may, in some cases, give rise to a nonspecific endometritis.

MORPHOLOGICAL SUBTYPES OF ENDOMETRITIS

MALAKOPLAKIA

Malakoplakia is an unusual inflammatory condition that may mimic a malignant neoplasm. It is associated with immunodeficiency states and thought to be caused by a defective macrophage response to bacterial infection. The bacteria most commonly implicated are coliforms. Malakoplakia involving the endometrium has only been reported infrequently. The patients have all been postmenopausal and presented with postmenopausal bleeding with, in some cases, tumor-like masses.

Microscopically, malakoplakia is characterised by sheets of cytologically bland macrophages with granular, eosinophilic cytoplasm admixed with chronic inflammatory cells (Figures 4.13 and 4.14). Occasional macrophages contain Michaelis–Gutman bodies, iron-rich calcific intracytoplasmic inclusions thought to represent degenerate bacteria. Intracytoplasmic organisms are identified on electron microscopy.[14] The correct histopathological diagnosis of malakoplakia is important as the patients respond to appropriate antibiotic therapy obviating any need for surgery.

XANTHOGRANULOMATOUS ENDOMETRITIS

Also referred to as histiocytic endometritis, this is a rare variant of endometritis with some 21 cases documented

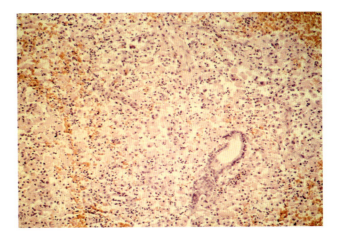

Figure 4.13 Malakoplakia: diffuse stromal infiltrate composed predominantly of histiocytes.

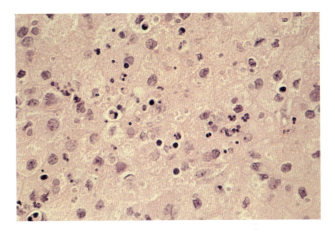

Figure 4.14 Malakoplakia: stromal infiltrate from the same case; the histiocytes have a granular cytoplasm and are admixed with a few neutrophils.

in the literature. Most women are postmenopausal. It may mimic malignancy clinically and radiologically.[15] On macroscopic examination, the endometrium is thickened and may have a friable yellow appearance. Histologically, there is a prominent stromal infiltrate of macrophages with regular small nuclei and abundant foamy cytoplasm (Figure 4.15). The foamy macrophages are admixed with chronic inflammatory cells and occasional multinucleate giant cells. In addition, there may be cholesterol clefts, endometrial necrosis and focal calcification. It is sometimes confused with metastatic adenocarcinoma, but the lack of immunoreactivity for epithelial cytokeratins and strong CD68 immunoreactivity of the foamy macrophages will rule out this diagnostic error. The commonest reported association is with endometrial adenocarcinoma that has been irradiated. It has been postulated that the xanthogranulomatous inflammation represents a response to necrotic tumor.

GRANULOMATOUS ENDOMETRITIS

Granulomatous endometritis is rare and, in our experience, occurs most commonly following transcervical resection

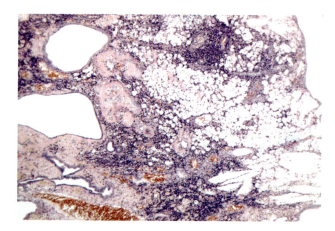

Figure 4.15 Xanthogranulomatous endometritis. There is a stromal infiltrate of foamy macrophages. Cholesterol clefts are seen at the top and bottom right.

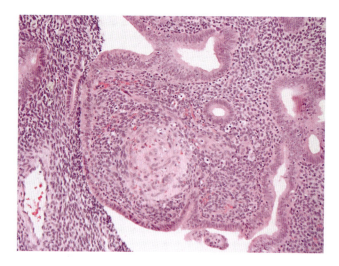

Figure 4.17 Tuberculous endometritis: epithelioid granuloma with Langhans giant cell and a surrounding lymphoplasmacytoid inflammatory infiltrate.

of the endometrium. This type of endometritis is discussed fully in Chapter 6.

Worldwide, tuberculosis is probably the commonest cause of granulomatous endometritis. The commonest reported clinical presentation of tuberculous endometritis is infertility (47%–68%), closely followed by menstrual disturbances (23%–42%); tuberculosis endometritis is much less common in the postmenopausal woman.[16,17] Tuberculous endometritis is more commonly seen as a component of widespread peritoneal and genital tuberculosis presenting with ascites and pelvic masses.

The typical epithelioid granulomas with Langhans giant cells are seen in some 60% of women with tuberculous endometritis (Figures 4.16 and 4.17).[17] Caseation is unusual and few or no acid-fast bacilli are identified. The background endometrium shows a lymphoplasmacytoid inflammatory infiltrate. In those cases where no granulomas are identified, the endometrium usually shows the features of a nonspecific endometritis with stromal lymphoplasmacytoid infiltrates and glandular destruction by neutrophils.[17]

Less commonly, granulomatous endometritis is caused by sarcoidosis and rare infectious diseases such as histoplasmosis and coccidiosis.

VIRAL ENDOMETRITIS

Viral infection is a rare cause of endometritis. The two viruses implicated to date are cytomegalovirus and herpes simplex virus. Cytomegalovirus is much more commonly isolated from endometrial samples of women with pelvic inflammatory disease than is herpes simplex virus.[18] The former is therefore more likely to be a significant endometrial pathogen than the latter.

Endometrial cytomegalovirus infection may occur as a consequence of immunosuppression, presumably due to reactivation of latent infection or as primary infection in non-immunocompromised women.[19] The endometrium shows a lymphoplasmacytoid stromal inflammatory infiltrate, occasional lymphoid follicles and characteristic owl's eye intranuclear inclusions in epithelial and stromal cells. Small, non-necrotising granulomas may also be seen.[19] Immunocytochemistry for cytomegalovirus antigens may be helpful in confirming the diagnosis, particularly in cases where viral inclusions are scanty.

There are few documented cases of herpes simplex endometritis. Reported cases have occurred as a component of fatal herpes simplex viremia, in conjunction with herpes simplex cervicitis and in endometrial specimens from women with miscarriages in whom there was no clinical suspicion of herpes simplex infection. On microscopic examination, herpes simplex endometritis is characterised by the finding of multinucleated epithelial and stromal cells with enlarged, ground-glass nuclei containing eosinophilic intranuclear inclusions. There may be focal necrosis

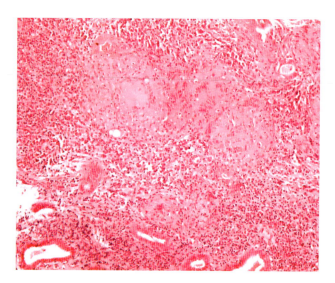

Figure 4.16 Tuberculous endometritis: epithelioid granulomas in tuberculous endometritis.

of endometrium associated with acute inflammation.[20] The diagnosis can be confirmed by demonstration of stromal and epithelial cells showing immunoreactivity to herpes simplex virus antigens.

MISCELLANEOUS

Other miscellaneous forms of endometritis that have been described include focal necrotising endometritis, ligneous endometritis and nodular histiocytic hyperplasia of the endometrium. All these are of uncertain clinical significance and are described briefly for completeness.

Focal necrotising endometritis occurs in premenopausal women with irregular vaginal bleeding. On microscopic examination, there is a sparse focal inflammatory infiltrate composed of lymphocytes and neutrophils centered on individual endometrial glands. It is not clear whether these features are the cause of the menstrual irregularities seen in these women or whether they represent an epiphenomenon.[21]

Ligneous inflammation has been described in the endometrium,[22] including women with type-1 congenital plasminogen deficiency.[23] The inflammation is characterised by the accumulation within the stroma of amorphous acellular hyaline material associated with patchy acute and chronic inflammation. The hyaline material is periodic acid–Schiff (PAS) positive and Congo red negative, but showed focal immunoreactivity for fibrin. Other parts of the female genital tract may be affected with the cervix being most often involved.[23]

Nodular histiocytic hyperplasia is a recently described lesion of uncertain etiology, comprising nodular aggregates of non-foamy histiocytes within the endometrium.[24] Fewer than 15 cases have been described, with all but one being associated with benign diseases, the exception being associated with an endometrial endometrioid carcinoma.[25] The histiocytic nodules may be mitotically active and, together with the presence of neutrophils and focal necrosis, may raise the possibility of a neoplastic proliferation. However, nodular histiocytic hyperplasia in the endometrium is considered to be a reactive process to necrotic tissue in the endometrial cavity, possibly related to a prior procedure (Summary Box 4.1).[24]

SUMMARY BOX 4.1: Endometritis

Endometritis is now rare in developed countries

- May be a cause of vaginal bleeding and infertility
- Most commonly seen postpartum, with residual placental tissue
- May be associated with endometrial polyps and malignancy
- May be associated with foreign material such as intrauterine devices

Diagnosis of chronic endometritis requires the presence of plasma cells

- Plasma cells are seen in normal endometrium and by themselves, especially if needing extensive high-power search for their presence, are of doubtful clinical significance
- The presence of eosinophils should prompt a histological search for plasma cells

Reactive endometritis

- Xanthogranulomatous endometritis, granulomatous endometritis and nodular histiocytic hyperplasia may be reactive processes to prior procedures on the endometrium

Specific forms of endometritis

- Endometritis caused by tuberculosis, herpes simplex, cytomegalovirus and sarcoidosis are rare

---

REFERENCES

1. Yeaman GR, Guyre PM, Fanger MW et al. Unique CD8+ T cell-rich lymphoid aggregates in human uterine endometrium. *J Leukoc Biol* 1997;61:427–35.
2. Pace D, Longfellow M, Bulmer JN. Characterization of intraepithelial lymphocytes in human endometrium. *J Reprod Fertil* 1991;91:165–74.
3. Jeziorska M, Salamonsen LA, Woolley DE. Mast cell and eosinophil distribution and activation in human endometrium throughout the menstrual cycle. *Biol Reprod* 1995;53:312–20.
4. Poropatich C, Rojas M, Silverberg SG. Polymorphonuclear leukocytes in the endometrium during the normal menstrual cycle. *Int J Gynecol Pathol* 1987;6:230–4.
5. Achilles SL, Amortegui AJ, Wiesenfeld HC. Endometrial plasma cells: Do they indicate subclinical pelvic inflammatory disease? *Sex Transm Dis* 2005;32:185–8.
6. Givan AL, White HD, Stern JE et al. Flow cytometric analysis of leukocytes in the human female reproductive tract: Comparison of fallopian tube, uterus, cervix, and vagina. *Am J Reprod Immunol* 1997;38:350–9.
7. Marshall RJ, Jones DB. An immunohistochemical study of lymphoid tissue in human endometrium. *Int J Gynecol Pathol* 1988;7:225–35.
8. Smith M, Hagerty KA, Skipper B, Bocklage T. Chronic endometritis: A combined histopathologic and clinical review of cases from 2002 to 2007. *Int J Gynecol Pathol* 2010;29:44–50.
9. McQueen DB, Perfetto CO, Hazard FK, Lathi RB. Pregnancy outcomes in women with chronic endometritis and recurrent pregnancy loss. *Fertil Steril* 2015;104:927–31.
10. Kiviat NB, Wolner-Hanssen P, Eschenbach DA et al. Endometrial histopathology in patients with

culture-proved upper genital tract infection and laparoscopically diagnosed acute salpingitis. *Am J Surg Pathol* 1990;14:167–75.
11. Adegboyega PA, Pei Y, McLarty J. Relationship between eosinophils and chronic endometritis. *Hum Pathol* 2010;41:33–7.
12. Bonet M, Ota E, Chibueze CE, Oladapo OT. Routine antibiotic prophylaxis after normal vaginal birth for reducing maternal infectious morbidity. *Cochrane Database Syst Rev* 2017;11:CD012137.
13. Paavonen J, Aine R, Teisala K et al. Chlamydial endometritis. *J Clin Pathol* 1985;38:726–32.
14. Kawai K, Fukuda K, Tsuchiyama H. Malacoplakia of the endometrium. An unusual case studied by electron microscopy and a review of the literature. *Acta Pathol Jpn* 1988;38:531–40.
15. Dogan-Ekici AI, Usubutun A, Kucukali T, Ayhan A. Xanthogranulomatous endometritis: A challenging imitator of endometrial carcinoma. *Infect Dis Obstet Gynecol* 2007;2007:34763.
16. Agarwal J, Gupta JK. Female genital tuberculosis—A retrospective clinico-pathologic study of 501 cases. *Indian J Pathol Microbiol* 1993;36:389–97.
17. Bazaz-Malik G, Maheshwari B, Lal N. Tuberculous endometritis: A clinicopathological study of 1000 cases. *Br J Obstet Gynaecol* 1983;90:84–6.
18. Clarke LM, Duerr A, Yeung KH et al. Recovery of cytomegalovirus and herpes simplex virus from upper and lower genital tract specimens obtained from women with pelvic inflammatory disease. *J Infect Dis* 1997;176:286–8.
19. Frank TS, Himebaugh KS, Wilson MD. Granulomatous endometritis associated with histologically occult cytomegalovirus in a healthy patient. *Am J Surg Pathol* 1992;16:716–20.
20. Duncan DA, Varner RE, Mazur MT. Uterine herpes virus infection with multifocal necrotizing endometritis. *Hum Pathol* 1989;20:1021–4.
21. Bennett AE, Rathore S, Rhatigan RM. Focal necrotizing endometritis: A clinicopathologic study of 15 cases. *Int J Gynecol Pathol* 1999;18:220–5.
22. Scurry J, Planner R, Fortune DW, Lee CS, Rode J. Ligneous (pseudomembranous) inflammation of the female genital tract. A report of two cases. *J Reprod Med* 1993;38:407–12.
23. Baithun M, Freeman-Wang T, Chowdary P, Kadir RA. Ligneous cervicitis and endometritis: A gynaecological presentation of congenital plasminogen deficiency. *Haemophilia* 2018;24:359–65.
24. Parkash V, Domfeh AB, Fadare O. Nodular histiocytic aggregates in the endometrium: A report of 7 cases. *Int J Gynecol Pathol* 2014;33:52–7.
25. Akhter S, Lawrence WD, Quddus MR. Polypoid nodular histiocytic hyperplasia associated with endometrioid adenocarcinoma of the endometrium: Report of a case. *Diagn Pathol* 2014;9:93.

5

Functional abnormal uterine bleeding

Dysfunctional uterine bleeding	43
Anovulatory cycles	44
Luteal phase defect	44
Irregular shedding	45
Estrogen deficiency	45
References	46

Abnormal uterine bleeding is defined as uterine bleeding that is abnormal in duration, volume, frequency and/or regularity and has been present for the majority of the previous six months.[1] Management of abnormal uterine bleeding has been advanced by the introduction of the International Federation of Gynecology and Obstetrics (FIGO) classifications. The first defines and brings nosological clarity to normal and abnormal bleeding while the second, known by the acronym PALM-COEIN, delineates the causes of abnormal uterine bleeding.

In the FIGO definition, uterine bleeding is described as being normal or abnormal based on frequency (normal being every 24–38 days, and abnormal as being absent (amenorrhea), frequent being occurring every less than 24 days, or infrequent being occurring every more than 38 days); duration (normal being up to 8 days, and abnormal being prolonged beyond 8 days); regularity (normal being a variation between shortest and longest period of less than 9 days, and abnormal as a variation being more than 9 days) and flow volume (where abnormal is either light or heavy). These descriptive terms replace previous terms that were poorly defined such as menorrhagia, metrorrhagia, polymenorrhea, menometrorrhagia and dysfunctional uterine bleeding (Table 5.1).

The second classification, PALM-COEIN, stands for polyp, adenomyosis, leiomyoma, malignancy and hyperplasia, coagulopathy, ovulatory disorders, endometrium, iatrogenic and not otherwise classified. It is a classification of potential causes of abnormal uterine bleeding but recognises that although women may have one or more entities, those may be asymptomatic and not contribute to the abnormal bleeding. The first group of causes – PALM – are structural and diagnosable by imaging and/or histopathology, while the second group of causes – COEIN – are nonstructural.

The FIGO group of ovulatory disorders overlap what would be 'functional endometrial disorders' that are abnormalities of endometrial morphology that have been attributed to ovarian dysfunction.[2] Some of these 'abnormalities' could be regarded as physiological, e.g. endometrial atrophy

Table 5.1 FIGO definitions and nomenclature for normal and abnormal uterine bleeding

	Normal	Abnormal
Frequency	Every 24–38 days	Absent Frequent (less than 24 days) Infrequent (more than 38 days)
Duration	Up to 8 days	Prolonged (more than 8 days)
Regularity	Regular variation (shortest to longest is less than 9 days)	Irregular variation (shortest to longest is greater than 10 days)
Flow volume	Normal	Light Heavy

due to estrogen deficiency, alterations in tissue sensitivity to endogenous hormones around the time of menopause and luteal phase defect. The morphological picture on its own may be inadequate for a definitive diagnosis. Accurate diagnosis necessitates a full clinical history, including a history of current and recent drug use/hormonal manipulation as well as factors that may affect the hypothalamic–pituitary–ovarian axis, such as mental stress, obesity, anorexia, weight loss and extreme aerobic exercise.

DYSFUNCTIONAL UTERINE BLEEDING

In a normal ovulatory cycle, menstruation follows the secretory phase and lasts for up to eight days. Prolonged or excessive bleeding in reproductive-age women without organic disease (such as polyps, hyperplasia or carcinoma, for example) is termed 'dysfunctional uterine

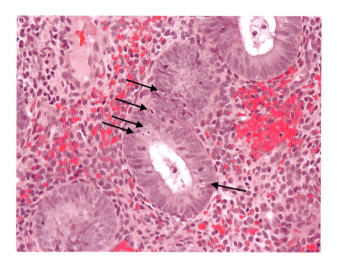

Figure 5.1 Increased amount of apoptosis (arrows) in proliferative-phase endometrial gland; a mitotic figure nearby is evident.

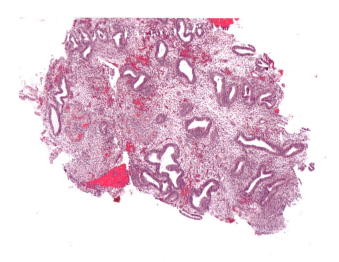

Figure 5.2 Proliferative endometrium with features of anovulation showing focal crowding of irregularly shaped and slightly cystic glands.

bleeding'. This is a diagnosis of exclusion. There are no specific morphological features attributable to dysfunctional uterine bleeding and the cause of bleeding in these women remains obscure. Dysregulation of proliferation and apoptosis may contribute to an increase in apoptosis in the proliferative phase of the endometrium (Figure 5.1) of some women with abnormal uterine bleeding of unknown cause.[3]

ANOVULATORY CYCLES

Many factors can affect the hypothalamic–pituitary–ovarian axis to result in failure to ovulate in a particular cycle. The frequency of anovulatory cycles is unknown, but they are common at the extremes of reproductive age just after the onset of menarche and in the perimenopausal period.[4,5]

During an anovulatory cycle, there is follicular development without ovulation and subsequent corpus luteum formation. The follicle may persist for some time before eventually undergoing atresia. The endometrium in an anovulatory cycle is subjected to the stimulus of a relative estrogen excess that is unopposed by progesterone. Thus, the endometrium shows persistent proliferative activity at a time of the cycle when a secretory a pattern would be expected, even at the time of menstruation. Caution must be exercised as the proliferative phase can be as long as 22 days in some women. The endometrial glands are similar to those seen in the proliferative phase, and there may be a mild degree of simple hyperplasia that may be difficult to diagnose (Figure 5.2). This has led some to use the term disordered proliferative endometrium or, preferably, proliferative endometrium with features of anovulation (see Chapter 8).

LUTEAL PHASE DEFECT

Luteal phase defect is reported in 3%–5% of infertile women. The luteal phase inadequacy may be spontaneous or induced by endocrine manipulation strategies such as those used for ovulation induction.[6] Affected women ovulate but recruit follicles early in the luteal phase, resulting in a relative deficiency of progesterone to high circulating levels of estradiol and a substandard response to progesterone by the endometrium.[7]

Luteal phase defect should be suspected when the endometrium is out of phase by more than two days, that is at least three days, and the difference is present in two successive cycles. A reason for performing endometrial biopsies in two different menstrual cycles is that they can be at variance: an out-of-phase biopsy followed by an in-phase biopsy or vice versa can be seen in about 50% of women being investigated for infertility. Chronological dating should be assigned prospectively rather than retrospectively to avoid inaccuracies caused by the variable length of the luteal phase and the accelerated onset of menses induced by the procedure. Sampling performed during the window of implantation (i.e. 6–8 days post ovulation) is more sensitive for identifying altered patterns of endometrial maturation.

Most commonly, the endometrium shows a general lag in glandular and stromal maturation in relation to the presumed day of ovulation. Less commonly, there may be an intimate admixture of proliferative- and secretory-phase endometrium, the so-called irregular ripening of the endometrium (Figure 5.3). However, similar changes sometimes occur in the endometrium of normal women. Even in these cases, caution is advised in making this diagnosis given that there is significant observer variation in endometrial dating and considerable anatomical variation in endometrial morphology.

Estrogen deficiency 45

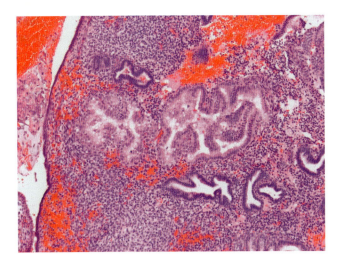

Figure 5.3 So-called irregular ripening of the endometrium with intimate admixture of proliferative- and secretory-phase endometrium.

IRREGULAR SHEDDING

In this situation, the endometrial biopsy contains fragments of menstrual-type endometrium, with portions also showing secretory activity and other portions showing early proliferative phase (Figure 5.4). These appearances are thought to be due to persistence of the corpus luteum with continued progesterone production resulting in delayed and prolonged menstrual bleeding. It has been suggested that many of these cases of irregular shedding of the endometrium are in fact nothing more than very early pregnancy losses occurring at the time of menstruation or the loss of the endometrium prepared for a blastocyst that did not implant, the blastocyst being responsible for the luteotrophic maintenance of the corpus luteum.

ESTROGEN DEFICIENCY

Proliferation of the endometrium is dependent upon an adequate supply of estrogen from the ovaries. The resultant endometrial morphology depends on the state of the endometrium at the time this estrogen supply is compromised. If no estrogen has been forthcoming from menarche, a hypoplastic endometrium will result. The loss of estrogen stimulus for a long time in a previously normal endometrium will result in an atrophic endometrium. If estrogen levels are low, the endometrium may be weakly proliferative or inactive.

A diminished estrogen supply is caused by abnormalities in the hypothalamus–pituitary–ovary axis. Women with Turner syndrome, for example, are born with nonfunctional ovaries. Primary ovarian disease such as premature ovarian failure or ovarian failure secondary to irradiation or ovariectomy will also result in a lack of estrogen. Hypopituitarism and other endocrine disorders such as hyperprolactinemia, which leads to suppression of luteinizing hormone so that ovarian follicles mature but fail to rupture, will also result in low estrogen levels. Hypothalamic dysfunction can result from severe malnutrition, anorexia nervosa, severe stress and other debilitating illness; athletes, particularly those involved in endurance events, have abnormal hypothalamic pulsatility. The presentation of these women may differ according to their age, duration and severity of disease. Commonly, they may have delayed puberty, delayed menarche, absent or infrequent periods or infertility.

The hypoplastic endometrium is indistinguishable from the atrophic endometrium. In both, the uterus may appear smaller. The endometrium resembles that seen in the immediate postmenstrual phase. It is thinned with cuboidal or flattened surface epithelium and small sparse glands by weakly proliferative or inactive cuboidal or low columnar epithelium set in a spindly fibroblast-like stroma (Figure 5.5).

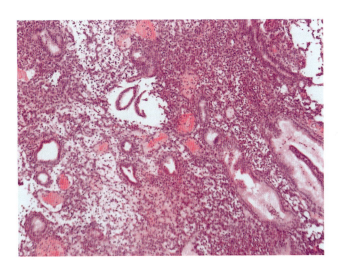

Figure 5.4 Irregular shedding of the endometrium: fragments of secretory, menstrual and proliferative endometrium are seen.

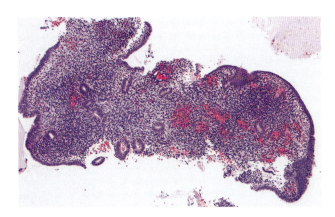

Figure 5.5 Hypoplastic endometrium with sparse, widely-spaced glands, set in a spindly stroma.

REFERENCES

1. Munro MG. Practical aspects of the two FIGO systems for management of abnormal uterine bleeding in the reproductive years. *Best Pract Res Clin Obstet Gynaecol* 2017;40:3–22.
2. Dallenbach-Hellweg G. Changes in the endometrium caused by endogenous hormonal dysfunction. *Verh Dtsch Ges Pathol* 1997;81:213–8.
3. Stewart CJ, Campbell-Brown M, Critchley HO, Farquharson MA. Endometrial apoptosis in patients with dysfunctional uterine bleeding. *Histopathology* 1999;34:99–105.
4. Rosenfield RL. Clinical review: Adolescent anovulation: Maturational mechanisms and implications. *J Clin Endocrinol Metab* 2013;98:3572–83.
5. Hale GE, Robertson DM, Burger HG. The perimenopausal woman: Endocrinology and management. *J Steroid Biochem Mol Biol* 2014;142:121–31.
6. Tavaniotou A, Smitz J, Bourgain C, Devroey P. Ovulation induction disrupts luteal phase function. *Ann N Y Acad Sci* 2001;943:55–63.
7. Baerwald A, Vanden Brink H, Hunter C et al. Age-related changes in luteal dynamics: Preliminary associations with antral follicular dynamics and hormone production during the human menstrual cycle. *Menopause* 2018;25:399–407.

6

Iatrogenic disease

Contraception	47	Other hormone treatment	60
Hormone therapy	53	References	61
Endometrial ablation	59		

CONTRACEPTION

COMBINED ORAL CONTRACEPTIVE PILL

The combined oral contraceptive pill (COP, commonly called the pill) contains an estrogen component (ethinylestradiol, mestranol, estradiol or its prodrug estradiol valerate) and a progestin (levonorgestrel, norethisterone, gestodene, desogestrel, drospirenone, nomegestrol, dienogest or cyproterone).[1] It works mainly by stopping ovulation, which means that a pregnancy cannot begin. Formulations of the oral contraceptive pill may be monophasic, delivering the same amount of estrogen and progestin; biphasic, delivering the same amount of estrogen each day while the progestin dose is increased halfway through cycle; triphasic, with three different doses of progestin and estrogen that change approximately every seven days; or quadriphasic which has an estrogen step-down and progestin step-up sequence. Most formulations have 21 active and 7 inactive pills, to mimic the menstrual cycle, with withdrawal bleeding occurring in the last 7 days.

Combined oral contraceptive use results in an endometrium with narrow, straight glands separated by pseudodecidualized stroma (Figures 6.1 and 6.2). The glands are lined by cuboidal epithelial cells lacking nuclear pseudostratification and mitotic activity. Stromal blood vessels are thin-walled, dilated and sinusoid-like. Occasionally, the stromal vessels may contain a thrombus.[2]

PROGESTINS

Progestins (or progestogens) are synthetic forms of progesterone and are widely used for the management of women with abnormal uterine bleeding, although their efficacy in this context is doubtful. They are also used in the management of endometriosis and for contraception in women for whom estrogens are contraindicated. Progestin contraception is administered orally, parenterally as subdermal implants or as a medicated intrauterine device. Low dose

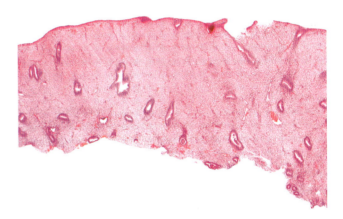

Figure 6.1 Combined oral contraceptive: endometrium showing narrow, straight glands separated by pseudodecidualized stroma.

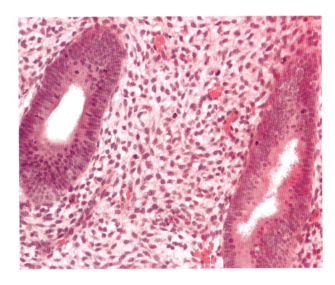

Figure 6.2 Combined oral contraceptive: glands are lined by cuboidal epithelial cells lacking nuclear pseudostratification and mitotic activity.

progestin-only contraceptives work mainly through thickening the cervical mucus and thinning the endometrium and are inconsistent in inhibiting ovulation. High-dose progestin-only contraception, such as the injectable depot medication, inhibits follicular development and ovulation as well as having effects on cervical mucus and endometrial thickness.

The progestin-only contraceptive pill (POP, commonly called the minipill) contains a low dose of progestin, such as levonorgestrel or norethisterone, and is taken every day with no breaks; the women experience light bleeds which may be irregular initially. Progestin-only contraceptive pills that contain 1.5 mg levonorgestrel ('morning after pill', emergency contraceptive pill, ECP) are taken within three days of unprotected sex. Intermediate-dose progestin-containing implants are inserted subdermally and can be left *in situ* and are effective for up to three years. Progestin-only contraception can be delivered also through intramuscular injection of a higher dose of a progestin, such as medroxyprogesterone acetate. A low dose of progestin can also be delivered topically through progestin-medicated intrauterine contraceptive devices (IUCD), such as Mirena®.

The effects of progestin treatment on the endometrium depend partly on duration of treatment, partly on the dose and type of progestin used. Progestin treatment is characterised by suppression of endometrial growth, variable endometrial stromal pseudodecidualization and increase in the number of granulated lymphocytes within the endometrium.[3]

On macroscopic examination, progestin-treated endometrium may be thickened and polypoid (Figure 6.3). Microscopic examination in the early stages of treatment shows endometrial glands without mitotic activity and secretory features while the stroma may be edematous. Prolonged use leads to profound endometrial glandular atrophy and florid stromal pseudodecidualization.[2] The endometrial glands are narrow and widely spaced with a single-layered, low cuboidal to flattened epithelium. Numerous dilated, thin-walled blood vessels and CD56+ granulated lymphocytes are seen in the stroma, which may show focal necrosis (Figures 6.4 through 6.10).

The effects of subdermal progestin implants on endometrial histology are similar but, less commonly, secretory changes have been described (Figures 6.11 through 6.13). Depomedroxyprogesterone acetate results in endometrial atrophy after six months use.

Various levonorgestrel-releasing intrauterine contraceptive devices are licensed for use as contraceptives and also used for treatment of heavy periods for which no underlying abnormality has been found. The dose of levonorgestrel released directly into the endometrium differs between the different products, which can be left *in situ* for between three and six years, depending on the product, although likely to be effective beyond the approved duration.[4] Local delivery of the progestin avoids the development of systemic progestogenic side effects. The morphological effects are those of a progestin combined with those of an inert

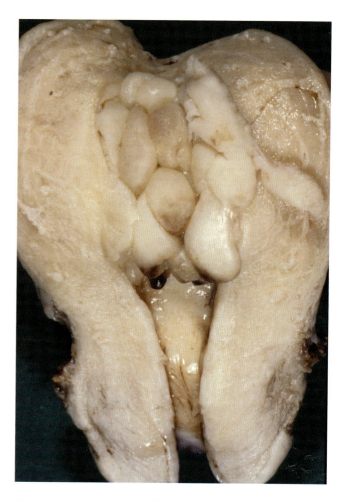

Figure 6.3 Endometrial effects of progestin treatment: hysterectomy specimen showing diffuse endometrial thickening with multiple polypoid projections.

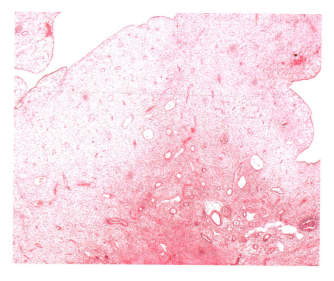

Figure 6.4 Endometrial effects of progestin treatment: scanty narrow glands within relatively abundant pseudo-decidualized stroma.

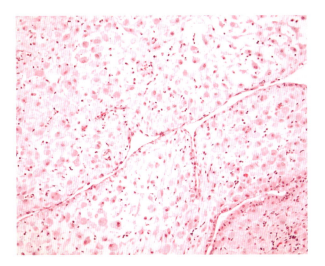

Figure 6.5 Endometrial effects of progestin treatment: pseudodecidualized stroma with numerous granulated lymphocytes and thinned surface epithelium.

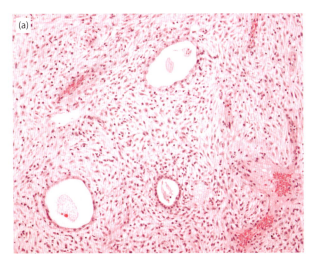

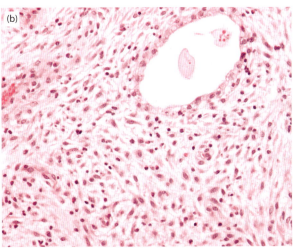

Figure 6.6 (a, b) Endometrial effects of progestin treatment: narrow glands lined by low cuboidal epithelium and rather spindly pseudodecidualized stroma with numerous granulated lymphocytes.

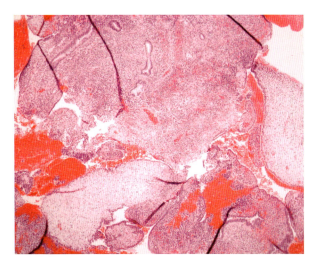

Figure 6.7 Endometrial effects of progestin treatment: much of the endometrium comprises dense, spindly stroma with scanty narrow glands. There are a few foci of stromal pseudodecidualization.

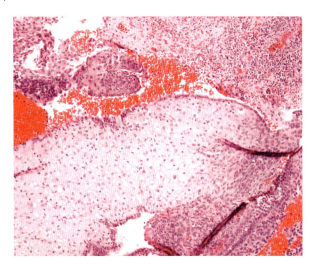

Figure 6.8 Endometrial effects of progestin treatment: high-power view showing the abrupt demarcation between pseudodecidualized and non-decidualized stroma.

mechanical device. The endometrium shows stromal pseudodecidualization, glandular atrophy, increased numbers of CD56+ lymphocytes, increase in stromal inflammatory cells including macrophages and a surface papillary pattern. Vacuolar stromal edema in the surface epithelium and hemosiderin deposition, necrosis and calcifications have also been observed (Figures 6.14 through 6.20).[5]

INTRAUTERINE CONTRACEPTIVE DEVICES

Progestin-releasing intrauterine devices have been described in the section 'Progestins'.

Nonmedicated intrauterine contraceptive devices made of plastic or copper and plastic have long been used for contraception. These devices elicit an endometrial inflammatory response combined with surface indentations or a

50 Iatrogenic disease

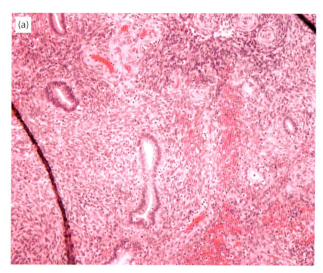

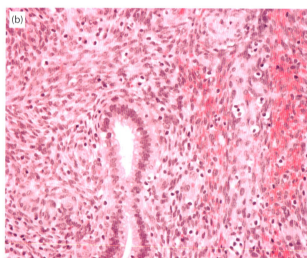

Figure 6.9 (a, b) Endometrial effects of progestin treatment: dense spindly stroma with numerous granulated lymphocytes. The few narrow glands show some secretory features.

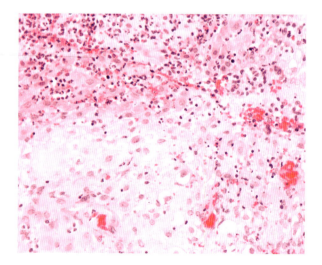

Figure 6.10 Endometrial effects of progestin treatment: pseudodecidualized stroma with focal necrosis.

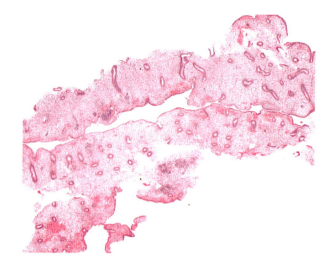

Figure 6.11 Endometrial effects of medroxyprogesterone acetate: narrow glands and relatively abundant stroma.

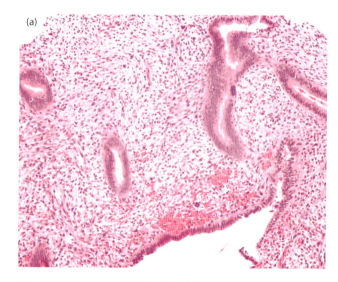

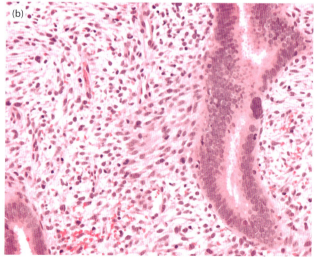

Figure 6.12 (a, b) Endometrial effects of medroxyprogesterone acetate: spindly and pseudodecidualized stroma with many granulated lymphocytes. The glands show some secretory features and one contains a giant nucleus.

Contraception / Selective progesterone receptor modulators 51

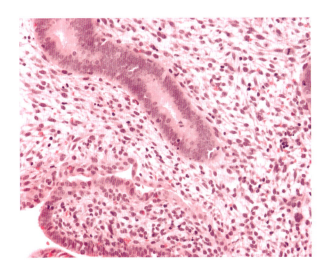

Figure 6.13 Endometrial effects of medroxyprogesterone acetate: scanty mitoses in glands and stroma.

papillary appearance at the contact site.[6] The endometrial stroma contains an infiltrate of neutrophils and chronic inflammatory cells, mainly within superficial endometrium. Microabscesses may be seen (Figures 6.21 and 6.22). There may be ulceration of surface epithelium, and adjacent glands may show epithelial regenerative changes.[6] With increasing duration of use, the stromal chronic inflammatory infiltrate may become more prominent (Figure 6.23).

SELECTIVE PROGESTERONE RECEPTOR MODULATORS

A selective progesterone receptor modulator (SPRM) is an agent that exerts agonist and antagonist activity at the progesterone receptor, depending on the target tissue.

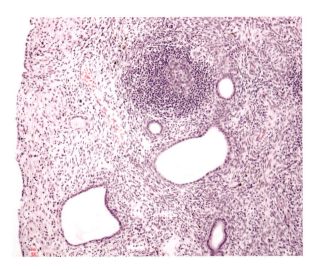

Figure 6.14 Endometrial effects of levonorgestrel-releasing intrauterine devices: endometrial atrophy with scanty narrow glands lined by cuboidal epithelial cells. There is pseudodecidualization of surface but not basal stroma. The stroma contains a reactive lymphoid follicle and chronic inflammatory cells.

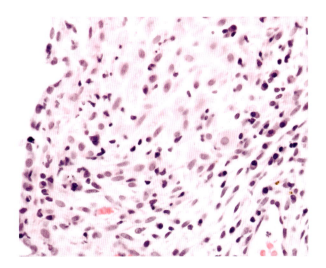

Figure 6.15 Endometrial effects of levonorgestrel-releasing intrauterine devices: pseudodecidualized surface stroma infiltrated by lymphocytes and plasma cells.

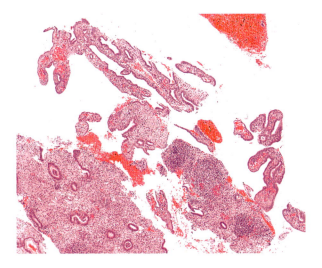

Figure 6.16 Endometrial effects of levonorgestrel-releasing intrauterine devices: pseudopapillary projections in surface epithelium, glandular atrophy and stromal chronic inflammation.

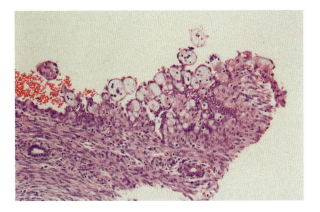

Figure 6.17 Endometrial effects of levonorgestrel-releasing intrauterine devices: surface epithelial cells show stromal edema, accentuating the micropapillary appearance.

52 Iatrogenic disease

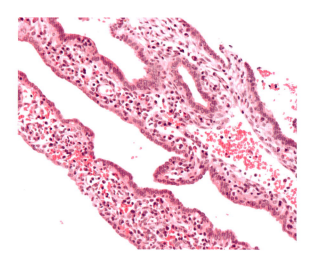

Figure 6.18 Endometrial effects of levonorgestrel-releasing intrauterine devices: subtle stromal pseudodecidualization and infiltration by plasma cells.

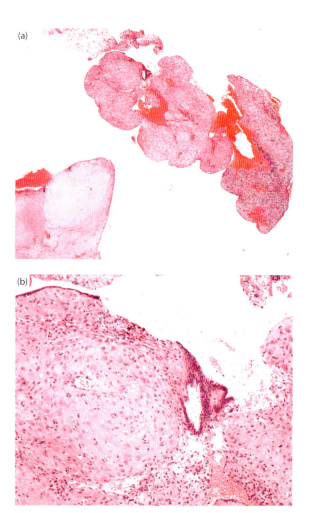

Figure 6.19 **(a, b)** Endometrial effects of levonorgestrel-releasing intrauterine devices: **(a)** pronounced stromal pseudodecidualization and focal necrosis (bottom left), **(b)** high power view showing pseudodecidualized stroma and inactive epithelium.

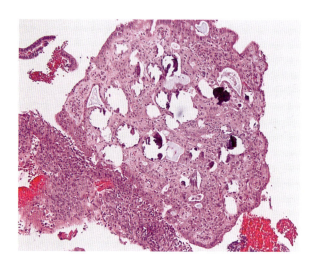

Figure 6.20 Endometrial effects of levonorgestrel-releasing intrauterine devices: calcification within stroma.

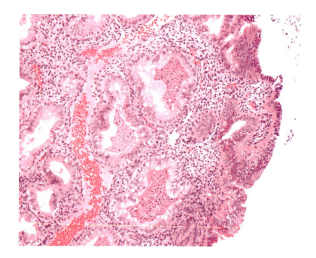

Figure 6.21 Endometrial effects of non-medicated intrauterine devices: glandular luminal abscess; neutrophils are also seen within the luminal epithelium and superficial stroma.

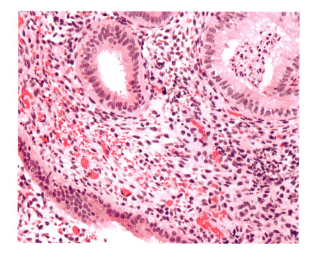

Figure 6.22 Endometrial effects of non-medicated intrauterine devices: microabscess and subepithelial neutrophils (bottom left).

Hormone therapy 53

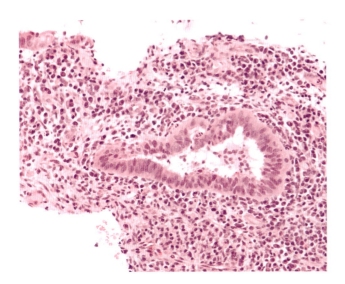

Figure 6.23 Endometrial effects of non-medicated intrauterine devices: dense stromal chronic inflammatory infiltrate with prominent plasma cells.

Two SPRMs, mifepristone and ulipristal acetate, are used as emergency contraception following unprotected intercourse, working by delaying or preventing ovulation depending on the time of the menstrual cycle. They are also used for treatment of uterine leiomyoma. At the time of writing, the European Medicines Agency was reviewing the benefits and risks with ulipristal acetate, following reports of serious liver injury. Reversible effects on the endometrium that might differ by agent and dose over time, labeled as progesterone receptor modulator-associated endometrial changes (PAEC), have been described.[7] The changes consisted of irregular, cystic glands showing a flattened secretory-like epithelium with vacuolation, coexisting mitoses and apoptosis, dyssynchrony between the secretory glands and stroma absent of pre-decidualization, and clusters of thick-walled vessels, prominent anastomosing capillary networks or vascular ectasia (Figures 6.24 and 6.25).[8–10]

HORMONE THERAPY

Hormone therapy, also known as hormone replacement therapy (HRT) and menopausal hormone therapy (MHT), has been used extensively in peri- and postmenopausal women to alleviate menopausal symptoms and to prevent diseases considered related to estrogen deficiency such as osteoporosis and ischemic heart disease. The history of hormone therapy was use of estrogen alone when first introduced in the 1960s and then with added progestin in the mid-1970s to minimise or eliminate the risk of endometrial carcinoma in women with an intact uterus. The widespread use of hormone replacement therapy was abruptly curtailed in the early 2000s following the publication of the Women's Health Initiative (WHI) trials that reported an increased risk of invasive breast cancer, ischemic heart disease, cerebrovascular disease and pulmonary embolism associated with hormone therapy.[11]

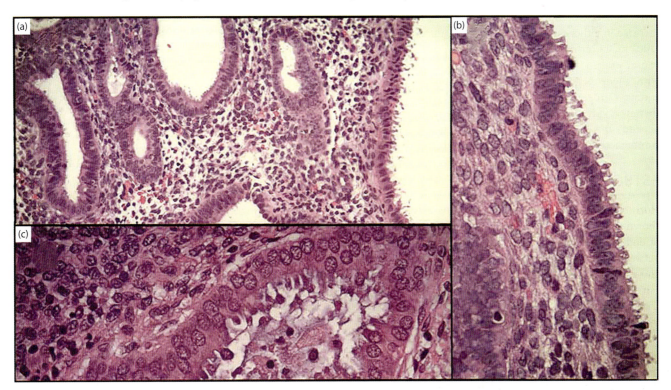

Figure 6.24 (a–c) Endometrial effects of selective progesterone receptor modulator, ulipristal acetate: most areas show a low columnar to weakly secretory epithelium; ciliated metaplasia shown in (b). (Reproduced with permission from Donnez J et al. *Expert Opin Drug Saf* 2016;15:1679–86.)

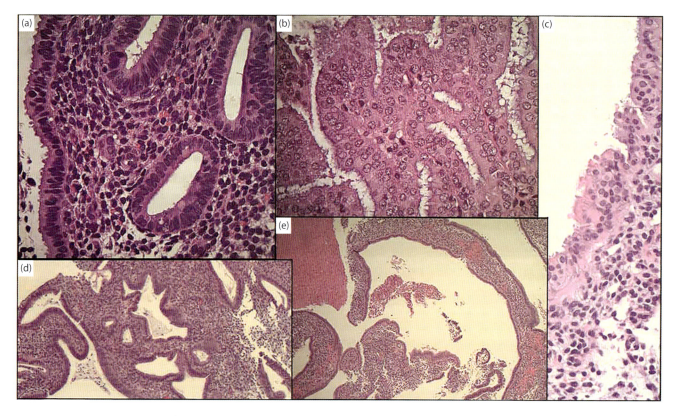

Figure 6.25 (a–e) Endometrial effects of selective progesterone receptor modulator, ulipristal acetate: (a) inactive to weakly proliferative epithelium with few mitoses and apoptosis; (b) ciliated metaplasia; (c) unusual secretory changes; (d, e) glands are folded or stellate and in the disrupted biopsy, stromal pillars line both sides with epithelium indicating large cystic spaces. (Reproduced with permission from Donnez J et al. *Expert Opin Drug Saf* 2016;15:1679–86.)

A re-evaluation of those WHI trials did not show a long-term increase in either all-cause mortality or cause-specific mortality, including cardiovascular mortality, among postmenopausal women taking combined conjugated equine estrogen with medroxyprogesterone acetate or taking conjugated equine estrogen alone.[12] The interplay between hormone therapy and health outcomes is complex and appears to also depend on age, time since menopause, when the therapy is commenced, dose, formulation and duration of treatment.

ESTROGEN-ONLY HORMONE THERAPY

Hormone therapy consisting of estrogens alone has been shown to be associated with a significantly increased risk of endometrial hyperplasia. There is a direct relationship between the risk of developing endometrial hyperplasia and carcinoma and increasing daily dose and duration of estrogen therapy.[13] Odds ratios for developing endometrial hyperplasia in estrogen-only hormone therapy range from 5.4 for 6 months of treatment to 16.0 for 36 months of treatment with moderate-dose estrogen.[14] The reported risk ratios for endometrial carcinoma in estrogen-treated women have ranged from 3.5 to 10.[15,16] The risk of endometrial cancer remains significantly elevated for 15 or more years after cessation of estrogen treatment.[15]

Endometrial carcinoma associated with estrogen treatment shows no specific morphological features. It does, however, have a relatively good prognosis. Affected women present at a younger age, with earlier-stage, lower-grade tumors and have higher survival rates when compared with non-estrogen-treated women who develop endometrial carcinoma.[17]

COMBINED HORMONE-THERAPY REGIMES

These combine progestins with estrogens in order to minimise the undesirable endometrial effects of prolonged unopposed estrogen treatment. The progestin may be given continuously with estrogen throughout the cycle (usually for postmenopausal women) or it may be added to the estrogen in a sequential (cyclical) fashion (usually for perimenopausal women). The combined hormone therapy preparations may be administered orally, topically, intradermally or a combination thereof. However, the hormones are most commonly administered orally, and the subsequent discussion refers to oral combined hormone-therapy preparations.

In sequential hormone-therapy regimes, estrogen is given continuously and progestin is added for 10–14 days per cycle or calendar month. In continuous combined hormone-therapy regimes, a progestin and an estrogen are administered daily throughout the cycle.

Adding progestins eliminates, at least for three years, the increased risk of endometrial hyperplasia associated with long-term estrogen treatment.[18] A systematic review of 46 studies found no significant difference in the risk of endometrial hyperplasia between women on combined hormone therapy and placebo at two years.[13] The addition of progestins also reduces the endometrial-cancer risk associated with prolonged estrogen treatment. One study described no significant increase in endometrial-cancer risk between women who used continuous combined hormone therapy or sequential moderate-dose estrogen-combined hormone therapy, when compared with nonusers, despite three years of therapy.[13]

Combined hormone therapy results in a combination of proliferative and secretory changes both in endometrial glands and stroma.[2] Thus, there is often an admixture of proliferative and secretory pattern glands separated by stroma showing varying degrees of stromal edema, mitotic activity and pseudodecidualization (Figures 6.26 through 6.28). In some cases, menstrual type changes may be observed. Interpretation of these biopsies may be made more difficult by the coexistent finding of various epithelial metaplasias and features of hyperplasia such as mitoses and glandular crowding.

There was more unassessable, inactive or atrophic endometrium in continuous hormone therapy compared with sequential combined therapy (59% versus 21%, respectively). Proliferative pattern endometrium was seen in 2% of the continuous combined hormone-therapy group compared with 17% of the sequential combined hormone-therapy group.[19]

Endometrial polyps are common among symptomatic and asymptomatic hormone therapy–treated women, particularly those receiving sequential hormone therapy. It is not clear whether hormone therapy confers an increased risk of endometrial polyps, although this would seem likely given its growth-stimulating effects on the endometrium. The higher expression of bcl-2 in endometrial polyps from women on combined continuous hormone therapy compared with those polyps from nontreated women would suggest that hormone therapy may inhibit apoptotic activity and

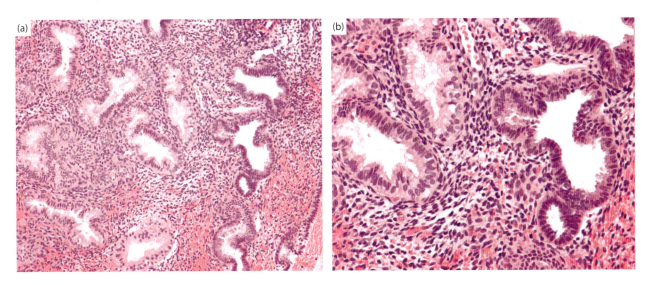

Figure 6.26 (a, b) Hormone therapy: secretory glands and inactive stroma.

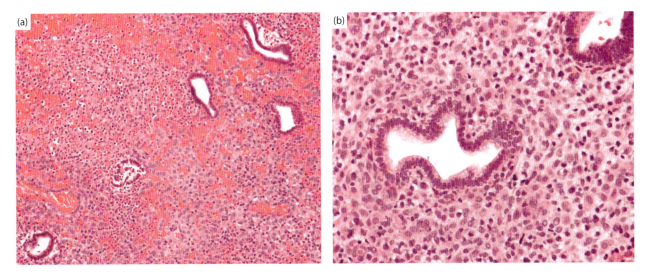

Figure 6.27 (a, b) Hormone therapy: narrow secretory-pattern glands within abundant pseudodecidualized stroma.

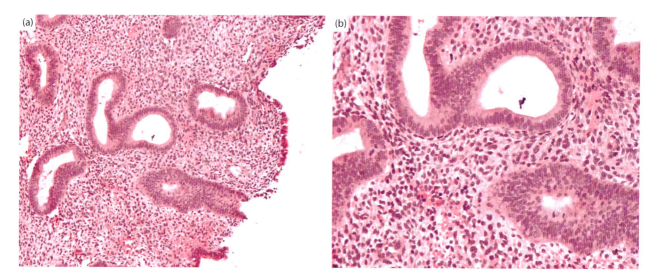

Figure 6.28 (a, b) Sequential hormone therapy: proliferative pattern endometrium.

may influence polyp growth.[20] Hormone therapy–associated endometrial polyps have a higher frequency of hyperplasia than non-hormone therapy–associated polyps (Summary Box 6.1).[21]

PROGESTIN-ONLY HORMONE THERAPY

Progestin-only hormone therapy is used by women who prefer to avoid estrogen. This form of treatment is used for treating vasomotor symptoms.[22] It is administered as oral micronized progesterone, transdermal cream, vaginal gel or nasal spray. Large safety trials of progesterone as postmenopausal monotherapy are lacking, and there is scant literature on the effects of progestin-only therapy on the endometrium. A small study showed that progesterone administered nasally did not induce secretory changes.[23]

SELECTIVE ESTROGEN RECEPTOR MODULATORS

Selective estrogen receptor modulators (SERMs) are agents that exert agonist and antagonist activity at estrogen receptors depending on the target tissue. The first-generation triphenylethylene derivatives, tamoxifen and toremifene, are used for treating premenopausal women with hormone receptor–positive breast cancer and, in the case of tamoxifen, in the prevention of breast cancer. Tamoxifen use can be extended, lasting up to ten years. Tamoxifen also improves bone density. Clomiphene (clomifene) is also a first-generation triphenylethylene derivative and is indicated for ovulation induction. The second generation benzothiopene derivative SERM, raloxifene, is indicated for the treatment and prevention of postmenopausal osteoporosis and for reducing the risk of breast cancer while bazedoxifene, a third-generation SERM, is indicated for the treatment of osteoporosis.[24]

Unlike tamoxifen, which has an estrogenic effect on the uterus, raloxifene and bazedoxifene have an anti-estrogenic effect on the uterus and thus can be used in combination with conjugated estrogens as hormone therapy (see 'Tissue-selective estrogen complex' section).[24] Effects of SERMs on the endometrium have been most extensively studied in women treated with tamoxifen, which exerts a proliferative effect on the endometrium.

Prolonged treatment with tamoxifen in postmenopausal women is associated with increased prevalence of endometrial pathology that includes polyps, hyperplasia, metaplasia and cancer, of which polyp is the most common.[25] There is less information about the effects of tamoxifen on the endometrium of premenopausal women, but polyps appear to predominate.[26]

> **SUMMARY BOX 6.1: Effects of most commonly used hormone therapy**
>
> Estrogens alleviate menopausal hot flushes and genitourinary symptoms as well as reduce bone loss but increase risk of endometrial hyperplasia and cancer.
> - Effects of estrogen only hormone therapy – endometrial glandular and stromal proliferation
>
> Progestins protect against endometrial cancer but increase vaginal bleeding risk, breast tenderness and potentially breast cancer.
> - Effects of continuous combined estrogen-progestin hormone therapy – tend to have more unassessable biopsies due to atrophy; atrophic changes or inactive endometrium
> - Effects of sequential combined estrogen-progestin hormone therapy – weak secretory changes, pseudodecidualization, may display proliferative activity, fewer atrophic biopsies
> - Metaplasias are common
> - Polyps are common, especially in sequential hormone therapy

Hormone therapy / Selective estrogen receptor modulators 57

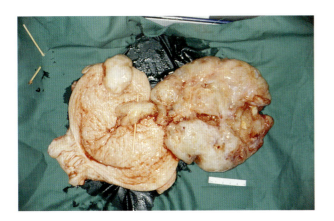

Figure 6.29 A hysterectomy specimen from a tamoxifen-treated woman. The uterus contains a pedunculated 15 cm polyp and a second smaller polyp (top).

The commonest endometrial pathology associated with prolonged tamoxifen treatment is occurrence of polyps, occurring in as many as a third of those women.[27] They are often multiple, and considerably larger (mean diameter of 50 mm) than sporadic polyps (mean diameter 20 mm) (Figure 6.29). Histologically, the polyps are composed of glands in abundant fibromyxoid connective tissue. Tamoxifen-associated polyps have a characteristic focal periglandular stromal condensation (Figure 6.30) and

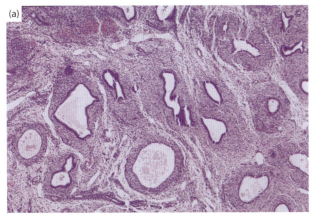

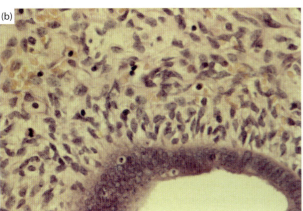

Figure 6.30 (a, b) Endometrial effects of tamoxifen treatment: periglandular stromal condensation in a tamoxifen-associated polyp.

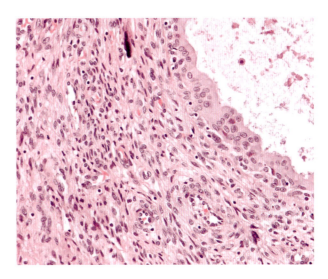

Figure 6.31 Endometrial effects of tamoxifen treatment: scattered atypical stromal cells in a tamoxifen-associated polyp.

diverse glandular epithelial metaplasia, including apocrine, mucinous, squamous, clear cell and papillary eosinophilic metaplasias.[28] Scattered atypical stromal cells with enlarged hyperchromatic nuclei may be seen in rare cases (Figure 6.31). The presence of mitotic activity and periglandular condensation within the stroma of tamoxifen-associated polyps may lead to a suspicion of adenosarcoma; tamoxifen-associated polyps are distinguished from adenosarcomas by the focal nature of periglandular stromal changes, relatively low mitotic activity within the stroma and lack of significant stromal atypia. The glands may show polarization along the long axis of the polyp with focal branching or budding. Cystic dilatation of glands is also frequently observed. Proliferative activity is common in both the epithelial and stromal elements. There is a relatively high prevalence of carcinoma developing within tamoxifen-associated endometrial polyps (Figure 6.32), which should thus be extensively sampled, whereas this is rare in sporadic polyps. The precise risk of endometrial carcinoma developing in tamoxifen-associated endometrial polyps remains uncertain as many studies are relatively small.

Hysterectomy specimens from tamoxifen-treated women with gynecological symptoms show a variable degree of diffuse endometrial thickening. The cut surface of the endometrium may have a 'Swiss cheese' appearance caused by cystic dilatation of endometrial glands (Figure 6.33).[28] Histology reveals features similar to those seen in tamoxifen-associated polyps: complex glandular branching, focal glandular crowding, epithelial metaplasias and stromal fibrosis (Figure 6.34). In the majority of cases, both the epithelial and stromal components of the endometrium show low mitotic activity. These morphological findings are best regarded as those of tamoxifen-induced endometrial hyperplasia.

The increased risk of developing endometrial cancer for women taking tamoxifen is well established; this risk

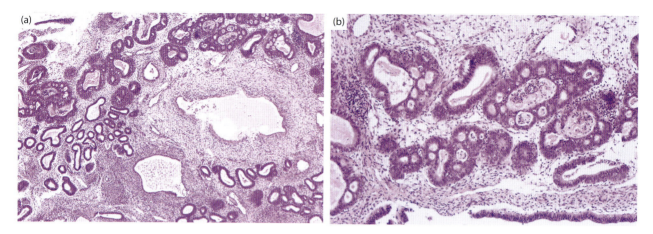

Figure 6.32 (a, b) Endometrioid adenocarcinoma in a tamoxifen-associated polyp.

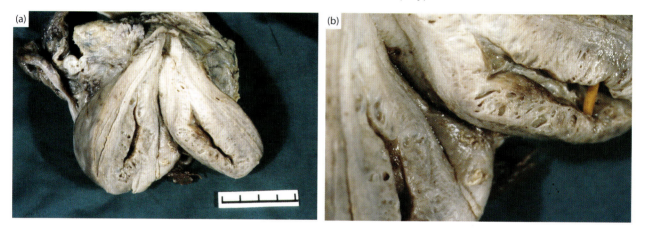

Figure 6.33 (a, b) Macroscopic features of tamoxifen-associated diffuse endometrial hyperplasia; there is a characteristic 'Swiss cheese' appearance.

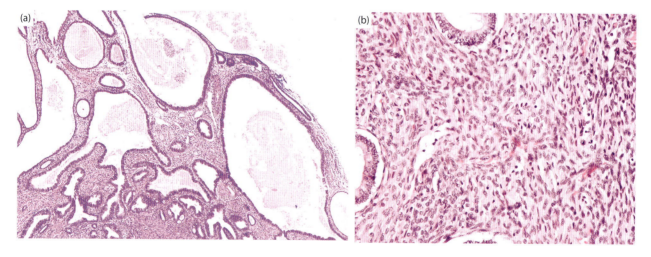

Figure 6.34 (a, b) Tamoxifen-associated endometrial hyperplasia: (a) there is complex glandular branching and focal glandular crowding; (b) collagen bundles between stromal cells.

increases with cumulative dose and duration of treatment.[29] Many studies have found that the stage, grade, histology and biology of tumors that develop in tamoxifen-treated women are no different from those that arise in the general population. Some smaller series studies have reported a worse prognosis for tamoxifen-treated women with endometrial malignancies due to the finding of more aggressive subtypes such as endometrial stromal sarcomas, adenosarcoma, malignant mixed Müllerian tumors or later stage endometrioid carcniomas.[30] Women using raloxifene demonstrate a lower risk of endometrial cancer when compared with those who used tamoxifen and with SERM nonusers,[31] while women treated with bazedoxifene alone for postmenopausal osteoporosis had a lower rate of endometrial carcinoma and no increase in endometrial hyperplasia.[32] There may be an increased risk of endometrial cancer in subfertile women exposed to clomiphene, but the quality of evidence and the confounding factors underlying subfertility for which clomiphene is used render the association unclear.[33]

Phytoestrogens are naturally occurring SERMs, being nonsteroidal plant compounds that are found in many fruits, vegetables and grains. The most common types of phytoestrogens are coumestans, lignans and isoflavones. They have been proposed as a natural alternative to treat menopausal symptoms, but their effects on breast cancer, cardiovascular disease, menopausal symptoms and osteoporosis are inconclusive. Phytoestrogen products do not appear to cause any stimulation on the endometrium when given for up to one year, and there is no evidence to suggest that phytoestrogens promote a proliferative endometrium.[34]

TISSUE-SELECTIVE ESTROGEN COMPLEX (TSEC)

A new alternative to the combined hormone therapy of estrogen-progestin is the tissue selective estrogen complex (TSEC), which partners a SERM with one or more estrogens. The principle is to balance the positive effects against the side effects and risks of the component SERM and estrogen.[35]

ENDOMETRIAL ABLATION

Endometrial ablation is an accepted alternative to hysterectomy in women with abnormal uterine bleeding whose symptoms have not responded to conservative management and who have no underlying uterine pathology. Endometrial ablation aims to destroy the endometrium and may be resectoscopic, such as laser ablation and electrosurgical resection, or nonresectoscopic, using a variety of energy sources to nonselectively destroy the endometrial lining.[36] Irrespective of the modality used for ablation, the post-ablation endometrium shows a range of abnormalities comprising necrosis, inflammation, foreign body giant cells, necrobiotic granulomas and fibrosis.[37] In the first three months following ablation, there is acute inflammation, necrosis, foreign body giant cells and a granulomatous response to necrotic tissue (Figures 6.35 and 6.36). The foreign body giant cells contain brown and black pigmented material (Figure 6.37). The necrobiotic granulomas are microscopically similar to rheumatoid nodules; they comprise a central zone of amorphous eosinophilic necrotic tissue surrounded by palisaded macrophages and an outer layer of fibrous tissue infiltrated by chronic inflammatory cells (Figures 6.38 and 6.39). Necrosis becomes less evident

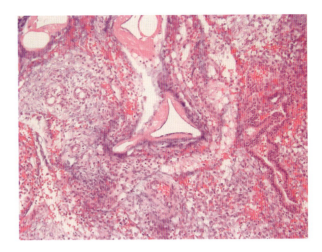

Figure 6.35 Post-laser ablation: acute on chronic endometritis with interstitial hemorrhage, coagulum and prominent necrosis of endometrial glands.

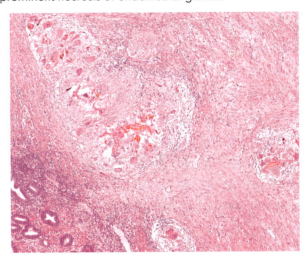

Figure 6.36 Post-laser ablation of uterus showing fibrosis extending to the myometrium. Foreign body granulomas are present within the fibrous tissue. Residual endometrium is seen bottom left.

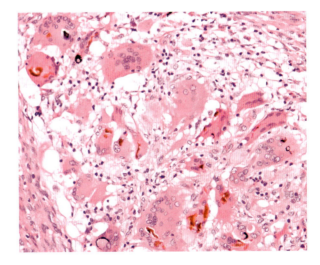

Figure 6.37 Endometrium following laser ablation: foreign body giant cells with brown and black pigment.

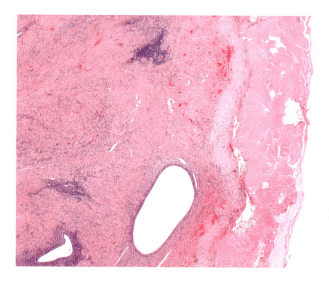

Figure 6.38 Endometrium following transcervical resection of the endometrium: on macroscopic examination, the endometrial cavity was lined by a 2 mm yellow membrane. The endometrial cavity is lined by a layer of eosinophilic amorphous necrotic tissue to which there is a granulomatous response, i.e. a necrobiotic granuloma.

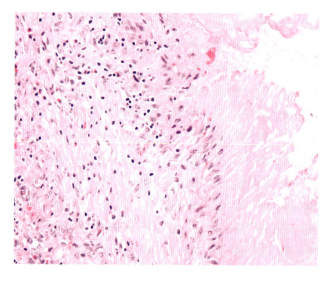

Figure 6.39 Endometrium following transcervical resection of the endometrium: palisaded histiocytes are seen between the necrotic tissue and the layer of fibrous tissue with scattered chronic inflammatory cells.

after the first few months, but the granulomatous response may persist and fibrosis develops. The fibrosis may extend into the myometrium and may be admixed with pigment-containing foreign body giant cells. Eventually the endometrial cavity may fuse either partially or completely (Figure 6.40).

Adenomyosis is frequent in treatment failure.[37,38] Where the ablation has been performed using a resectoscope, evaluation of the specimens suggests that specimen weight is inversely related to the need for further surgery with no further operations performed when more than 12 g of endometrium and myometrium had been resected.[39] Others did not find an association between volume (maximum aggregate dimension) and failure but did find that the number of myometrial fragments with endometrium on opposite sides was significantly associated with ablation failure and need for further surgery. The number of myometrial fragments with endometrium on three sides or number of fragments with myometrium completely surrounding endometrial islands did not differ between women who required or did not require subsequent surgery.[38]

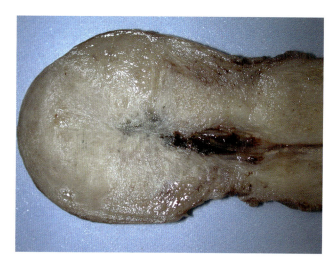

Figure 6.40 A uterus two years after laser ablation: the endometrial cavity is largely obliterated and replaced by fibrous tissue. Note the speckled dark pigmentation within the scar.

OTHER HORMONE TREATMENT

Other commonly used hormonal treatments that may cause alterations in endometrial morphology include gonadotrophin-releasing hormone (GnRH) agonists, danazol, gestrinone, tibolone and co-cyprindiol (cyproterone acetate with etinylestradiol).

Gonadotrophin-releasing hormone agonists are used for short periods in the management of endometriosis and adenomyosis to reduce the size of large leiomyomas prior to surgery and in assisted reproduction. They have also been used prior to endometrial ablation for heavy menstrual bleeding, especially in conjunction with the first-generation ablation methods. Commonly used drugs in this category include buserelin, goserelin, leuproreline and nafarelin.

Treatment with GnRH agonists results in a fall in gonadotrophin levels within 10–14 days, with consequent suppression of ovulation and ovarian hormone secretion. The end result is profound hypo-estrogenism associated with endometrial atrophy (Figure 6.41). Amenorrhea develops within eight weeks. Cyclical endometrial changes are resumed in parallel with normal ovarian function within three months of cessation of treatment.

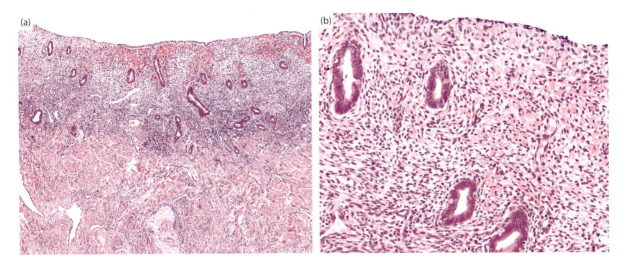

Figure 6.41 (a, b) Endometrial effects of GnRH agonist: the endometrium after three months course of subcutaneous goserelin is inactive and of basal type.

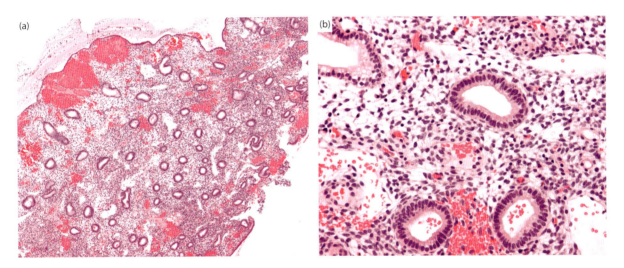

Figure 6.42 (a, b) Endometrial effects of Dianette® (cyproterone acetate with ethinylestradiol): the glands are narrow and mitotically inactive with some secretory features set in a rather myxoid stroma.

Danazol and gestrinone have combined androgenic, antiestrogenic and antiprogestogenic activity. Both are used in the treatment of endometriosis, and danazol is sometimes used for menorrhagia and other menstrual disorders. Both drugs cause endometrial atrophy, although danazol seems to induce atrophy earlier than gestrinone.

Tibolone has combined estrogenic and progestogenic activity as well as weak androgenic effects. It is used for alleviation of menopausal symptoms and for prevention of osteoporosis. Given to postmenopausal women, tibolone induces estrogen-like changes in the lower genital tract, but the endometrium remains inactive and does not induce endometrial hyperplasia or carcinoma in postmenopausal women.[40]

Cyproterone acetate with ethinylestradiol (Dianette®) combines an anti-androgen with an estrogen. It is licensed for use in women with severe acne unresponsive to antibacterial treatment and in the management of hirsutism. The endometrium of treated women shows changes similar to those induced by conventional low-dose combined oral contraceptives (Figure 6.42).

REFERENCES

1. Stewart M, Black K. Choosing a combined oral contraceptive pill. *Aust Prescr* 2015;38:6–11.
2. Deligdisch L. Hormonal pathology of the endometrium. *Mod Pathol* 2000;13:285–94.
3. Song JY, Fraser IS. Effects of progestogens on human endometrium. *Obstet Gynecol Surv* 1995;50: 385–94.
4. McNicholas C, Swor E, Wan L, Peipert JF. Prolonged use of the etonogestrel implant and levonorgestrel intrauterine device: 2 years beyond Food and Drug Administration-approved duration. *Am J Obstet Gynecol* 2017;216:586e1–6.

5. Hejmadi RK, Chaudhri S, Ganesan R, Rollason TP. Morphologic changes in the endometrium associated with the use of the Mirena coil: A retrospective study of 106 cases. *Int J Surg Pathol* 2007;15: 148–54.
6. Sheppard BL. Endometrial morphological changes in IUD users: A review. *Contraception* 1987;36:1–10.
7. Mutter GL, Bergeron C, Deligdisch L et al. The spectrum of endometrial pathology induced by progesterone receptor modulators. *Mod Pathol* 2008;21: 591–8.
8. Donnez J, Donnez O, Dolmans MM. Safety of treatment of uterine fibroids with the selective progesterone receptor modulator, ulipristal acetate. *Expert Opin Drug Saf* 2016;15:1679–86.
9. Fiscella J, Bonfiglio T, Winters P, Eisinger SH, Fiscella K. Distinguishing features of endometrial pathology after exposure to the progesterone receptor modulator mifepristone. *Hum Pathol* 2011;42:947–53.
10. Nogales FF, Crespo-Lora V, Cruz-Viruel N, Chamorro-Santos C, Bergeron C. Endometrial changes in surgical specimens of perimenopausal patients treated with ulipristal acetate for uterine leiomyomas. *Int J Gynecol Pathol* 2017;37:575–80.
11. Rossouw JE, Anderson GL, Prentice RL et al. Risks and benefits of estrogen plus progestin in healthy postmenopausal women: Principal results From the Women's Health Initiative randomized controlled trial. *JAMA* 2002;288:321–33.
12. Manson JE, Aragaki AK, Rossouw JE et al. Menopausal hormone therapy and long-term all-cause and cause-specific mortality: The women's health initiative randomized trials. *JAMA* 2017;318: 927–38.
13. Furness S, Roberts H, Marjoribanks J, Lethaby A. Hormone therapy in postmenopausal women and risk of endometrial hyperplasia. *Cochrane Database Syst Rev* 2012;CD000402.
14. Lethaby A, Farquhar C, Sarkis A et al. Hormone replacement therapy in postmenopausal women: Endometrial hyperplasia and irregular bleeding. *Cochrane Database Syst Rev* 2000;CD000402.
15. Paganini-Hill A, Ross RK, Henderson BE. Endometrial cancer and patterns of use of oestrogen replacement therapy: A cohort study. *Br J Cancer* 1989;59: 445–7.
16. Shapiro S, Kelly JP, Rosenberg L et al. Risk of localized and widespread endometrial cancer in relation to recent and discontinued use of conjugated estrogens. *N Engl J Med* 1985;313:969–72.
17. Schwartzbaum JA, Hulka BS, Fowler WC Jr, Kaufman DG, Hoberman D. The influence of exogenous estrogen use on survival after diagnosis of endometrial cancer. *Am J Epidemiol* 1987;126:851–60.
18. The Writing Group for the PEPI Trial. Effects of hormone replacement therapy on endometrial histology in postmenopausal women. The Postmenopausal Estrogen/Progestin Interventions (PEPI) Trial. *JAMA* 1996;275:370–5.
19. Wells M, Sturdee DW, Barlow DH et al. Effect on endometrium of long term treatment with continuous combined oestrogen-progestogen replacement therapy: Follow up study. *BMJ* 2002;325:239–43.
20. McGurgan P, Taylor LJ, Duffy SR, O'Donovan PJ. An immunohistochemical comparison of endometrial polyps from postmenopausal women exposed and not exposed to HRT. *Maturitas* 2006;53:454–61.
21. Orvieto R, Bar-Hava I, Dicker D et al. Endometrial polyps during menopause: Characterization and significance. *Acta Obstet Gynecol Scand* 1999;78: 883–6.
22. Hitchcock CL, Prior JC. Oral micronized progesterone for vasomotor symptoms--a placebo-controlled randomized trial in healthy postmenopausal women. *Menopause* 2012;19:886–93.
23. Cicinelli E, Petruzzi D, Scorcia P, Resta L. Effects of progesterone administered by nasal spray on the human postmenopausal endometrium. *Maturitas* 1993;18:65–72.
24. Komm BS, Mirkin S. An overview of current and emerging SERMs. *J Steroid Biochem Mol Biol* 2014;143:207–22.
25. Deligdisch L, Kalir T, Cohen CJ et al. Endometrial histopathology in 700 patients treated with tamoxifen for breast cancer. *Gynecol Oncol* 2000;78: 181–6.
26. Jeon SJ, Lee JI, Lee M et al. Endometrial polyp surveillance in premenopausal breast cancer patients using tamoxifen. *Obstet Gynecol Sci* 2017;60: 26–31.
27. Lahti E, Blanco G, Kauppila A et al. Endometrial changes in postmenopausal breast cancer patients receiving tamoxifen. *Obstet Gynecol* 1993;81:660–4.
28. Ismail SM. Pathology of endometrium treated with tamoxifen. *J Clin Pathol* 1994;47:827–33.
29. American College of Obstetricians and Gynecologists. Committee Opinion No. 601: Tamoxifen and uterine cancer. *Obstet Gynecol* 2014;123:1394–7.
30. Ngô C, Brugier C, Plancher C et al. Clinico-pathology and prognosis of endometrial cancer in patients previously treated for breast cancer, with or without tamoxifen: A comparative study in 363 patients. *Eur J Surg Oncol* 2014;40:1237–44.
31. DeMichele A, Troxel AB, Berlin JA et al. Impact of raloxifene or tamoxifen use on endometrial cancer risk: A population-based case-control study. *J Clin Oncol* 2008;26:4151–9.
32. Parish SJ, Gillespie JA. The evolving role of oral hormonal therapies and review of conjugated estrogens/bazedoxifene for the management of menopausal symptoms. *Postgrad Med* 2017;129: 340–51.

33. Skalkidou A, Sergentanis TN, Gialamas SP et al. Risk of endometrial cancer in women treated with ovary-stimulating drugs for subfertility. *Cochrane Database Syst Rev* 2017;3:CD010931.
34. Lethaby A, Marjoribanks J, Kronenberg F et al. Phytoestrogens for menopausal vasomotor symptoms. *Cochrane Database Syst Rev* 2013;(12):CD001395.
35. Pickar JH, Boucher M, Morgenstern D. Tissue selective estrogen complex (TSEC): A review. *Menopause* 2018;25:1033–45.
36. Laberge P, Leyland N, Murji A et al. Endometrial ablation in the management of abnormal uterine bleeding. *J Obstet Gynaecol Can* 2015;37:362–79.
37. Tresserra F, Grases P, Ubeda A et al. Morphological changes in hysterectomies after endometrial ablation. *Hum Reprod* 1999;14:1473–7.
38. Busca A, Parra-Herran C. The role of pathologic evaluation of endometrial ablation resections in predicting ablation failure and adenomyosis in hysterectomy. *Pathol Res Pract* 2016;212:778–82.
39. Hellen EA, Coghill SB, Shaxted EJ. The histopathology of transcervical resection of the endometrium: An analysis of 200 cases. *Histopathology* 1993;22:361–5.
40. Archer DF, Hendrix S, Gallagher JC et al. Endometrial effects of tibolone. *J Clin Endocrinol Metab* 2007;92:911–8.

7

Benign tumors and tumor-like conditions, including metaplasia

Endometrial polyp	65	Adenofibroma	73
Adenomyomatous polyp	68	Other tumor-like lesions of the endometrium	74
Atypical polypoid adenomyoma (APA)	69	Endometrial metaplasia and related changes	76
Endometrial stromal nodule (ESN)	70	References	86

A number of benign lesions or metaplastic changes can arise in the endometrium, many of them potentially resembling malignant neoplasms due to morphologic overlap and variations. Some of these lesions, including the common endometrial polyps, are also infrequently associated with clinically significant premalignant or malignant lesions. Clear understanding of their diagnostic features and differential diagnosis is critical to avoid under- or overdiagnosis of malignancy.

ENDOMETRIAL POLYP

Endometrial polyps are commonly encountered in clinical practice. Although conventionally regarded as non-neoplastic, endometrial polyps have been reported as clonal proliferations of endometrial stromal cells with induced growth of endometrial glands, based on genetic studies.[1] They may occur at any age but tend to be more common in perimenopausal and postmenopausal women.[2] Small endometrial polyps may be asymptomatic and detected as endometrial thickening on ultrasound, while larger ones could present with abnormal uterine bleeding (including postmenopausal bleeding)[2] or protrusion through the cervical os, resembling an endocervical lesion. The size of endometrial polyps ranges from less than 1 cm to (uncommonly) over 5 cm, usually with a grossly smooth surface and firm fibrous consistency. Tamoxifen therapy has a known association with an increased chance of developing endometrial polyps which tend to be bigger than those in general population.[2]

DIAGNOSTIC FEATURES

The key histologic features of endometrial polyps include

- Cystically dilated or branching glands, often with inactive features but sometimes proliferative (Figure 7.1)
- Fibrous appearance of stroma (to variable extent), but sometimes cellular (with or without mitotic activity)
- Thick-walled vessels in the stroma (Figure 7.2)
- Polypoid or pedunculated configuration of tissue fragments

A helpful diagnostic clue that distinguishes endometrial polyps from background endometrium is the parallel arrangement of the long axis of endometrial glands to the surface epithelium,[3] but this feature is not always observed.

MORPHOLOGIC VARIATION

- **Bizarre stromal cells** are uncommonly present in endometrial polyps, similar to some other benign mesenchymal lesions in the lower genital tract.[4–6] These bizarre stromal cells (Figure 7.3) can demonstrate marked nuclear enlargement and hyperchromasia, occasionally multinucleated, but they typically show smudgy chromatin and absent mitotic activity, thereby distinguishing them from sarcomatous lesions.[4]
- **Morphologic features resembling adenosarcoma** are also occasionally noted in endometrial polyps,[7] which may generate significant diagnostic difficulty. Howitt et al. found that features overlapping with adenosarcoma (including phyllodes-like architecture, intraglandular polypoid projections and altered periglandular stroma) (Figure 7.4) were not infrequently found in endometrial polyps, and these cases followed a benign clinical course.[7] The relevant parameters that allow distinction from adenosarcoma include the size, stromal cell atypia and the extent of phyllodes-like architecture,[7] which will be discussed in the section on differential diagnosis.

66 Benign tumors and tumor-like conditions, including metaplasia

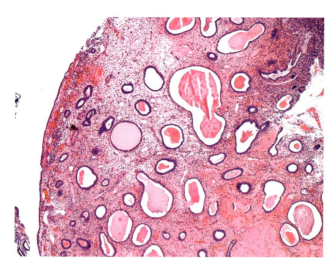

Figure 7.1 Endometrial polyp. Typical low-power view showing polypoid appearance with dilated glands in fibrous stroma.

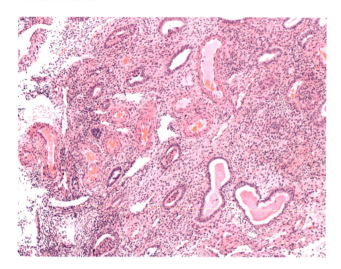

Figure 7.2 Endometrial polyp. Thick-walled vessels are commonly present.

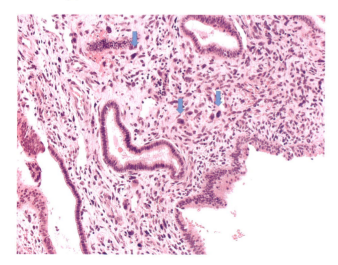

Figure 7.3 Endometrial polyp. Bizarre stromal cells (arrows) with hyperchromatic smudgy nuclei may be present. (Courtesy of Prof. Glenn McCluggage.)

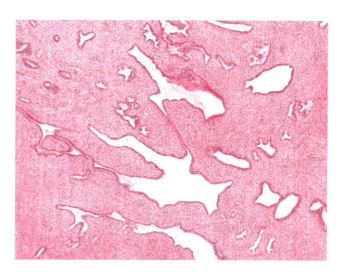

Figure 7.4 Endometrial polyp. Morphologic features resembling adenosarcoma may sometimes be observed, such as intraglandular polypoid projections as depicted here. (Courtesy of Prof. Glenn McCluggage.)

ASSOCIATION WITH HYPERPLASIA AND MALIGNANCY

Occasionally, endometrial polyps may harbor premalignant or malignant epithelial lesions such as endometrial hyperplasia, endometrioid adenocarcinoma or serous endometrial intraepithelial carcinoma.

- **Endometrial hyperplasia**, either complex without atypia or atypical, can be present in endometrial polyps. Simple hyperplasia is not diagnosed in endometrial polyps because dilated proliferative glands with mild crowding can be normally seen in endometrial polyps.[8] Complex hyperplasia can be diagnosed in endometrial polyp when there is significant glandular crowding with increased gland to stroma ratio, involving more than a few glands and exhibiting proliferative activity.[8] Atypical hyperplasia requires (in addition to the glandular crowding) the presence of cytologic atypia that is demarcated from the non-atypical glands, usually with nuclear rounding, loss of nuclear polarity and prominent nucleoli (Figure 7.5).[8] Kelly et al. studied 32 cases of endometrial polyps harboring endometrial hyperplasia and found that 52% had endometrial hyperplasia involving the nonpolypoid endometrium.[8] Another study has demonstrated that atypical complex hyperplasia in endometrial polyps was associated with hyperplasia in the nonpolyp endometrium in 66% of cases, and carcinoma in subsequent hysterectomy in 31% of cases.[9] These data suggest that endometrial hyperplasia identified in a polyp warrants further investigation and management.
- **Endometrioid adenocarcinoma** can be diagnosed in an endometrial polyp by applying the usual criteria (Figure 7.6). In the study by Mittal et al., eight out of

Endometrial polyp / Association with hyperplasia and malignancy 67

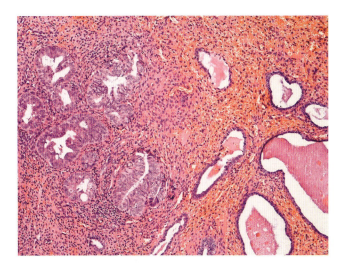

Figure 7.5 Endometrial polyp with atypical hyperplasia. Crowded branching glands with cytologic atypia (left) are seen coexisting with inactive dilated endometrial glands (right).

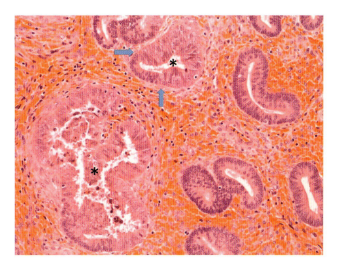

Figure 7.7 Endometrial polyp with serous endometrial intraepithelial carcinoma (EIC). The EIC component (*) typically exhibits prominent luminal tufting which serves as a low-power clue, in contrast with the surrounding glands. Abrupt transition between intraepithelial carcinoma and non-neoplastic epithelium is sometimes observed (arrows).

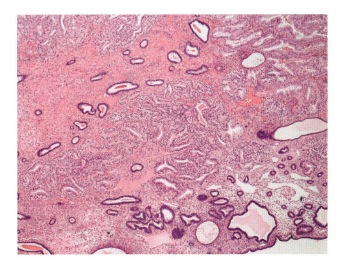

Figure 7.6 Endometrial polyp with endometrial adenocarcinoma. Confluent proliferation of closely packed glands (upper and middle) is present in this polyp, infiltrating among the non-neoplastic glands.

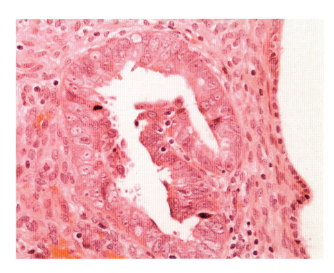

Figure 7.8 Endometrial polyp with serous endometrial intraepithelial carcinoma (EIC). High power showing marked nuclear pleomorphism with prominent nucleoli and mitotic activity in the EIC.

nine cases of endometrioid adenocarcinoma in endometrial polyps were associated with endometrial pathology on subsequent hysterectomy, including four cases with myoinvasive adenocarcinoma.[9]

- **Serous endometrial intraepithelial carcinoma** (serous EIC) is uncommon but typically identified in the context of endometrial polyp.[10–12] Serous EIC is recognised by an abrupt transition between benign epithelium and neoplastic cells, which exhibit pleomorphic nuclei with increased nuclear-to-cytoplasmic ratio, coarse chromatin and mitotic figures including atypical forms (Figures 7.7 and 7.8).[11] The diagnosis of serous EIC requires absence of stromal invasion, whereas cases with stromal invasion (based on confluent glands or infiltrative growth in desmoplastic stroma) should be diagnosed as uterine serous carcinoma. The diagnosis of serous EIC or uterine serous carcinoma may be supported by immunohistochemistry for p53, which shows mutation-type immunoprofile (diffusely positive or completely negative) in the neoplastic cells.[13] The presence of serous EIC or uterine serous carcinoma in an endometrial polyp not only implies possible involvement of the nonpolyp endometrium by serous carcinoma, but also in itself carries the risk of extrauterine involvement (even if entirely intraepithelial).[13]

DIFFERENTIAL DIAGNOSIS

The following conditions may sometimes be confused with an endometrial polyp, especially in endometrial aspirates with limited material.

- **Basalis layer of endometrium** could have thick-walled vessels within cellular spindly stroma, but the glands are generally tubular and inactive or weakly proliferative, and polypoid fragments are not seen.
- **Isthmic endometrium** in the lower uterine segment usually shows relatively fibrous stroma and few glands, but the absence of thick-walled vessels and admixture of endocervical mucinous epithelium and ciliated epithelium may aid distinction from an endometrial polyp.[14]
- **Adenomyomatous polyp** (or uterine adenomyoma) is distinguished from endometrial polyp by the presence of predominating smooth-muscle stroma.
- **Adenosarcoma** (or Müllerian adenosarcoma) may be distinguished from endometrial polyp by its size (usually >3 cm), typically well-developed and diffuse phyllodes-like architecture and the presence of stromal cell atypia (often diffuse, with coarse chromatin, nuclear enlargement and irregular nuclear membranes).[7] For endometrial polyps, the size is usually <3 cm, phyllodes-like architecture may be present but is usually poorly developed or focal, while stromal cell atypia is rare and usually focal and mild.[7]

ANCILLARY STUDIES

Although not necessary for diagnosis, p16 immunoreactivity has been found to be common in the stromal cells of endometrial polyps (Figure 7.9).[15,16] However, it should also be noted that focal p16 positivity could also be seen in the functional layers of normal endometrium.[16]

ADENOMYOMATOUS POLYP

Adenomyomatous polyp, also known as 'uterine adenomyoma', is a benign lesion composed of endometrial glands surrounded by endometrial stroma and smooth muscle. It has not been ascertained whether they represent clonal proliferations or localized forms of adenomyosis.[17] They are not considered to be associated with malignancy and polypectomy is adequate treatment.[18]

CLINICAL AND MACROSCOPIC FEATURES

Adenomyomatous polyps commonly present with abnormal uterine bleeding.[17,18] They may present as a polypoid lesion in the endometrium or located within the myometrium.[18] The cut surface is usually firm with cystic areas, sometimes with focal hemorrhage present.[18]

DIAGNOSTIC FEATURES

Adenomyomatous polyps have the following histological features:[17,18]

- Circumscribed nodular lesions composed of endometrial glands accompanied by periglandular endometrial stroma, which is surrounded by predominant component of smooth-muscle stroma (Figure 7.10)
- Endometrial glands lined by proliferative endometrial-type epithelium without cytologic atypia
- Variable glandular outlines (which may include tubular, irregular or cystically dilated glands) and density, but usually well separated without glandular crowding or back-to-back pattern

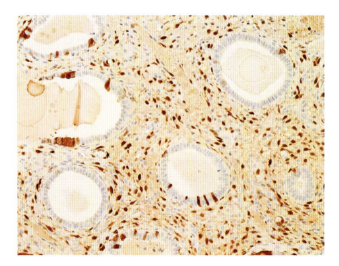

Figure 7.9 p16 immunohistochemistry in endometrial polyp. The stroma of endometrial polyp is typically positive for p16. Note also the mosaic pattern of positivity in the epithelium that is commonly seen in endometrial glands.

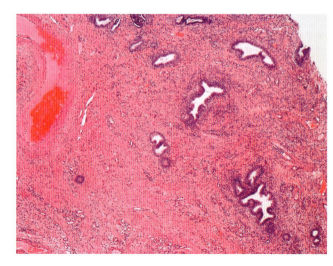

Figure 7.10 Adenomyomatous polyp. Branching endometrial glands are accompanied by endometrial stroma and well separated in a background of smooth-muscle stroma.

- Smooth-muscle stroma may demonstrate variable degree of cellularity, edema or hyalinization, commonly including thick-walled vessels, and sometimes merging with adjacent myometrium
- Mitotic activity and metaplastic changes can be present in the epithelium, sometimes in the stroma[19]

DIFFERENTIAL DIAGNOSIS

Lesions that may be confused with adenomyomatous polyp include

- **Endocervical-type adenomyoma:** Adenomyomas in the cervix may be of endocervical or endometrioid type.[18] Endocervical-type adenomyomas are characterised by lobular arrangement of large irregular glands that are mostly lined by endocervical-type mucinous epithelium.[17,18] In contrast, endometrioid-type adenomyomatous polyps are composed of mainly endometrial-type glands with nonlobular arrangement.[18]
- **Atypical polypoid adenomyoma** is distinguished from adenomyomatous polyp by the presence of glandular crowding and epithelial atypia, as well as squamous morules which are usually observed.[17,18]
- **Endometrial polyps** do not have the predominating smooth-muscle stroma that is found in adenomyomatous polyps, although minor smooth-muscle differentiation can be seen in endometrial polyps and a small amount of underlying myometrium may sometimes be included during polypectomy.
- **Adenosarcoma** is distinguished by the presence of stromal-cell atypia (which can be focal and mild) and phyllodes-like architecture. Smooth-muscle differentiation may be observed in the stroma of adenosarcomas but is usually not prominent.[18]

ATYPICAL POLYPOID ADENOMYOMA (APA)

Atypical polypoid adenomyoma (APA) was traditionally regarded as a benign lesion although it was well documented that some cases were associated with coexisting endometrial hyperplasia or malignancy.[20–22] Recent studies with genetic analysis have challenged the conventional paradigm and suggested that APA might represent a localized form of atypical hyperplasia.[23,24]

CLINICAL FEATURES

Most patients are in the reproductive age group, but reported cases ranged from 21 to 73 years of age.[20–22] The usual presentation was abnormal uterine bleeding, especially heavy bleeding.[20]

DIAGNOSTIC FEATURES

APA is diagnosed by a combination of histological features:[20,22]

- Endometrial glands with architectural complexity (irregular branching glands with variable crowding) and cytologic atypia, to a degree comparable to that observed in atypical hyperplasia (Figure 7.11)
- Morules are commonly seen (Figure 7.12)
- Background of myomatous (or myofibromatous) stroma (Figure 7.13) with intersecting bundles of smooth-muscle cells

The term 'APA of low malignant potential' has been used by Longacre et al. for APA with foci indistinguishable from well-differentiated endometrioid carcinoma.[22] While this term has gained popular usage, it is not included in the 2014

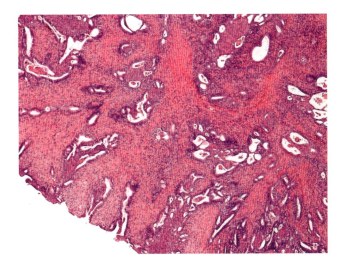

Figure 7.11 Atypical polypoid adenomyoma. Irregular branching glands with focal crowding are dispersed in myomatous stroma.

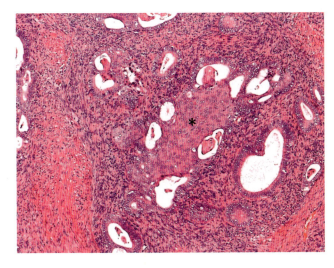

Figure 7.12 Atypical polypoid adenomyoma. Morular metaplasia is commonly seen in the glands.

70 Benign tumors and tumor-like conditions, including metaplasia

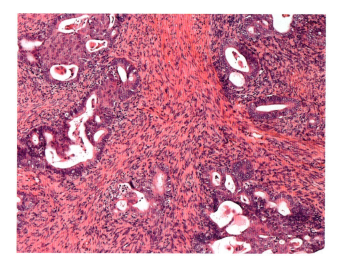

Figure 7.13 Atypical polypoid adenomyoma. The background stroma often has a myofibromatous appearance as shown here.

WHO Classification as a separate entity.[25] From a practical point of view, cases with areas that fulfil the diagnostic criteria of endometrioid carcinoma are probably best regarded as carcinoma arising in APA, in order to avoid undertreatment of malignancy.

PROGNOSIS

Based on the largest series of APA to date, about 45% of cases treated by polypectomy or curettage would develop recurrent or persistent APA.[22] A systematic review of 136 cases of APA suggested that 30% had residual or recurrent APA after local excision, and the risk of coexistent endometrial hyperplasia or carcinoma was estimated at approximately 9%.[26] Occasional cases of synchronous or metachronous endometrioid carcinoma (including those with myoinvasive disease) associated with APA have been documented.[21,22]

DIFFERENTIAL DIAGNOSIS

- **Adenomyomatous polyp** is distinguished from APA by the absence of architectural complexity and cytologic atypia in the endometrial glands.
- **Adenocarcinoma with myometrial invasion** may be considered as a differential when APA presents in curettage specimens. APA generally does not have the severe degree of architectural abnormality diagnostic of endometrioid carcinoma[20] (if present, this should raise suspicion of carcinoma arising in APA). It is also unusual for endometrioid carcinoma to present solely with a myoinvasive component without the exophytic portion that comprises mostly carcinoma cells.[20] The appearance of smooth-muscle stroma in APA is typically more cellular than normal myometrium.[20] Immunohistochemistry for h-caldesmon may offer some help for this distinction, as a study found negative h-caldesmon immunoreactivity in the stroma of APA, but positive in the myometrium invaded by endometrial carcinoma.[27]

ANCILLARY STUDIES

Immunohistochemically, nuclear expression of β-catenin has been observed in the epithelial component of APA for a majority of cases studied.[23,24] The extent and intensity of β-catenin staining was found to be greater in the squamous morules than the glandular elements.[23] This finding is congruent with the molecular studies demonstrating frequent mutations of *CTNNB1* (β-*catenin* gene) in APA.[24]

Other possible genetic alterations that have been identified in some cases of APA include *PTEN* deletion (which may be associated with lost or preserved PTEN expression by immunohistochemistry) and *KRAS* mutations.[24] These observations have led to the proposal that APA should be regarded as a localized form of atypical hyperplasia,[24] but this view is not yet universally accepted.

ENDOMETRIAL STROMAL NODULE (ESN)

Endometrial stromal nodules are rare benign mesenchymal tumors of endometrial stromal differentiation.

CLINICAL AND MACROSCOPIC FEATURES

ESN typically presents in the perimenopausal age group, although a wide age range (23–86 years) has been observed in reported cases.[28–30] The clinical presentation may be abnormal uterine bleeding, clinically enlarged uterus, abdominal pain or pelvic mass.[29] Grossly, ESN is usually a well-circumscribed mass with fleshy, diffusely or focally yellow cut surface, measuring 1–22 cm in size (average 7 cm).[29,30] ESN may involve the endometrium as a polypoid mass or be located in the myometrium as a submucosal or intramural lesion.[29,30] ESN is generally managed by hysterectomy and the outcome is benign.[29]

DIAGNOSTIC FEATURES

ESN is diagnosed by the following histologic features:

- Circumscribed pushing border with surrounding myometrium (Figure 7.14)
  - Focal irregularities with finger-like projections may be allowed if not more than 3 mm beyond the main border and less than three in number[29]
- Diffuse densely cellular proliferation of small cells resembling endometrial stroma is at least focally present, with or without other morphologic patterns typical of endometrial stromal tumors

Endometrial stromal nodule (ESN) / Differential diagnosis 71

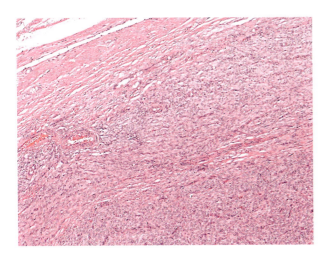

Figure 7.14 Endometrial stromal nodule. The tumor shows high cellularity and a circumscribed border with the underlying myometrium.

- Tumor cells usually have scant cytoplasm and small, uniform, round-to-oval nuclei with fine chromatin and inconspicuous nucleoli[29]
- Wide range of morphologic variations have been observed, including fibrous, hyalinized, myxoid or edematous foci, cells with abundant eosinophilic cytoplasm, hyaline plaques, smooth-muscle differentiation and sex cord-like differentiation[29]
- Mitotic count is typically low (usually less than five per 10 high-power fields), but higher mitotic count is possible[29,30]
- Cyst formation and infarct-type necrosis are sometimes observed[29]
- Arterioles are typically present in the vasculature (Figure 7.15)
   - Thick-walled vessels may be present but generally less prominent than in submucosal leiomyomas[29]

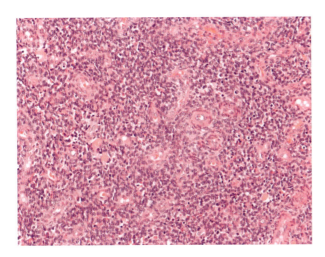

Figure 7.15 Endometrial stromal nodule. Arterioles are often present in the tumor.

Variant: Endometrial stromal tumor with limited infiltration

The term 'endometrial stromal tumor with limited infiltration' has been recommended for those endometrial stromal tumors with satellite nodules or irregularities of border extending up to 9 mm from the main border of the tumor, but lacking the typical permeative pattern or vascular invasion of endometrial stromal sarcoma.[29,30] Clinical data are limited in view of the small number of cases reported under this category, but these cases seem to follow a benign course similar to ESN.[29,30]

DIFFERENTIAL DIAGNOSIS

- **Low grade endometrial stromal sarcoma** (LG-ESS) is distinguished from ESN by its permeative growth pattern, characterised by infiltrative border (exceeding the degree allowed for ESN or endometrial stromal tumor with limited infiltration) and/or vascular invasion.[29,30] The cellular composition, vascular pattern, morphologic variations and immunoprofiles are similar for both LG-ESS and ESN.[30] The molecular finding of JAZF1-SUZ12 gene fusion has been identified in both LG-ESS and ESN,[31] so this is of no value in differential diagnosis.
- Submucosal cellular leiomyoma, being more common than ESN, is an important differential diagnosis which could exhibit similar cell morphology. Clues to the diagnosis of cellular leiomyoma include the presence of more typical spindle cells in fascicular pattern merged with surrounding myometrium and prominent thick-walled vessels (Figure 7.16).[28] Immunohistochemistry is helpful by demonstrating extensive positivity

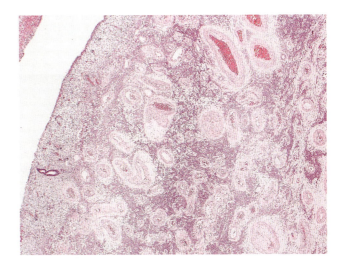

Figure 7.16 Submucosal cellular leiomyoma. The cellular morphology closely resembles that of endometrial stromal nodule, but the prominent thick-walled vessels would favor cellular leiomyoma, which could be confirmed by immunohistochemistry. (Courtesy of Prof. Glenn McCluggage.)

for smooth-muscle markers (such as desmin and h-caldesmon), but it should be emphasised that these markers could be focally positive in ESN with smooth-muscle differentiation.[30,32] CD10 is also commonly positive in leiomyomas.[30,32]

- UTROSCT (uterine tumor resembling ovarian sex cord tumor) can be confused with ESN with sex cord-like differentiation, as both are typically circumscribed and contain sex cord-like elements arranged in cords and tubules.[30] Immunohistochemistry is of limited value as both can have variable expression of CD10, inhibin, desmin and cytokeratin, but UTROSCT do not contain the typical endometrial stromal component with rich arterioles.[30]

IMMUNOHISTOCHEMISTRY

ESN is typically diffusely positive for CD10 (Figure 7.17), estrogen receptor (ER) and progesterone receptor (PR).[30] Positive staining for α-smooth-muscle actin is also common, but this is of limited value in differential diagnosis.[33] Desmin and h-caldesmon are often negative but focal positivity could be observed in ESN with or without morphologic evidence of smooth-muscle differentiation.[30,32,33] ESN is also usually positive for WT-1, but it should be noted that cellular leiomyomas are also commonly positive.[33]

MOLECULAR FINDINGS

The *JAZF1-SUZ12* gene fusion (previously known as *JAZF1-JJAZ1*) associated with the t(7;17)(p15;q21) translocation has been identified in about 65% of endometrial stromal nodules,[30] as detected by reverse transcriptase-polymerase chain reaction (RT-PCR) or fluorescence in-situ hybridization (FISH).[31,34,35] This genetic abnormality is also present in about 45% of LG-ESS, which suggests that this might represent an early event in the pathogenesis of endometrial stromal tumors. Although this genetic alteration is not helpful in the distinction between ESN and LG-ESS, its detection may help to distinguish ESN from smooth-muscle tumors, UTROSCT or other extrauterine tumors in difficult cases (Box 7.1).[30,36]

> **BOX 7.1: Approach to diagnosis of endometrial stromal tumor in biopsy or curettage**
>
> In daily practice, the initial recognition of endometrial stromal nodules commonly begins with an endometrial biopsy or curettage specimen which contains fragments composed of endometrial stromal cells with relative paucity of glands (Figure 7.18). The following diagnostic issues are commonly encountered.
>
> - Distinction from non-neoplastic endometrial stroma may sometimes be difficult in specimens containing mostly small tissue fragments.
>   - Possible causes of abundant endometrial stroma may include stromal breakdown (typically with compact stroma and associated fibrin) and gland-poor adenomyosis (usually atrophic stromal cells surrounded by hypertrophic smooth muscle).[30]
>   - In cases with indeterminate morphology, a comment could be added to the report stating that the possibility of endometrial stromal tumor could not be excluded and suggesting further endometrial sampling or curettage.
> - Distinction between ESN and LG-ESS in biopsy or curettage specimens is difficult and generally not feasible.
>   - Care should be taken not to confuse tangential sectioning or artifacts with infiltrative borders in curettage specimens.

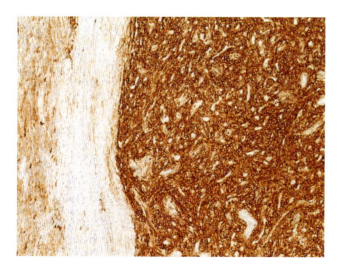

Figure 7.17 CD10 immunohistochemistry in endometrial stromal nodule. Diffuse strong positivity is typically seen.

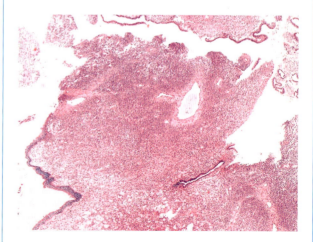

Figure 7.18 Endometrial stromal nodule. Large areas of endometrial stroma without glands are clues to the diagnosis in endometrial biopsies or curettings.

- In most cases, it is sufficient to diagnose 'endometrial stromal tumor' with a comment explaining the differential diagnosis of ESN and LG-ESS that would require a hysterectomy specimen for proper assessment of the tumor border.
- The presence of smooth-muscle cells within endometrial stromal tumors could raise the differential diagnosis of myometrial infiltration (which would suggest LG-ESS) and ESN with smooth-muscle differentiation.
  - Smooth-muscle differentiation in ESN usually appears relatively disorganised with a fibrillary and wispy pattern, commonly with myofibroblasts or whorls of hyalinized smooth muscle.[30]
  - Myometrium entrapped by LG-ESS generally comprises thick and organised smooth-muscle bundles as in normal myometrium.[30]
  - In curettage specimens displaying suspected myometrial infiltration, the report could be issued as 'endometrial stromal tumor, suspicious for low grade endometrial stromal sarcoma', while the definitive diagnosis could be deferred to the hysterectomy specimen.

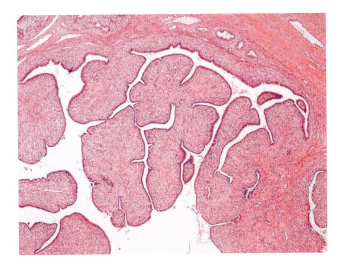

Figure 7.19 Adenofibroma. Papillary growths with fibromatous stroma covered by cytologically benign glandular epithelium is a typical histologic pattern traditionally regarded as typical of 'adenofibroma', although similar areas could also be found in adenosarcoma.

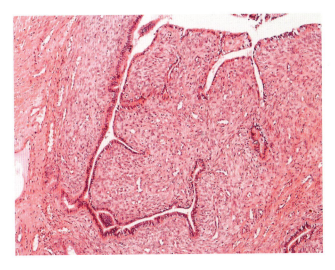

Figure 7.20 Adenofibroma. The stroma comprises bland spindly fibroblastic cells without stromal-cell atypia or periglandular condensation.

ADENOFIBROMA

Although still included in the 2014 WHO Classification,[25] whether or not adenofibroma exists as a pathologic entity in the endometrium is a subject of controversy.[37,38] As elaborated in the 'Diagnostic criteria and related problems' section, the major problem with the diagnosis of adenofibroma is the lack of reliable histopathologic criteria for distinguishing adenofibroma from adenosarcoma.[37,38] The diagnosis of adenofibroma is now extremely rarely made in the endometrium.

DIAGNOSTIC CRITERIA AND RELATED PROBLEMS

Traditionally, adenofibroma was described as a mixed tumor with bland epithelial and mesenchymal components which were sharply demarcated from the adjacent endometrium and myometrium.[39] The usual histologic pattern features broad papillary fronds covered by endometrial-type epithelium (Figure 7.19) overlying fibromatous stroma (Figure 7.20).[39] In addition, the absence of more than mild stromal cell atypia, periglandular stromal cuffing and significant mitotic activity (two or more mitotic figures per 10 high-power fields) were used as criteria to distinguish adenofibroma from adenosarcoma.[37–39]

While earlier studies suggested that adenofibromas diagnosed by these criteria generally had benign clinical outcome following hysterectomy,[39] there have been reported cases of 'adenofibroma' which developed recurrence, myometrial invasion or vascular invasion.[40,41] Metastasis has also been noted for occasional cases diagnosed as adenofibromas, with only mild stromal atypia and less than two mitotic figures per 10 high-power fields.[37] In light of these findings, it has been argued that the conventional diagnostic criteria for adenofibroma could not reliably predict a benign clinical behavior, implying that some cases of 'adenofibromas' diagnosed by these criteria could represent well-differentiated adenosarcomas.[37] It is now widely held that adenofibroma and adenosarcoma are part of a spectrum, analogous to benign, borderline and malignant phyllodes tumors of the breast (Box 7.2).[38]

BOX 7.2: Practical approach to the differential diagnosis of an 'adenofibroma-like' lesion

Lesions with adenofibroma-like features are occasionally encountered in endometrial biopsies, curettage or hysterectomy specimens. In view of the questionable validity of diagnostic criteria for adenofibroma, a pragmatic approach to the differential diagnosis is presented.

- **Adenosarcoma** should always be considered for any adenofibroma-like lesion, especially with phyllodes-like architecture, because the diagnostic features of adenosarcoma (stromal atypia, periglandular cuffing and mitotic activity) are often focal and subtle.[38] Careful assessment of stromal cell atypia is required to detect subtle nuclear hyperchromasia and irregularity, which is an important diagnostic clue.
- **Endometrial polyps** with unusual morphologic patterns may sometimes contain foci resembling adenofibroma.[7] Areas typical of endometrial polyp with thick-walled vessels are normally present in such cases.
- **Endocervical-type adenomyoma** is an uncommon lesion that occasionally harbors adenofibroma-like foci.[42] Apart from the location in the cervix, the presence of endocervical mucinous epithelium and lobular arrangement of glands could aid the diagnosis.
- Definitive diagnosis of adenofibroma should not be rendered in endometrial biopsies or curettage specimens because the possibility of adenosarcoma could not be excluded unless the whole tumor is available for assessment.[37,38]
- The diagnosis of adenofibroma should only be reserved for hysterectomy specimens with complete sampling of the lesion and careful assessment for morphologic features of adenosarcoma. If this diagnosis was ever made, a comment could be included to convey the uncertainty about its clinical behavior.

OTHER TUMOR-LIKE LESIONS OF THE ENDOMETRIUM

LYMPHOMA-LIKE LESION

Lymphoma-like lesions are florid reactive inflammatory lesions presenting in the female genital tract that may be confused with lymphoma.[43,44] They are usually found in women of reproductive age, more commonly recognised in the cervix but occasionally in the endometrium.[43,44] Most cases are believed to represent reactive changes in a background of chronic cervicitis or endometritis.[43,44] The typical histologic picture shows dense inflammatory infiltrate with admixed large lymphoid cells exhibiting variable atypia and mitotic activity, which could raise suspicion for lymphoma (Figures 7.21 and 7.22).[43] They are usually superficial lesions associated with surface erosions and mixed inflammatory infiltrate, including plasma cells and neutrophils.[44] The key features that help distinguish lymphoma-like lesions from lymphoma are the absence of mass lesion, deep invasion and sclerosis.[43] Immunohistochemical studies typically show a mixture of B and T cells without immunoglobulin light-chain restriction.[43] Clonal rearrangement of the *IGH* gene

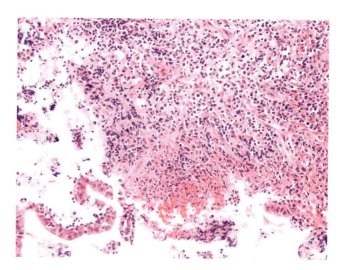

Figure 7.21 Chronic endometritis with prominent lymphoid infiltrate. Such cases of endometritis sometimes exhibit prominent reactive atypia in the lymphoid cells raising the suspicion of lymphoma, which may be referred to as 'lymphoma-like lesion'.

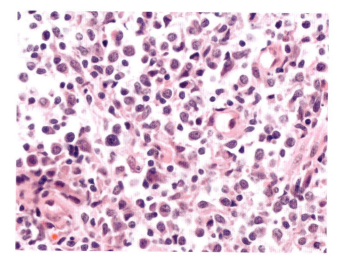

Figure 7.22 Chronic endometritis with prominent lymphoid infiltrate. High-power view may demonstrate a spectrum of nuclear enlargement and distinct nucleoli, which could possibly mimic lymphoma.

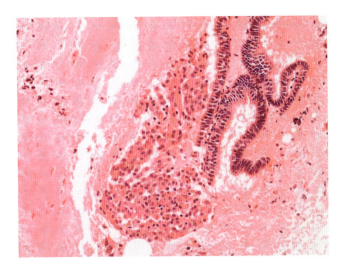

Figure 7.23 Nodular histiocytic hyperplasia. A compact aggregate of histiocytes are present admixed with endometrial glandular epithelium.

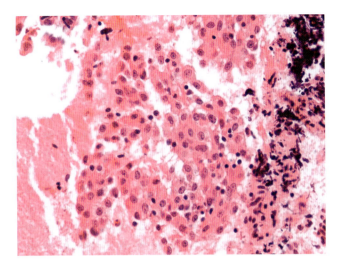

Figure 7.24 Nodular histiocytic hyperplasia. The histiocytes in these lesions may appear somewhat cohesive and mimic decidualized endometrial stroma. However, the nuclei are typical of histiocytes with oval to reniform shape and fine chromatin.

(immunoglobulin heavy-chain gene) has been identified in a few cases from the cervix, suggesting a potential pitfall in diagnosis.[43]

NODULAR HISTIOCYTIC HYPERPLASIA

Nodular histiocytic hyperplasia could be regarded as the endometrial equivalent of nodular histiocytic/mesothelial hyperplasia involving serosal cavities.[45] This is usually an incidental finding with detached nodular aggregates of histiocytes in endometrial biopsies or curettings (Figure 7.23),[45] but it may also present as an endometrial nodule in a hysterectomy specimen.[46] The characteristic morphology of histiocytes in nodular histiocytic hyperplasia has been described as round or polygonal cells with lobulated, ovoid, reniform or crescent-shaped nuclei.[45,46] These histiocytes possess a moderate amount of pale, granular or amphophilic cytoplasm, often with distinct cell borders (Figure 7.24).[45,46] Some cases may demonstrate prominent cytoplasmic vacuoles with eccentric nuclei, thus mimicking signet ring cells.[46,47] Immunohistochemically, the histiocytes are positive for CD68 (Figure 7.25) and lysozyme, while negative for cytokeratin, S-100, hormone receptors and CD10.[45,46] Nodular histiocytic hyperplasia is believed to represent a reaction to intracavity debris with no known clinical significance.[45] Awareness of this lesion could avoid misdiagnosis as other conditions such as xanthogranulomatous endometritis, Langerhans cell histiocytosis, malakoplakia, decidualized endometrial stroma or signet ring cell carcinoma.[45,46]

PLEXIFORM TUMORLET OF UTERUS

The term 'plexiform tumorlet' was used to describe a distinctive benign lesion in the endometrium or myometrium, measuring 1 cm or less, characterised by a trabecular or cord-like arrangement of epithelioid cells in a plexiform pattern (Figures 7.26 through 7.28).[48,49] Most reported cases

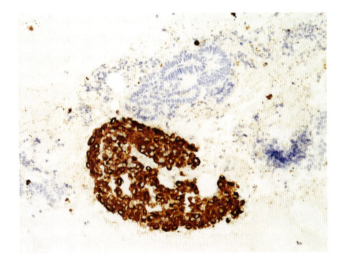

Figure 7.25 CD68 immunohistochemistry in nodular histiocytic hyperplasia. Positive staining for CD68 will confirm the histiocytic nature.

are incidental microscopic findings, which may be solitary or multiple, with circumscribed or ill-defined borders. The lesion was believed to show smooth-muscle differentiation based on earlier studies which demonstrated ultrastructural evidence of myoid features[48] and immunohistochemical expression of smooth-muscle markers.[49,50]

The major differential diagnosis is UTROSCT (uterine tumor resembling ovarian sex cord tumor), which could have identical morphology[49] and also is known to have variable expression of smooth-muscle markers.[51] A study by Nogales et al. demonstrated that plexiform tumorlets expressed smooth-muscle markers (smooth-muscle actin, desmin and h-caldesmon), as well as CD56, estrogen receptor and progesterone receptor, while inhibin, calretinin, CD10 and epithelial membrane antigen were negative.[49] The authors thus

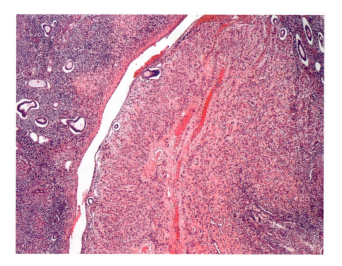

Figure 7.26 Plexiform tumorlet. A small lesion comprising cords of eosinophilic cells is present in the endometrial stroma.

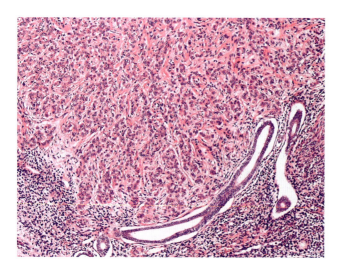

Figure 7.27 Plexiform tumorlet. The cords of epithelioid cells show a plexiform growth pattern.

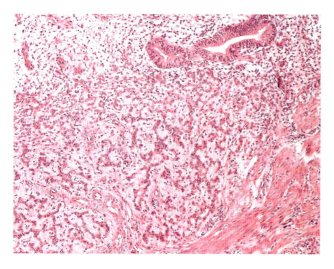

Figure 7.28. Plexiform tumorlet. This lesion is situated at the endomyometrial junction.

proposed that plexiform tumorlets should be regarded as small UTROSCTs with predominant myoid differentiation.[49] Whether plexiform tumorlets are biologically distinct from UTROSCTs is still an unresolved issue.[49,52] From a practical point of view, for lesions displaying morphologic features of plexiform tumorlet, immunohistochemical studies for sex cord markers (inhibin, calretinin, WT1 and melan-A) should be attempted. Lesions expressing sex cord markers (with or without expression of smooth-muscle markers) are best regarded as UTROSCTs, while those expressing smooth-muscle markers and negative for sex cord markers could be reported as plexiform tumorlets.

ENDOMETRIAL METAPLASIA AND RELATED CHANGES

The term 'metaplasia' as applied to the endometrium encompasses a broad range of epithelial and stromal changes.[53–55] While some of these changes fall within the original meaning of 'metaplasia', which refers to the transformation from one to another mature cell type, many of them may be better considered as cytoplasmic or architectural changes.[53,54] However, it has become conventional to refer to these changes collectively as 'endometrial metaplasia', with new entities being continuously introduced to the list. Some of the following entities do not explicitly carry the word 'metaplasia', but by their nature are most appropriately considered together as a form of cellular changes. These conditions are grouped into epithelial (Table 7.1) and stromal (Table 7.2) changes for clarity of discussion.

ENDOMETRIAL EPITHELIAL METAPLASIAS

Squamous metaplasia and morules

Squamous metaplasia and morules are currently regarded as two different types of endometrial metaplasias,[53,54] but they are often considered together because morules were traditionally believed to represent an immature form of squamous metaplasia.[53–55]

SQUAMOUS METAPLASIA

Use of the term 'squamous metaplasia' is preferably restricted to the presence of typical squamous elements in the endometrium, featuring keratinization, intercellular bridges and/or prominent cell membranes, with bland nuclei in the squamous cells (Figure 7.29).[55,56]

Squamous metaplasia may be associated with endometrial hyperplasia or carcinoma, but is also sometimes associated with endometritis or chronic pyometra.[56]

ICHTHYOSIS UTERI

When extensive squamous metaplasia is present in the endometrial surface epithelium and glands, the term 'ichthyosis uteri' could be applied.[57]

Table 7.1 Types of endometrial epithelial metaplasia

	Key morphologic features and ancillary studies	Clinical significance and possible associations
Squamous metaplasia (with typical squamous elements)	Squamous epithelium with keratinization, intercellular bridges and/or prominent cell membranes Bland nuclei	Risk of endometrial hyperplasia or carcinoma Associated with endometritis or chronic pyometra
Morules	Rounded aggregates or syncytial sheets of cells with eosinophilic cytoplasm Indistinct cell borders Bland nuclei CDX2 positive	Risk of endometrial hyperplasia or carcinoma Sometimes seen in normal endometrium or benign endometrial lesions
Tubal metaplasia	Large number of ciliated cells with bland nuclei present in endometrial glands p16 mosaic pattern	Occasionally associated with anovulatory cycles or other high estrogen states
Eosinophilic metaplasia	Cells with abundant eosinophilic cytoplasm Bland nuclei	Nonspecific; may be found in normal endometrium, benign endometrial lesions, endometrial hyperplasia or carcinoma
Mucinous metaplasia	Cells with intracytoplasmic mucin Bland nuclei Simple architecture (without the architectural complexity of atypical/malignant mucinous proliferations)	May be associated with hormone replacement therapy Common in tamoxifen-associated endometrial polyps
Intestinal metaplasia (subtype of mucinous metaplasia)	Intestinal-type epithelium with goblet cells and neuroendocrine cells CK20, CDX2 and villin positive	May be associated with intestinal metaplasia in other gynecologic sites
Gastric metaplasia (subtype of mucinous metaplasia)	Resembles benign gastric-type lesions of cervix MUC6 and/or HIK1083 positive	May be associated with synchronous and multifocal mucinous lesions of the female genital tract
Papillary syncytial metaplasia	Syncytial aggregates of cells with eosinophilic cytoplasm and indistinct cell borders Pseudopapillae with cellular tufting and stratification Neutrophil infiltration	Reactive change associated with endometrial breakdown
Hobnail metaplasia	'Hobnail' appearance (rounded apical blebs with nuclei bulging toward luminal side) Bland nuclei	Probably reactive change May occur after curettage or radiotherapy
Clear-cell metaplasia	Cells with clear cytoplasm rich in glycogen Bland nuclei Nongestational endometrium	May be associated with tamoxifen usage
Papillary proliferation	True papillary structures with fibrovascular stromal cores Variable degree of branching No significant cytologic atypia	Risk of endometrial hyperplasia or carcinoma (especially for cases with complex or extensive lesions) Typically identified in association with endometrial polyp and coexisting with various types of metaplasia

Ichthyosis uteri is typically associated with chronic inflammatory conditions like endometritis or pyometra, but ichthyosis uteri–like changes with dysplasia have also been reported in association with cervical squamous neoplasia.[58]

MORULES (MORULAR METAPLASIA)

Morule refers to a characteristic morphologic pattern in which rounded aggregates or syncytial sheets of cells with eosinophilic cytoplasm, indistinct cell borders and bland nuclei fill the glandular lumina (Figures 7.30 and 7.31).[55,56] Overt morphologic evidence of squamous differentiation (keratinization and/or intercellular bridges) is absent from morules, although they may coexist and merge with foci of squamous metaplasia.[55] Central necrosis may be present in morules (Figure 7.32), but mitotic figures are sparse and nuclear pleomorphism minimal.[55] The term 'squamous

Table 7.2 Types of endometrial stromal metaplasia and other stromal changes

	Key morphologic features	Clinical significance and possible associations
Osseous metaplasia	Bone tissue blending with endometrial stroma	Associated with infertility and previous abortion
Cartilaginous metaplasia	Islands of benign-appearing cartilage blending with endometrial stroma	Not known
Adipose metaplasia	Clusters of mature adipocytes which blend with endometrial stroma	Not known
Smooth-muscle metaplasia	Isolated short fascicles or small nodules of smooth-muscle cells in endometrial stroma	Not known
Pseudorosette-like proliferation	Small discrete foci of spindly cells in short fascicles, arranged radially around an eosinophilic central region resembling pseudorosettes	Not known
Synovial-like metaplasia	Eroded surface epithelium Synovial-like cells in a palisaded arrangement oriented perpendicular to the endometrial surface	Associated with the levonorgestrel-releasing intrauterine system
Glial tissue in the endometrium	Nodules or polyps of glial tissue in the endometrium	Often presumed to represent retained fetal tissue
Extramedullary hematopoiesis in the endometrium	Hematopoietic cells of different lineages in the endometrium	May be associated with hematologic diseases

morules' was commonly used, but they are now preferably known as 'morules' or 'morular metaplasia', because current evidence suggests that morules may not exhibit genuine squamous differentiation.[56] Houghton et al. demonstrated that morules were usually diffusely positive for CDX2, with nuclear and cytoplasmic positivity for β-catenin, and negative for p63, an immunophenotype that was partially overlapping but often distinct from typical squamous metaplasia.[56] However, whether morules represent immature squamous differentiation has not been unanimously agreed upon among authorities.[53,54,56]

Similar to typical squamous metaplasia, the presence of morules is also associated with endometrial hyperplasia and carcinoma;[54,56] in such cases, extensive morular metaplasia may create difficulties with architectural assessment.[54] Unlike typical squamous metaplasia, morules are sometimes seen in normal endometrium or benign endometrial lesions.[56]

Tubal metaplasia (ciliated-cell metaplasia)

As scattered ciliated cells are present in normal endometrial epithelium, tubal metaplasia (or ciliated-cell metaplasia) is

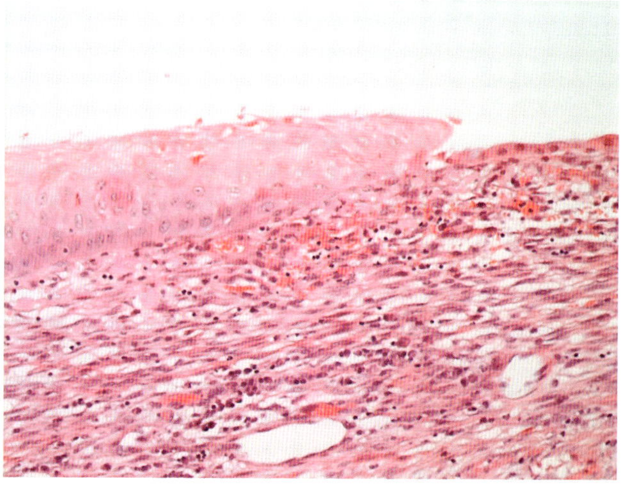

Figure 7.29 Squamous metaplasia (with typical squamous elements). The endometrial surface epithelium is replaced by nonkeratinizing squamous epithelium with intercellular bridges and bland nuclei.

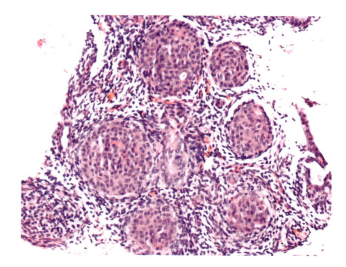

Figure 7.30 Morules. Solid cellular proliferation with berry-like configuration replaces most of the glandular epithelium in this focus.

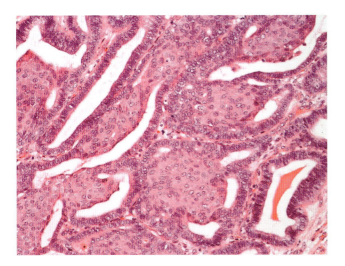

Figure 7.31 Morules in endometrial hyperplasia. Crowded glands with foci of syncytial cellular proliferation continuous with the glandular epithelium.

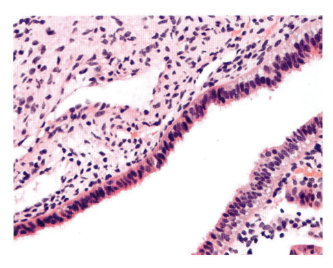

Figure 7.33 Tubal metaplasia (ciliated-cell metaplasia).

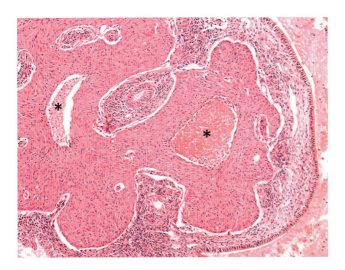

Figure 7.32 Morules. Central necrosis (*) is a possible finding in morules.

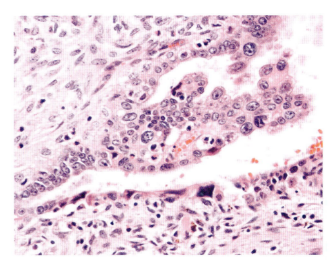

Figure 7.34 Tubal metaplasia with cytologic atypia. Nuclear enlargement with hyperchromasia, distinct nucleoli and smudgy chromatin is occasionally present in tubal metaplasia but generally believed to represent a degenerative phenomenon.

diagnosed only when a large number of cytologically bland ciliated cells are present in endometrial glands (Figure 7.33).[54,55] Strictly speaking, tubal metaplasia is used when all three cell types of tubal epithelium (ciliated, secretory and intercalated peg cells) are present, while ciliated-cell metaplasia is used when the epithelium is predominantly replaced by ciliated cells, but the two terms are often applied interchangeably.[53] The ciliated cells in tubal metaplasia often have eosinophilic cytoplasm, but some cells with clear cytoplasm and more vesicular nuclei are also not uncommon.[55] The epithelium could be stratified or show bridge-like tufts, but mitotic figures are uncommon.[55] Simon et al. studied cases of tubal metaplasia with cytologic atypia (defined as enlarged pleomorphic hyperchromatic nuclei with small to prominent nucleoli and increased nuclear-to-cytoplasmic ratio) (Figure 7.34), and the clinical follow-up found no increased risk of endometrial hyperplasia or malignancy.[59]

This suggests that cytologic atypia of reactive or degenerative nature can be seen in tubal metaplasia.

Immunohistochemically, tubal metaplasia commonly exhibits p16 expression but in a mosaic pattern.[60]

Tubal metaplasia may be occasionally associated with anovulatory cycles or other conditions with high estrogen levels.[53–55]

Eosinophilic metaplasia

Eosinophilic metaplasia broadly refers to the endometrial epithelium composed of cells with abundant eosinophilic cytoplasm and bland nuclei (Figure 7.35).[55,61] There may be variable degrees of cytoplasmic vacuolation or granularity.[54,61] The nuclei are typically round and uniform with no significant nuclear pleomorphism and rare mitotic

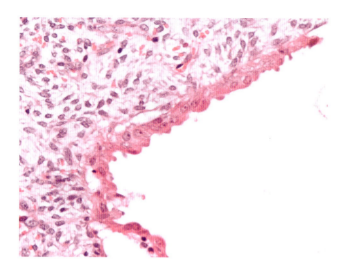

Figure 7.35 Eosinophilic metaplasia. Abundant eosinophilic cytoplasm in the endometrial glandular epithelium is a relatively nonspecific change.

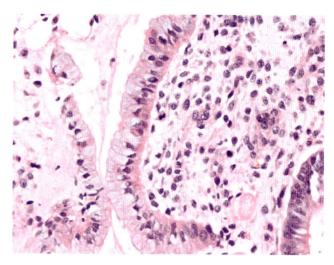

Figure 7.36 Mucinous metaplasia. Intracytoplasmic mucin is present in the metaplastic foci with basally located banal nuclei.

activity.[54,55] A small subgroup of cases may be specifically labeled as oncocytic metaplasia, characterised histologically by granular eosinophilic cytoplasm with ultrastructural presence of abundant mitochondria.[61,62] However, most cases of eosinophilic metaplasia do not have overt oncocytic features, and it has been postulated that many of these cases represent a form of immature mucinous differentiation.[61] Frequent coexistence of eosinophilic metaplasia with mucinous metaplasia, coupled with MUC5AC expression in eosinophilic metaplasia, have been cited as evidence for this postulation.[61]

Eosinophilic metaplasia is relatively nonspecific, which may be found in normal endometrium, benign endometrial lesions, as well as endometrial hyperplasia and carcinoma.[53,61]

Mucinous metaplasia

Mucinous metaplasia refers to the replacement of endometrial glandular epithelium by cells which contain intracytoplasmic mucin, have cytologically bland nuclei and simple architecture, without the architectural features that warrant the diagnosis of atypical mucinous glandular proliferation or mucinous carcinoma.[54,55,63,64] The mucinous epithelium typically resembles endocervical epithelium with columnar cells, basally located uniform nuclei and low nuclear-to-cytoplasmic ratio, as well as rare mitotic activity (Figures 7.36 and 7.37).[55] In contrast to other types of metaplasia, the architectural assessment is a critical part of evaluating any mucinous proliferations in the endometrium, because atypical and malignant mucinous proliferations commonly display no or minimal nuclear atypia.[63,64] A practical diagnostic approach to mucinous proliferations of the endometrium is presented in Box 7.3.

Although usually not necessary, the intracytoplasmic mucin may be demonstrated by histochemical stains such as periodic acid-Schiff with diastase digestion or mucicarmine.[54]

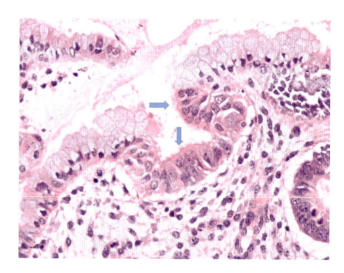

Figure 7.37 Mucinous metaplasia and tubal metaplasia. Mucinous metaplasia coexists with tubal metaplasia (arrows) in this area.

Mucinous metaplasia often occurs in perimenopausal or postmenopausal women and it may be associated with hormone replacement therapy.[53] Mucinous metaplasia is commonly found in tamoxifen-associated endometrial polyps.[65]

VARIANT: INTESTINAL METAPLASIA

Rare cases of intestinal metaplasia have been reported in the endometrium, characterised by intestinal-type epithelium with goblet cells and neuroendocrine cells.[66,67] Immunohistochemically, the intestinal-type epithelium is generally positive for CK20, CDX2 and villin, with scattered chromogranin-positive cells.[66] The few reported cases suggest a possible association with intestinal metaplasia in other sites of the female genital tract, such as the cervix.[66]

VARIANT: GASTRIC METAPLASIA

Gastric metaplasia is another exceedingly rare subgroup of mucinous metaplasia, which has been recognised in the context of synchronous and multifocal mucinous lesions of the female genital tract.[68] Morphologically, these lesions may resemble lobular endocervical glandular hyperplasia or pyloric gland metaplasia of the cervix (Figure 7.38), with the evidence of gastric differentiation supported by MUC6 and/or HIK1083 immunohistochemistry.[68]

Papillary syncytial metaplasia

Papillary syncytial metaplasia (also known as surface papillary syncytial change or eosinophilic syncytial change)[73] refers to the morphologic change in endometrial epithelium characterised by syncytial aggregates of cells with eosinophilic cytoplasm and indistinct cell borders, pseudopapillae formed by cellular tufting and stratification and commonly infiltrated by neutrophils (Figure 7.43).[54] The nuclei are round to oval with fine chromatin, occasionally displaying mild reactive atypia and mitotic activity.[54]

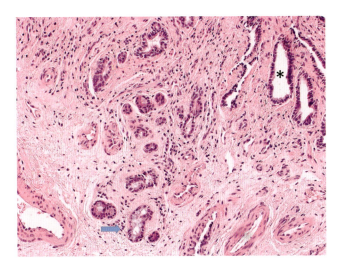

Figure 7.38 Gastric metaplasia in an endometrial polyp. A mucinous gland (arrow) is present together with lobular arrangement of glands with amphophilic cytoplasm, resembling pyloric glands. Inactive endometrial glands (*) are also noted in a fibrous stroma with thick-walled vessels. (Courtesy of Prof. Glenn McCluggage.)

BOX 7.3: Approach to the diagnosis of endometrial mucinous proliferations and the utility of *KRAS* mutation analysis

Mucinous proliferations of the endometrium could be conceptually divided into three types: benign mucinous metaplasia, atypical mucinous glandular proliferation and mucinous adenocarcinoma. This paradigm has been largely adopted by the 2014 WHO Classification,[25] although different terminology has been proposed in the literature.[63,64,69,70]

- **Benign mucinous metaplasia** comprises mucinous epithelium involving endometrial surface epithelium or glands with normal architecture (at most small tufts of mucinous cells), with no cytologic atypia.[63]

- Benign mucinous metaplasia has no significant association with malignancy.[63,64,70]
- **Mucinous adenocarcinoma** is diagnosed by the presence of confluent or cribriform architecture (as the criteria applied to endometrioid adenocarcinoma), even with minimal cytologic atypia (Figures 7.39 and 7.40).[25,64]
  - The diagnosis of mucinous adenocarcinoma requires mucinous cells accounting for more than 50% of tumor cells.[25] Focal mucinous differentiation in endometrioid adenocarcinoma is not

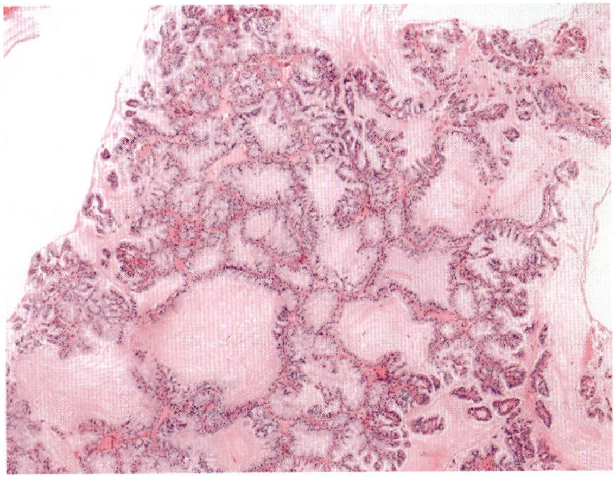

Figure 7.39 Mucinous adenocarcinoma. Confluent proliferation of mucinous glands with papillary tufting and minimal intervening stroma characterises malignancy.

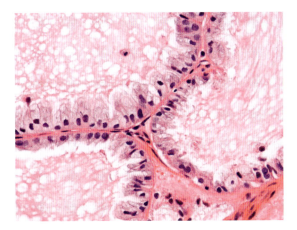

Figure 7.40 Mucinous adenocarcinoma (same case as Figure 7.39). High-power view of these crowded mucinous glands demonstrates the minimal degree of nuclear atypia that could be seen in malignant mucinous proliferations.

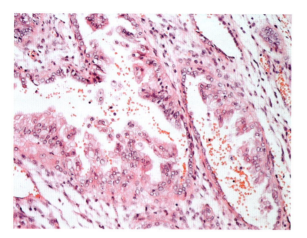

Figure 7.41 Atypical mucinous glandular proliferation. Crowded glands lined by mucinous epithelium with cellular tufting and mild degree of nuclear atypia.

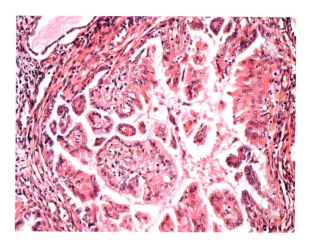

Figure 7.42 Atypical mucinous glandular proliferation. The architecture of this mucinous gland is complex with branching papillary structures.

uncommon and should be considered in cases with less-extensive mucinous change.[64]
- **Atypical mucinous glandular proliferation (AMGP)** is the term endorsed by the 2014 WHO Classification for mucinous proliferations in which the architectural complexity exceeds that of benign mucinous metaplasia but is insufficient for a definitive diagnosis of mucinous adenocarcinoma.[25,64]
    - Possible histologic features include papillary architecture, microglandular pattern (resembling microglandular hyperplasia of cervix), extensive branching and budding or moderate to severe cytologic atypia (Figures 7.41 and 7.42).[63,64]
    - Rawish et al. studied 41 cases of biopsy-detected AMGP and found that, among 29 cases with hysterectomy performed, 17% had no residual AMGP or carcinoma, 38% had AMGP and 45% had adenocarcinoma in the uteri.[64]
    - Studies have shown that the adenocarcinomas associated with atypical mucinous proliferations are usually of endometrioid or mucinous types, mostly low grade and early stage.[63,64,70]
    - Morphologic features are generally not helpful for predicting the outcome of cases diagnosed as AMGP in biopsies or curettings,[64] so *KRAS* mutation analysis has been proposed by some authors as an adjunct for risk stratification.[71,72]
- The clinical management of AMGP has not been universally standardised, although many cases are managed by repeating curettage or biopsy, followed by hysterectomy for persistent mucinous proliferations.[70]
- ***KRAS* mutation analysis** may be employed in cases of AMGP to predict the risk of significant neoplastic lesions in subsequent hysterectomy, but it should be stressed that even AMGP without detectable *KRAS* mutation may have atypical hyperplasia or carcinoma in subsequent specimens.[71,72]
    - In the study by Alomari et al., *KRAS* mutation was detected in 55% of cases (18 of 33) diagnosed as 'complex mucinous lesions' but absent from all five cases diagnosed as 'simple mucinous lesions'.[71] Among the complex mucinous lesions with *KRAS* mutations, 10 of 15 cases had atypical hyperplasia or carcinoma in follow-up curettage or hysterectomy, while five of 12 cases of *KRAS* wild-type complex mucinous lesions developed atypical hyperplasia or carcinoma.

The changes typically involve the surface epithelium or superficial glands.[54]

Papillary syncytial metaplasia is considered a reactive process associated with endometrial breakdown, representing either regenerative or degenerative ischemia-induced changes.[73] Morphologic features of breakdown such as stromal aggregates, fibrinoid material, neutrophilic infiltration and apoptotic bodies are often present.[73]

Immunohistochemically, papillary syncytial metaplasia was found to exhibit decreased ER expression compared with adjacent endometrium, wild-type (but increased) p53 expression and diffuse p16 positivity. Awareness of the immunoprofile could avoid misdiagnosis of serous carcinoma in cases with prominent reactive atypia.

Hobnail metaplasia

Hobnail metaplasia features glandular epithelium dominated by cells with 'hobnail' appearance (rounded apical blebs with nuclei bulging toward luminal side), scanty clear

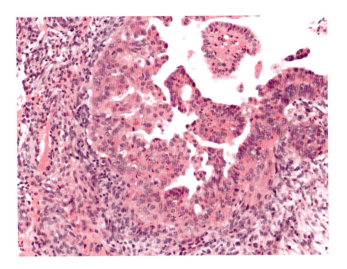

Figure 7.43 Papillary syncytial metaplasia. Superficial epithelium with syncytial pseudopapillae composed of eosinophilic cells, accompanied by rich neutrophilic infiltrate.

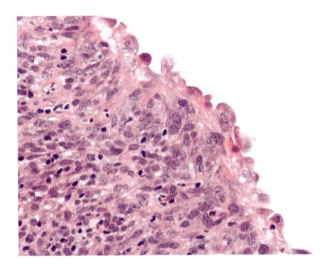

Figure 7.44 Hobnail metaplasia. The 'hobnail' appearance refers to rounded apical border with nuclei bulging toward the luminal side.

or eosinophilic cytoplasm and cytologically bland nuclei (Figure 7.44).[53–55] This is an uncommon phenomenon of presumably reactive nature, which may occur after curettage or radiotherapy.[53,54]

Conditions that may resemble hobnail metaplasia include Arias-Stella reaction, clear-cell carcinoma and serous carcinoma.[53,54] Bland nuclear morphology, absent or rare mitotic activity and focal nature of metaplastic changes are of help for distinction from malignancy.[54]

Clear-cell metaplasia

Clear-cell metaplasia refers to epithelial cells with clear cytoplasm rich in glycogen and cytologically bland nuclei in the nongestational endometrium.[54,55] This is very uncommon but some cases may be associated with tamoxifen usage.[54]

The differential diagnosis may include Arias-Stella reaction and clear-cell carcinoma,[54] which could usually be resolved by finding their respective histologic features.

Papillary proliferation

Papillary proliferation refers to a morphologically distinctive lesion in the endometrium, comprising true papillary structures with fibrovascular stromal cores and variable degrees of branching but lacking significant cytologic atypia (Figures 7.45 and 7.46).[74,75] Mitotic activity is generally rare.[74] These lesions are typically found in postmenopausal patients and often identified within or associated with an endometrial polyp.[74,75] Many cases are found to coexist with various

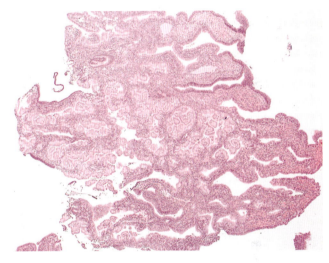

Figure 7.45 Papillary proliferation of the endometrium. Low-power view demonstrating the focal transformation of endometrial glands into papillary structures. (Courtesy of Prof. Glenn McCluggage.)

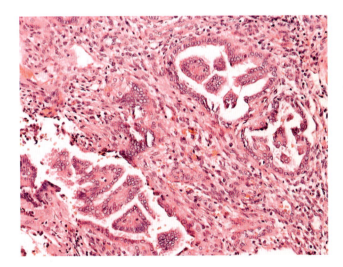

Figure 7.46 Papillary proliferation of the endometrium. The papillary structures are generally short with fibrovascular cores and variable branching, but there is no cytologic atypia in the epithelium.

types of metaplasia (especially mucinous, eosinophilic and ciliated-cell metaplasias).[74,75] An approach to assessing and stratifying papillary proliferations of the endometrium has been proposed by Ip et al.,[75] which is presented in Box 7.4.

> **BOX 7.4: Approach to papillary proliferation of the endometrium**
>
> - Papillary proliferations of the endometrium could be conceptually divided into two groups: simple and complex, based on the degree of architectural complexity and the extent of the proliferation.[75]
>   - Simple papillary proliferation refers to papillae with short, predominantly nonbranching stalks, including those with occasional secondary branches. The extent is localized with one or two foci or <50% of an endometrial polyp.
>   - Complex papillary proliferation refers to papillae with frequent secondary and complex branches. Cases with extensive involvement (three or more foci in a specimen) or involving >50% of an endometrial polyp are also placed in this group.
> - Based on the study by Ip et al., most cases (22 of 25 cases) classified as 'simple papillary proliferation' have benign outcome, although one case developed atypical hyperplasia and two developed grade 1 endometrioid adenocarcinoma.[75] Among 21 cases classified as 'complex papillary proliferation' in the study, endometrial hyperplasia or carcinoma were diagnosed concurrently or in subsequent specimens in 17 of them (eight with non-atypical hyperplasia, five with atypical hyperplasia and four with grade 1 or 2 endometrioid adenocarcinoma).
> - From a practical point of view, papillary proliferations that are localized and architecturally simple, present within a hysterectomy specimen or confined to a completely removed polyp, could be regarded as benign.[75] Curettage should be considered when there is uncertainty about whether the lesion has been completely removed.[75]
> - Papillary proliferations with architecturally complex papillae, multifocality (three or more foci) or extensive involvement (>50%) of an endometrial polyp could be referred to as 'complex papillary hyperplasia', and they are regarded as having significant associated risk of concurrent or subsequent atypical hyperplasia or endometrial carcinoma.[75]
> - In view of the practical difficulties in evaluating the architecture of papillae as well as cytologic atypia in biopsies, repeat biopsies or curettage may be recommended for cases with suspicion of complex papillae or focal cytologic atypia.

The differential diagnosis of papillary proliferation may include papillary syncytial metaplasia, endometrioid carcinoma with villoglandular pattern or small nonvillous papillae, as well as serous carcinoma.[54,74,75] Papillary syncytial metaplasia may have small papillary tufts, but these lack fibrovascular cores.[75] Endometrioid carcinomas with villoglandular pattern usually have longer slender papillae rather than the short branching papillae in papillary proliferations, while carcinomas with small nonvillous papillae exhibit no fibrovascular cores.[75] Serous carcinoma (especially serous EIC) could have similar architecture as that of papillary proliferation, but the marked cytologic atypia and brisk mitotic activity are keys to the diagnosis.

ENDOMETRIAL STROMAL METAPLASIAS AND OTHER STROMAL CHANGES

Endometrial stromal metaplasias are less commonly identified than epithelial metaplasias. Most present as incidental findings of little clinical significance.[53]

Osseous metaplasia

Osseous metaplasia is an uncommon condition with bone in the endometrium, which may be seen to blend with endometrial stroma (Figure 7.47).[54] Most patients have previous history of abortion, and the typical clinical presentation is infertility.[76,77] Sonographic or hysteroscopic evidence of bone within the uterine cavity may be observed.[76,77] Genotyping analysis has demonstrated that osseous metaplasia represents a true metaplastic process rather than retained fetal bone from a previous miscarriage.[78] Osseous metaplasia may be rarely identified in association with endometrial carcinoma.[79] For any case with bone tissue identified in the endometrium, the differential diagnosis of heterologous elements in a carcinosarcoma or adenosarcoma should be carefully evaluated, looking for any atypical features in the bone tissue or underlying sarcomatous component.[54]

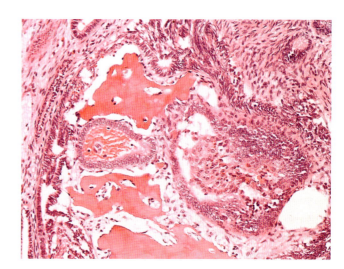

Figure 7.47 Osseous metaplasia. Islands of osteoid matrix are present within endometrial stroma.

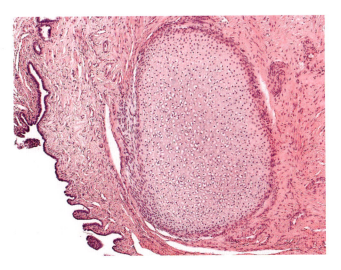
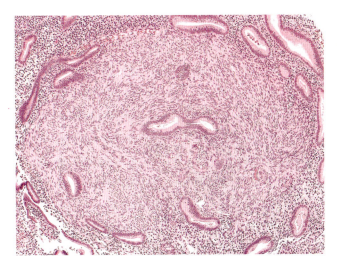

Figure 7.48 Cartilaginous metaplasia in an endometrial polyp. Mature cartilage is present within the fibrous stroma of an endometrial polyp, focally covered by endometrial glandular epithelium (left). (Courtesy of Prof. Glenn McCluggage.)

Figure 7.49 Pseudorosette-like proliferation. The endometrial stroma is transformed into short fascicles of spindly cells arranged radially around eosinophilic material. (Courtesy of Prof. Glenn McCluggage.)

Cartilaginous metaplasia

Islands of benign-appearing cartilage which blend with the surrounding endometrial stroma constitute cartilaginous metaplasia (Figure 7.48), which is a rare finding.[53] Like osseous metaplasia, the possibility of heterologous chondroid elements in a carcinosarcoma or adenosarcoma should always be carefully excluded.[54]

Adipose metaplasia

Adipose metaplasia (or fatty change) in the endometrium exists as clusters of mature adipocytes which blend with endometrial stroma.[53,80] Awareness of this uncommon reactive change could avoid misinterpretation as evidence of uterine perforation.[54]

Smooth-muscle metaplasia

Smooth-muscle metaplasia may manifest as isolated short fascicles or small nodules of smooth-muscle cells in the endometrial stroma, presumably of metaplastic origin, although possibly representing extension from myometrium.[53]

Pseudorosette-like proliferation

Pseudorosette-like proliferation is a recently recognised microscopic lesion in the endometrial stroma, characterised by small discrete foci of spindly cells in short fascicles, which are arranged radially around an eosinophilic central region resembling pseudorosettes (Figure 7.49).[81] Immunohistochemistry demonstrates that pseudorosette-like proliferations are usually positive for smooth-muscle actin, occasionally positive for CD10, but negative for cytokeratin, S-100 and h-caldesmon.[81] While no clinical significance has been documented for this lesion, it has been postulated to represent a benign lesion displaying smooth-muscle differentiation.[81]

Synovial-like metaplasia

Synovial-like metaplasia is another newly described morphologic alteration in the endometrial stroma, which is typically associated with the levonorgestrel-releasing intrauterine system.[82] The histologic appearance is characterised by areas with eroded surface epithelium and the presence of synovial-like cells in a palisaded arrangement oriented perpendicular to the endometrial surface. Immunohistochemically, the synovial-like cells are vimentin positive and variably positive for CD68, focally CD10 positive, but negative for ER, PR or cytokeratin. This is believed to represent an endometrial stromal reaction to surface erosion induced by an intrauterine foreign body.[82]

Glial tissue in the endometrium

Mature glial tissue has been rarely identified in the endometrium, typically in women of reproductive age with a history of abortion.[83,84] The glial tissue may present as nodules or polyps in the endometrium, immunohistochemically highlighted by glial fibrillary acidic protein.[83,84] The origin of the glial tissue is usually presumed to be retained fetal tissue.[84]

Extramedullary hematopoiesis in the endometrium

Extramedullary hematopoiesis is rarely identified in the endometrium, featuring variable admixture of hematopoietic cells of erythroid, myeloid and megakaryocytic lineages.[85–87] Some of the reported cases were associated with underlying hematologic diseases (such as myeloproliferative disorders),[85] but other cases had unknown etiology.[86,87] Their recognition should trigger clinical investigations for any hematologic conditions.[87]

REFERENCES

1. Tallini G, Vanni R, Manfioletti G, Kazmierczak B, Faa G, Pauwels P, Bullerdiek J, Giancotti V, Van Den Berghe H, Dal Cin P. HMGI-C and HMGI(Y) immunoreactivity correlates with cytogenetic abnormalities in lipomas, pulmonary chondroid hamartomas, endometrial polyps, and uterine leiomyomas and is compatible with rearrangement of the HMGI-C and HMGI(Y) genes. *Lab Invest* 2000;80:359–69.
2. Reslová T, Tosner J, Resl M, Kugler R, Vávrová I. Endometrial polyps. A clinical study of 245 cases. *Arch Gynecol Obstet* 1999;262:133–9.
3. Kim KR, Peng R, Ro JY, Robboy SJ. A diagnostically useful histopathologic feature of endometrial polyp: The long axis of endometrial glands arranged parallel to surface epithelium. *Am J Surg Pathol* 2004;28:1057–62.
4. Tai LH, Tavassoli FA. Endometrial polyps with atypical (bizarre) stromal cells. *Am J Surg Pathol* 2002;26: 505–9.
5. Heller D, Barrett T. Bizarre stromal cells in an endometrial polyp. *Int J Surg Pathol* 2016;24:320–1.
6. Russell P, Lynnhtun K, James D, Obermair A. Endometrial polyp and endometriosis with atypical stromal cells. *Pathology* 2013;45:191–3.
7. Howitt BE, Quade BJ, Nucci MR. Uterine polyps with features overlapping with those of Müllerian adenosarcoma: A clinicopathologic analysis of 29 cases emphasizing their likely benign nature. *Am J Surg Pathol* 2015;39:116–26.
8. Kelly P, Dobbs SP, McCluggage WG. Endometrial hyperplasia involving endometrial polyps: Report of a series and discussion of the significance in an endometrial biopsy specimen. *BJOG* 2007;114:944–50.
9. Mittal K, Da Costa D. Endometrial hyperplasia and carcinoma in endometrial polyps: Clinicopathologic and follow-up findings. *Int J Gynecol Pathol* 2008;27:45–8.
10. Wheeler DT, Bell KA, Kurman RJ, Sherman ME. Minimal uterine serous carcinoma: Diagnosis and clinicopathologic correlation. *Am J Surg Pathol* 2000;24:797–806.
11. McCluggage WG, Sumathi VP, McManus DT. Uterine serous carcinoma and endometrial intraepithelial carcinoma arising in endometrial polyps: Report of 5 cases, including 2 associated with tamoxifen therapy. *Hum Pathol* 2003;34:939–43.
12. Hui P, Kelly M, O'Malley DM, Tavassoli F, Schwartz PE. Minimal uterine serous carcinoma: A clinicopathological study of 40 cases. *Mod Pathol* 2005;18:75–82.
13. Rabban JT, Zaloudek CJ. Minimal uterine serous carcinoma: Current concepts in diagnosis and prognosis. *Pathology*. 2007;39:125–33.
14. McCluggage WG. My approach to the interpretation of endometrial biopsies and curettings. *J Clin Pathol* 2006;59:801–12.
15. Moritani S, Ichihara S, Hasegawa M, Iwakoshi A, Murakami S, Sato T, Okamoto T, Mori Y, Kuhara H, Silverberg SG. Stromal p16 expression differentiates endometrial polyp from endometrial hyperplasia. *Virchows Arch* 2012;461:41–8.
16. Stewart CJ, Bharat C, Crook M. p16 immunoreactivity in endometrial stromal cells: Stromal p16 expression characterises but is not specific for endometrial polyps. *Pathology* 2015;47:112–7.
17. Tahlan A, Nanda A, Mohan H. Uterine adenomyoma: A clinicopathologic review of 26 cases and a review of the literature. *Int J Gynecol Pathol* 2006;25:361–5.
18. Gilks CB, Clement PB, Hart WR, Young RH. Uterine adenomyomas excluding atypical polypoid adenomyomas and adenomyomas of endocervical type: A clinicopathologic study of 30 cases of an underemphasized lesion that may cause diagnostic problems with brief consideration of adenomyomas of other female genital tract sites. *Int J Gynecol Pathol* 2000;19:195–205.
19. Kenny SL, McCluggage WG. Adenomyomatous polyp of the endometrium with prominent epithelioid smooth muscle differentiation: Report of two cases of a hitherto undescribed lesion. *Int J Surg Pathol* 2014;22:358–63.
20. Young RH, Treger T, Scully RE. Atypical polypoid adenomyoma of the uterus. A report of 27 cases. *Am J Clin Pathol* 1986;86:139–45.
21. Fukunaga M, Endo Y, Ushigome S, Ishikawa E. Atypical polypoid adenomyomas of the uterus. *Histopathology* 1995;27:35–42.
22. Longacre TA, Chung MH, Rouse RV, Hendrickson MR. Atypical polypoid adenomyofibromas (atypical polypoid adenomyomas) of the uterus. A clinicopathologic study of 55 cases. *Am J Surg Pathol* 1996;20:1–20.
23. Němejcová K, Kenny SL, Laco J, Škapa P, Staněk L, Zikán M, Kleiblová P, McCluggage WG, Dundr P. Atypical polypoid adenomyoma of the uterus: An immunohistochemical and molecular study of 21 cases. *Am J Surg Pathol* 2015;39:1148–55.
24. Takahashi H, Yoshida T, Matsumoto T, Kameda Y, Takano Y, Tazo Y, Inoue H, Saegusa M. Frequent β-catenin gene mutations in atypical polypoid adenomyoma of the uterus. *Hum Pathol* 2014;45:33–40.
25. Kurman RJ, Carcangiu ML, Herrington CS, Young RH (eds), *WHO Classification of Tumours of Female Reproductive Organs*. International Agency for Research on Cancer. Lyon, 2014.
26. Heatley MK. Atypical polypoid adenomyoma: A systematic review of the English literature. *Histopathology* 2006;48:609–10.

27. Horita A, Kurata A, Maeda D, Fukayama M, Sakamoto A. Immunohistochemical characteristics of atypical polypoid adenomyoma with special reference to h-caldesmon. *Int J Gynecol Pathol* 2011;30:64–70.
28. Oliva E, Young RH, Clement PB, Bhan AK, Scully RE. Cellular benign mesenchymal tumors of the uterus. A comparative morphologic and immunohistochemical analysis of 33 highly cellular leiomyomas and six endometrial stromal nodules, two frequently confused tumors. *Am J Surg Pathol* 1995;19:757–68.
29. Dionigi A, Oliva E, Clement PB, Young RH. Endometrial stromal nodules and endometrial stromal tumors with limited infiltration: A clinicopathologic study of 50 cases. *Am J Surg Pathol* 2002;26:567–81.
30. Conklin CM, Longacre TA. Endometrial stromal tumors: The new WHO classification. *Adv Anat Pathol* 2014;21:383–93.
31. Nucci MR, Harburger D, Koontz J, Dal Cin P, Sklar J. Molecular analysis of the JAZF1-JJAZ1 gene fusion by RT-PCR and fluorescence in situ hybridization in endometrial stromal neoplasms. *Am J Surg Pathol* 2007;31:65–70.
32. Oliva E, Young RH, Amin MB, Clement PB. An immunohistochemical analysis of endometrial stromal and smooth muscle tumors of the uterus: A study of 54 cases emphasizing the importance of using a panel because of overlap in immunoreactivity for individual antibodies. *Am J Surg Pathol* 2002;26:403–12.
33. Sumathi VP, Al-Hussaini M, Connolly LE, Fullerton L, McCluggage WG. Endometrial stromal neoplasms are immunoreactive with WT-1 antibody. *Int J Gynecol Pathol* 2004;23:241–7.
34. Oliva E, de Leval L, Soslow RA, Herens C. High frequency of JAZF1-JJAZ1 gene fusion in endometrial stromal tumors with smooth muscle differentiation by interphase FISH detection. *Am J Surg Pathol* 2007;31:1277–84.
35. Huang HY, Ladanyi M, Soslow RA. Molecular detection of JAZF1-JJAZ1 gene fusion in endometrial stromal neoplasms with classic and variant histology: Evidence for genetic heterogeneity. *Am J Surg Pathol* 2004;28:224–32.
36. Chiang S, Oliva E. Cytogenetic and molecular aberrations in endometrial stromal tumors. *Hum Patho.* 2011;42:609–17.
37. Gallardo A, Prat J. Mullerian adenosarcoma: A clinicopathologic and immunohistochemical study of 55 cases challenging the existence of adenofibroma. *Am J Surg Pathol* 2009;33:278–88.
38. McCluggage WG. Mullerian adenosarcoma of the female genital tract. *Adv Anat Pathol* 2010;17:122–9.
39. Zaloudek CJ, Norris HJ. Adenofibroma and adenosarcoma of the uterus: A clinicopathologic study of 35 cases. *Cancer* 1981;48:354–66.
40. Seltzer VL, Levine A, Spiegel G, Rosenfeld D, Coffey EL. Adenofibroma of the uterus: Multiple recurrences following wide local excision. *Gynecol Oncol* 1990;37:427–31.
41. Clement PB, Scully RE. Müllerian adenofibroma of the uterus with invasion of myometrium and pelvic veins. *Int J Gynecol Pathol* 1990;9:363–71.
42. Casey S, McCluggage WG. Adenomyomas of the uterine cervix: Report of a cohort including endocervical and novel variants. *Histopathology* 2015;66:420–9.
43. Geyer JT, Ferry JA, Harris NL, Young RH, Longtine JA, Zukerberg LR. Florid reactive lymphoid hyperplasia of the lower female genital tract (lymphoma-like lesion): A benign condition that frequently harbors clonal immunoglobulin heavy chain gene rearrangements. *Am J Surg Pathol* 2010;34:161–8.
44. Young RH, Harris NL, Scully RE. Lymphoma-like lesions of the lower female genital tract: A report of 16 cases. *Int J Gynecol Pathol* 1985;4:289–99.
45. Kim KR, Lee YH, Ro JY. Nodular histiocytic hyperplasia of the endometrium. *Int J Gynecol Pathol* 2002;21:141–6.
46. Fukunaga M, Iwaki S. Nodular histiocytic hyperplasia of the endometrium. *Arch Pathol Lab Med* 2004;128:1032–4.
47. Iezzoni JC, Mills SE. Nonneoplastic endometrial signet-ring cells. Vacuolated decidual cells and stromal histiocytes mimicking adenocarcinoma. *Am J Clin Pathol* 2001;115:249–55.
48. Kaminski PF, Tavassoli FA. Plexiform tumorlet: A clinical and pathologic study of 15 cases with ultrastructural observations. *Int J Gynecol Pathol* 1984;3:124–34.
49. Nogales FF, Nicolae A, García-Galvis OF, Aneiros-Fernández J, Salas-Molina J, Stolnicu S. Uterine and extrauterine plexiform tumourlets are sex-cord-like tumours with myoid features. *Histopathology* 2009;54:497–500.
50. Balaton AJ, Vuong PN, Vaury P, Baviera EE. Plexiform tumorlet of the uterus: Immunohistological evidence for a smooth muscle origin. *Histopathology* 1986;10:749–54.
51. de Leval L, Lim GS, Waltregny D, Oliva E. Diverse phenotypic profile of uterine tumors resembling ovarian sex cord tumors: An immunohistochemical study of 12 cases. *Am J Surg Pathol* 2010;34:1749–61.
52. Pradhan D, Mohanty SK. Uterine tumors resembling ovarian sex cord tumors. *Arch Pathol Lab Med* 2013;137:1832–6.
53. Nicolae A, Preda O, Nogales FF. Endometrial metaplasias and reactive changes: A spectrum of altered differentiation. *J Clin Pathol* 2011;64:97–106.
54. Stringfellow HF, Elliot VJ. Endometrial metaplasia. *Diagn Histopathology* 2017;23:303–10.

55. Hendrickson MR, Kempson RL. Endometrial epithelial metaplasias: Proliferations frequently misdiagnosed as adenocarcinoma. Report of 89 cases and proposed classification. *Am J Surg Pathol* 1980; 4:525–42.
56. Houghton O, Connolly LE, McCluggage WG. Morules in endometrioid proliferations of the uterus and ovary consistently express the intestinal transcription factor CDX2. *Histopathology* 2008;53:156–65.
57. Brown D Jr, Spjut HJ. Extensive squamous metaplasia of the endometrium (ichthyosis uteri). *South Med J* 1982;75:593–5.
58. Fadare O. Dysplastic Ichthyosis uteri-like changes of the entire endometrium associated with a squamous cell carcinoma of the uterine cervix. *Diagn Pathol* 2006;1:8.
59. Simon RA, Peng SL, Liu F, Quddus MR, Zhang C, Steinhoff MM, Lawrence WD, Sung CJ. Tubal metaplasia of the endometrium with cytologic atypia: Analysis of p53, Ki-67, TERT, and long-term follow-up. *Mod Pathol* 2011;24:1254–61.
60. Horree N, Heintz AP, Sie-Go DM, van Diest PJ. p16 is consistently expressed in endometrial tubal metaplasia. *Cell Oncol* 2007;29:37–45.
61. Moritani S, Kushima R, Ichihara S, Okabe H, Hattori T, Kobayashi TK, Silverberg SG. Eosinophilic cell change of the endometrium: A possible relationship to mucinous differentiation. *Mod Pathol* 2005;18:1243–8.
62. Silver SA, Cheung AN, Tavassoli FA. Oncocytic metaplasia and carcinoma of the endometrium: An immunohistochemical and ultrastructural study. *Int J Gynecol Pathol* 1999;18:12–9.
63. Nucci MR, Prasad CJ, Crum CP, Mutter GL. Mucinous endometrial epithelial proliferations: A morphologic spectrum of changes with diverse clinical significance. *Mod Pathol* 1999;12:1137–42.
64. Rawish KR, Desouki MM, Fadare O. Atypical mucinous glandular proliferations in endometrial samplings: Follow-up and other clinicopathological findings in 41 cases. *Hum Pathol* 2017;63:53–62.
65. Deligdisch L, Kalir T, Cohen CJ, de Latour M, Le Bouedec G, Penault-Llorca F. Endometrial histopathology in 700 patients treated with tamoxifen for breast cancer. *Gynecol Oncol* 2000;78:181–6.
66. Nicolae A, Goyenaga P, McCluggage WG, Preda O, Nogales FF. Endometrial intestinal metaplasia: A report of two cases, including one associated with cervical intestinal and pyloric metaplasia. *Int J Gynecol Pathol* 2011;30:492–6.
67. Wells M, Tiltman A. Intestinal metaplasia of the endometrium. *Histopathology* 1989;15:431–3.
68. Mikami Y, Kiyokawa T, Sasajima Y, Teramoto N, Wakasa T, Wakasa K, Hata S. Reappraisal of synchronous and multifocal mucinous lesions of the female genital tract: A close association with gastric metaplasia. *Histopathology* 2009;54:184–91.
69. Yoo SH, Park BH, Choi J, Yoo J, Lee SW, Kim YM, Kim KR. Papillary mucinous metaplasia of the endometrium as a possible precursor of endometrial mucinous adenocarcinoma. *Mod Pathol* 2012;25:1496–507.
70. Turashvili G, Childs T. Mucinous metaplasia of the endometrium: Current concepts. *Gynecol Oncol* 2015;136:389–93.
71. Alomari A, Abi-Raad R, Buza N, Hui P. Frequent KRAS mutation in complex mucinous epithelial lesions of the endometrium. *Mod Pathol* 2014; 27:675–80.
72. He M, Jackson CL, Gubrod RB, Breese V, Steinhoff M, Lawrence WD, Xiong J. KRAS mutations in mucinous lesions of the uterus. *Am J Clin Pathol* 2015;143: 778–84.
73. McCluggage WG, McBride HA. Papillary syncytial metaplasia associated with endometrial breakdown exhibits an immunophenotype that overlaps with uterine serous carcinoma. *Int J Gynecol Pathol* 2012;31:206–10.
74. Lehman MB, Hart WR. Simple and complex hyperplastic papillary proliferations of the endometrium: A clinicopathologic study of nine cases of apparently localized papillary lesions with fibrovascular stromal cores and epithelial metaplasia. *Am J Surg Pathol* 2001;25:1347–54.
75. Ip PP, Irving JA, McCluggage WG, Clement PB, Young RH. Papillary proliferation of the endometrium: A clinicopathologic study of 59 cases of simple and complex papillae without cytologic atypia. *Am J Surg Pathol* 2013;37:167–77.
76. Khan SN, Modi M, Hoyos LR, Imudia AN, Awonuga AO. Bone in the endometrium: A review. *Int J Fertil Steril* 2016;10:154–61.
77. Garg D, Bekker G, Akselrod F, Narasimhulu DM. Endometrial osseous metaplasia: An unusual cause of infertility. *BMJ Case Rep* 2015.
78. Parente RC, Patriarca MT, de Moura Neto RS, de Oliveira MA, Lasmar RB, de Holanda Mendes P, de Sá PG, Cardeman L, Silva R, de Freitas V. Genetic analysis of the cause of endometrial osseous metaplasia. *Obstet Gynecol* 2009;114:1103–8.
79. Nogales FF, Gomez-Morales M, Raymundo C, Aguilar D. Benign heterologous tissue components associated with endometrial carcinoma. *Int J Gynecol Pathol* 1982;1:286–91.
80. Nogales FF, Pavcovich M, Medina MT, Palomino M. Fatty change in the endometrium. *Histopathology* 1992;20:362–3.
81. Lomme MM, Lin LW, Sung CJ, Lawrence WD, Quddus MR. Pseudorosette-like proliferations of the endometrium. *Int J Gynecol Pathol* 2015;34:590–4.
82. Stewart CJ, Leake R. Endometrial synovial-like metaplasia associated with levonorgestrel-releasing intrauterine system. *Int J Gynecol Pathol* 2015;34: 570–5.

83. Brown LJ, Wells M. Heterotopic adipose and glial tissue in the endometrium with staining for glial fibrillary acidic protein. Case report. *Br J Obstet Gynaecol* 1986;93:637–9.
84. Russell P, de Costa C, Yeoh G. Fetal glial allograft in the endometrium: Case report of a recurrent pseudo-tumor. *Pathology* 1993;25:247–9.
85. Creagh TM, Bain BJ, Evans DJ, Reid CD, Young RH, Flanagan AM. Endometrial extramedullary haemopoiesis. *J Pathol* 1995;176:99–104.
86. Sirgi KE, Swanson PE, Gersell DJ. Extramedullary hematopoiesis in the endometrium. Report of four cases and review of the literature. *Am J Clin Pathol* 1994;101:643–6.
87. Valeri RM, Ibrahim N, Sheaff MT. Extramedullary hematopoiesis in the endometrium. *Int J Gynecol Pathol* 2002;21:178–81.

Endometrial premalignant lesions

Precursors of endometrioid carcinoma	91
Precursors of endometrial serous carcinoma	101
Putative precursor for endometrial clear-cell carcinoma	107
References	109

Endometrial cancers encompass tumors with a range of morphologies that display a spectrum of clinical presentations. Endometrial premalignant lesions, which are commonly referred as precursors or precancers of the endometrium, are less illustrated compared to those malignant counterparts. Among all the endometrial precursor lesions, the most common and better understood is endometrial intraepithelial neoplasia (EIN) or atypical hyperplasia (AH), which has been accepted as a precancerous lesion of endometrial endometrioid carcinoma. In contrast to EIN, endometrial glandular dysplasia (EmGD) as the precancerous lesion of endometrial serous carcinoma is far less encountered in daily practice. Although EmGD is less common, it is clinically important to be recognised before it develops into its cancerous status, no matter with or without myometrial invasion, which will have a very poor prognosis. Putative precursors of endometrial clear-cell carcinoma have been briefly described in the past. There is no precursor of endometrial mucinous, poorly differentiated or undifferentiated or de-differentiated carcinomas described. In this chapter, we will focus on the precursors of endometrioid and serous cancers.

PRECURSORS OF ENDOMETRIOID CARCINOMA

In the WHO 1994 classification of endometrial precancerous lesions, endometrial hyperplasias are divided into four categories depending on the presence or absence of cytologic atypia and complicated architecture, including hyperplasia (simple and complex hyperplasia without atypia) and atypical hyperplasia (simple and complex atypical hyperplasia). Unfortunately, this classification system has been dropped due to its poor reproducibility even among gynecological pathologists.[1,2] The current WHO 2014 classification dropped previous arbitrary architectural criteria and adopted a simple two-tiered system, which includes benign hyperplasia or hyperplasia without atypia and EIN/AH. In the WHO 1994 classification system, cytologic atypia was defined by the presence of loss of nuclear polarity, irregular

Table 8.1 Comparison between 1994 and 2014 WHO classification of endometrial precancerous lesion

1994/2003 WHO classification	2014 WHO classification
Simple endometrial hyperplasia	Endometrial hyperplasia without atypia
Complex endometrial hyperplasia	
Simple atypical endometrial hyperplasia	Atypical hyperplasia (AH)/Endometrioid intraepithelial neoplasia(EIN)
Complex atypical endometrial hyperplasia	

nuclear shape, irregular nuclear contours, vesicular chromatin, hyperchromatic chromatin and prominent nucleoli. While similar criteria are still used in the WHO 2014 system, the comparison of possible foci of EIN/AH with the background endometrium has increased the diagnostic reproducibility among pathologists and resulted in better prediction for the presence of concurrent endometrioid carcinoma as well as future development of cancer in subsequent years.[3] The previous and current WHO classification systems are summarized in Table 8.1.

BENIGN HYPERPLASIA (HYPERPLASIA WITHOUT ATYPIA)

Definition

Endometrial hyperplasia is characterised by an abnormal increase in the amount of endometrium that, on microscopic examination, shows architectural abnormalities without cytological abnormalities. Simply put, the endometrial glandular-to-stroma ratio is over 1 in a defined endometrial tissue sample.

Etiology and genetic profile

Prolonged unopposed exposure to estrogen is the major known etiological factor for endometrial hyperplasia. Obesity, chronic anovulation, hormone replacement and an estrogen-secreting ovarian tumor remain the main causes of excessive estrogen production. Over time, excessive unopposed estrogen exposure leads to irregular endometrial cycles, retention and sustained growth of the endometrium, which in turn can progress to non-atypical hyperplasia and set the stage for possible neoplastic transformation. Remodeling of the endometrium in this manner is a spectrum of disease, first manifesting in disordered (anovulatory) endometrium, followed by benign hyperplasia, EIN/AH and eventually endometrioid carcinoma.[4] Hyperplasia without atypia tends to be polyclonal and harbors only low levels of somatic mutations in the scattered endometrial glands.[5]

Prognosis and predictive factors

Prolonged and unopposed estrogen exposure can lead to a 2–10 fold increased risk of endometrial carcinoma.[6,7] From 1% to 3% of patients with 'untreated' endometrial hyperplasia without atypia may progress to well-differentiated endometrioid carcinoma.[8] From this perspective, unopposed estrogen therapy is not used for women with intact uteri.

Histopathology

Endometrial hyperplasia without atypia is defined by an exaggerated glandular proliferation, with increased gland-to-stroma ratio compared with proliferative endometrium, yet without significant cytologic atypia.[9] As estrogen overstimulation continues, the global glandular-to-stromal ratio of the endometrium will increase, which is the cardinal difference between disordered proliferative endometrium and hyperplasia without atypia. In hysterectomy specimens, cysts of varying size may be visible within the thickened endometrium. Under microscopic examination, the glands are well spaced and separated by a reasonable amount of stroma, but the glandular-to-stromal ratio is over 1. The microscopic features of benign endometrial hyperplasia are summarized as follows.

- This is best appreciated at low magnification (2–4X) as a 'regularly-irregular' (diffuse growth) pattern of crowded, small, proliferative glands alternating with pockets of even more crowded, dilated or branched glands (Figure 8.1).
- The glands show marked variation in size and shape. Some glands are of normal size, while many are cystically dilated.
- The glandular outline may be round or irregular, and occasionally intraluminal papillary fronds (infolding), budding and branching can be present (Figure 8.2).
- The epithelium lining the glands closely resembles proliferative endometrium (Figure 8.3). The epithelial cells are commonly columnar, pseudostratified and may be arranged with the long axis of their nuclei roughly at right angles to the basement membrane.
- There is no cytological atypia or epithelial disorganization. The nuclei show evenly dispersed chromatin and inconspicuous nucleoli.

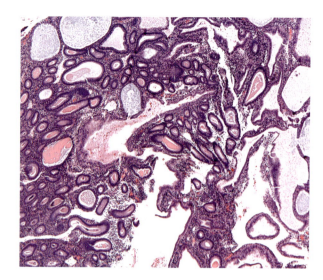

Figure 8.1 Hyperplasia without atypia. Note the regularly irregular distribution of crowded glands. Focally more condensed area is frequently seen.

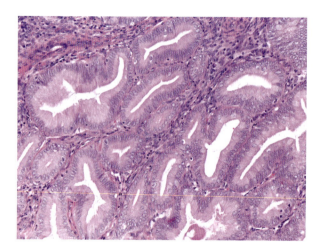

Figure 8.2 Hyperplasia without atypia. There are many crowded glands with tubular and focal cystic formation.

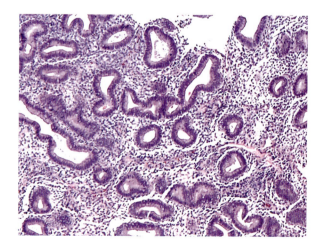

Figure 8.3 Hyperplasia without atypia. Lining epithelia resemble those of proliferative endometrium. Focal secretory areas can be seen.

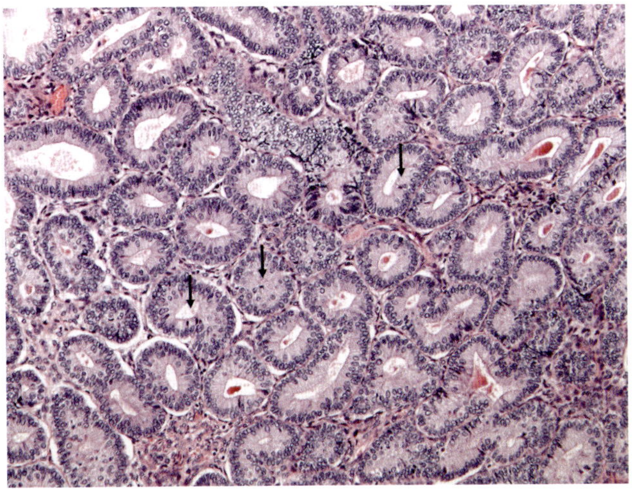

Precursors of endometrioid carcinoma / Benign hyperplasia 93

Figure 8.4 Hyperplasia without atypia. Non-atypical hyperplasia can have packed proliferative-type endometrial glands. Mitotic figures are frequently seen (arrows). However, no atypical mitotic figure is present. Compared to the background proliferative glands, there is no dramatic cytologic difference (not shown in this field).

- There is little or no variation in nuclear shape or size.
- Epithelial mitotic figures are frequent due to estrogen dominant status, but are not atypical (Figure 8.4).
- The stroma in hyperplasia without atypia is more cellular than that seen in a normal proliferative endometrium. The stromal cells resemble those seen in the proliferative phase and have small oval nuclei with very scanty cytoplasm and poorly demarcated cytoplasmic margins. Variable mitotic activity is also seen within the stroma.

More importantly, no discernable cytologic changes typically seen in EIN/AH should be seen throughout the entirety of the tissue even at high magnification. This lack of 'cytologic demarcation' compared to those background proliferative endometrial glands is the key histologic feature to set non-atypical hyperplasia apart from EIN/AH. Stromal breakdown, hemorrhage and associated reactive epithelial changes are not uncommon and are typically a consequence of microthrombi.[9,10]

Differential diagnosis

The differential diagnosis of benign hyperplasia includes disordered proliferative endometrium, secretory endometrium and EIN/AH.

DISORDERED PROLIFERATIVE ENDOMETRIUM (DPE)

The earliest histologic manifestation of estrogen excess is so-called 'DPE'. At this stage of development, a normal gland-to-stroma ratio is usually retained (Figure 8.5). Occasionally dilated glands are interspersed in a background of otherwise unremarkable proliferative endometrium (Figure 8.6). The quantity and complexity of abnormally dilated endometrial

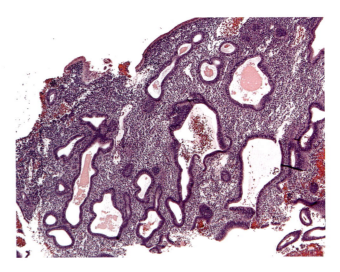

Figure 8.5 Disordered proliferative endometrium. A normal gland-to-stroma ratio is less than 1, but dilated glands are present.

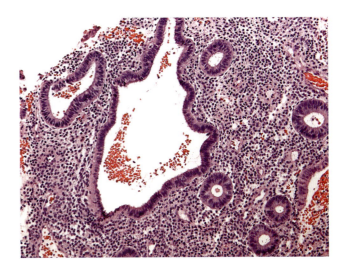

Figure 8.6 Disordered proliferative endometrium. Dilated glands are interspersed in a background of otherwise unremarkable proliferative endometrium.

glands vary from case to case, including microcystic or cystic growth patterns (Figure 8.7). Occasionally, multilobular growth patterns may be seen. When these histologic features are present, a diagnosis of DPE or 'proliferative endometrium with features of anovulation' is appropriate. That is to say, cases of DPE may contain small areas of glandular crowding, similar to that seen in benign hyperplasia; however, these areas are limited and will not be as widely distributed as in cases of hyperplasia. We use less than 10% of dilated or abnormally shaped glands as a dividing line to separate proliferative endometrium from DPE, although a minor degree of abnormal-looking glands in the proliferative phase of the endometrium is acceptable.

SECRETORY ENDOMETRIUM

Secretory endometrium may display a global increase in the gland-to-stroma ratio throughout the specimen, causing

94 Endometrial premalignant lesions

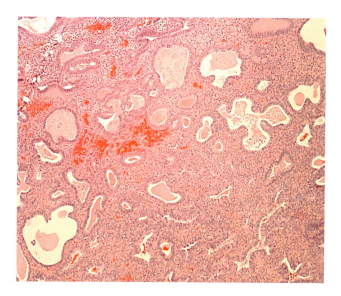

Figure 8.7 Disordered proliferative endometrium. Disordered proliferative glands can be microcystic and/or cystic.

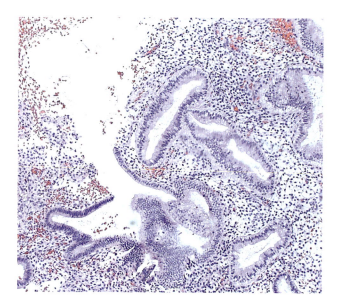

Figure 8.8 Secretory endometrium. Epithelial secretory vacuoles as well as stromal pseudodecidualization are characteristic of secretory endometrium, although the glandular to stroma ratio can be greater than 1.

concern for benign hyperplasia. Epithelial secretory vacuoles, as well as stromal pseudodecidualization, can help to identify secretory endometrium (Figure 8.8). Rare cases of the secretory type of EIN may occur, and PAX2 loss in these cases can help to identify these subtle lesions (see the section 'Endometrial intraepithelial neoplasia (EIN)/atypical hyperplasia (AH)' for more details).

EIN/AH

Cases of oversized EIN/AH, which is sometimes also called over-run EIN/AH, may lack a discernable background endometrium, making it difficult to identify cytologic demarcation (see the section 'Endometrial intraepithelial neoplasia (EIN)/atypical hyperplasia (AH)' for more details). These cases may closely resemble benign hyperplasia; however, EIN/AH typically displays a greater degree of glandular crowding and will generally lack the low-power 'regularly-irregular' pattern of benign hyperplasia. Careful application of PAX2 may be helpful in such cases.[11]

ENDOMETRIAL INTRAEPITHELIAL NEOPLASIA (EIN)/ATYPICAL HYPERPLASIA (AH)

Definition

Cytologic atypia superimposed on endometrial hyperplasia defines the EIN/AH. It is considered as a precancer for endometrioid carcinoma of the endometrium.

Etiology and genetic profile

Risk of EIN/AH and endometrial cancers includes hormonal imbalances (including obesity) and genetic defects. Endometrial cancers and their precursors are known to be driven by increases in estrogen and dampened by relative decreases in progestin.[12] Patients with hereditary nonpolyposis colorectal cancer syndrome (HNPCC or Lynch syndrome)[13] or Cowden syndrome[14] are known to have an increased risk of developing endometrial cancers. A well-described risk factor for development of precancerous lesions is tamoxifen therapy. Patients on tamoxifen are prone to developing endometrial polyps, hyperplasia and premalignant and malignant endometrioid lesions.[15,16] Unlike hyperplasia without atypia, EIN/AH represents a *de novo* monoclonal population that is genetically distinct from the background endometrium, but which is similar to the subsequent adenocarcinoma.[5,17-19] Epigenetic inactivation of the *MLH1* through hypermethylation of its promoter region has been identified in a subset of precancerous lesions.[20] Moreover, similar mismatch repair protein loss of expression is observed in both precancerous and adjacent malignant endometrial lesions.[21] Inactivation of *PAX2*[22] and genetic mutations of *PTEN*,[23-25] *K-RAS*[26-28] and *CTNNB1*(β-catenin)[29] have been associated with EIN/AH.

Prognosis and predictive factors

Patients with a diagnosis of EIN/AH carry a significant risk of progression to endometrioid adenocarcinoma. Up to 40% of patients with a diagnosis of EIN/AH have either concurrent endometrioid carcinoma within the uterus demonstrated by immediate hysterectomy or subsequent cancer found in the first year of follow-up.[8,30,31] It is believed that some of the cancers found in subsequent hysterectomies represent the development of precancerous lesions of EIN/AH.[32] Patients in their first year after diagnosis of EIN/AH carry approximately a 45-fold increased risk of developing low-grade endometrioid carcinoma compared with those with a diagnosis of non-atypical hyperplasia.[33]

Histopathology

The diagnostic criteria of EIN/AH in the WHO 2014 system include the following components, which are required to make the diagnosis.

- Architectural glandular crowding
- Cytologic demarcation from the background endometrium
- Size greater than 1 mm
- Exclusion of benign mimics and carcinoma

The above diagnostic criteria are summarized in Table 8.2.

Architectural glandular crowding is defined by overall gland-to-stroma ratio greater than 1 (Figure 8.9). In typical cases of EIN/AH, the stroma makes up about 10%–30% of the volume of the tissue. Of note, glands should still be separated by stroma and a diagnosis of focal adenocarcinoma may be entertained if the area exceeds the level of EIN/AH. The crowded glands are typically tubular or branching, but sometimes infolding, budding and dilatation may occur. Usually, the glands of EIN/AH are more condensed at the 'epicenter' of the lesion, and more diluted at the periphery (Figure 8.10), mainly due to clonal growth process. Normal background glands may be seen admixed with precancerous glands at the periphery of the lesion (Figure 8.11).

Nuclear atypia used to be the only criterion to distinguish between non-atypical and atypical hyperplasia in the WHO 1994 system. The nuclear atypia is defined by the presence of loss of nuclear polarity, irregular nuclear shape, irregular nuclear contours, vesicular chromatin, hyperchromatic chromatin and prominent nucleoli. However, nuclear atypia can be variable both qualitatively and quantitatively, and somewhat subjective. They are also commonly influenced by hormone levels of individual patients. In addition, the presence of metaplasia further adds to the difficulty of interpreting nuclear atypia. Thus, the introduction of 'cytologic demarcation' in the WHO 2014 system becomes an important histologic feature for diagnosing EIN/AH. This

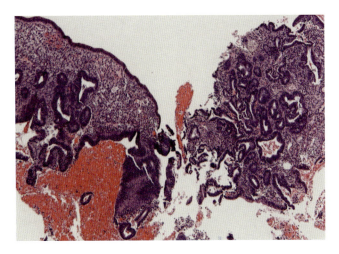

Figure 8.9 EIN/AH. Overall gland-to-stroma ratio greater than 1.

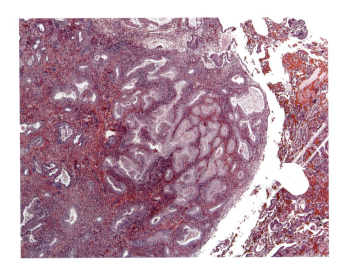

Figure 8.10 EIN/AH. This EIN lesion presents a typical 'clonal' growth appearance (center). The background nonhyperplastic proliferative endometrial glands surround the EIN lesion.

Table 8.2 Diagnostic criteria for EIN/AH

Criteria	Definition	Tips for application
Gland crowding	The gland-to-stroma ratio should exceed 1:1	In practice, 55% of the tissue should be composed of glands vs. stroma. This is best determined at low power.
Cytologic demarcation	Crowded glands should differ cytologically from the background endometrium	Once an area of crowded glands is noted, carefully analyze the cytology of the crowded focus to see if it differs from the adjacent normal. Best performed at 10–20x.
Size	The size of the lesion should be greater than 1 mm	The 10x objective on most microscopes fives a field of view of approximately 2 mm; therefore, if the lesion is greater than 1/2 a 10x field, it is likely larger than 1 mm.
Exclusion of mimics	Benign and malignant mimics should be excluded	Confirm that benign mimics such as endometrium with metaplasia, secretory endometrium, polyps, endometrial basalis, as well as carcinoma are not present.

Abbreviations: AH, atypical hyperplasia; EIN, endometrioid intraepithelial neoplasia.

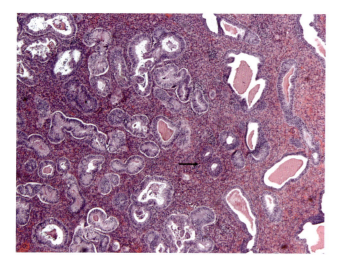

Figure 8.11 EIN/AH. Normal background glands (arrow) are present adjacent to the EIN lesion. Cytologically, the background glands are apparently different from those EIN glands.

demarcation can be differences in cytologic and/or nuclear features. Since metaplastic changes in cytology do not eliminate the difference in appearance between the precancer lesion and normal endometrium, the diagnosis of EIN/AH can be facilitated by comparison of glands of interest with background normal glands, when present. The presence of classically defined nuclear atypia does not necessarily need to be met for cytologic demarcation to be identified. Often, cytologic demarcation can be identified at low magnification along with glandular crowding and/or complexity, but in small samples, or samples with extensive glandular crowding, closer inspection for single or a few isolated background glands can be helpful (Figure 8.12). However, based on our experience, selection of the background non-hyperplastic endometrial glands can be biased by those benign glands from endometrial basalis, which commonly show apparent different nuclear features compared to the

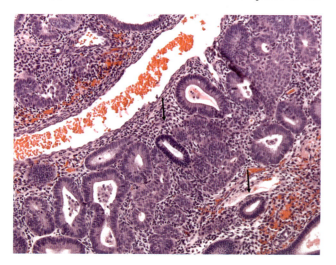

Figure 8.12 EIN/AH. There is an isolated background gland (arrow) in an EIN lesion. Focal squamous metaplasia is present in the upper right corner.

endometrial glands of functionalis. Keeping this concept in mind can avoid such bias in the majority of situations.

The minimum size of the crowded, cytologically altered focus is defined as 1 mm. Of note, separate foci of glandular crowding, spread across different tissue fragments, are not additive to generate a lump-sum size of the lesion. Lesions that demonstrate true cytologic demarcation and crowding, but are less than 1 mm in size, should be given a descriptive diagnosis with a comment to explain the features of the lesion and what are the reasons for the lesion not reaching to the point of EIN/AH. Appropriate recommendations may be made if appropriate. Alternatively, a discussion with the clinician about the special situation is usually fruitful.

Differential diagnosis

Before the diagnosis of EIN/AH is made, we have to exclude many benign lesions and endometrial cancers, which morphologically may resemble this endometrioid precancerous lesion. Some of those more common benign mimics include telescoping artifact, shearing of stroma leading to artifactual gland crowding, polyps, reactive epithelial changes (which may appear as cytologic demarcation), atypical polypoid adenomyoma, endometrial basalis and non-atypical hyperplasia. The cancerous lesions fall into the differential diagnosis including endometrioid carcinoma and glandular-type endometrial serous carcinoma.

ENDOMETRIAL POLYPS

Unless removed piecemeal, polyps have a polypoid architecture on macroscopic examination. On microscopic examination, they are covered by surface epithelium except at the base and may be ulcerated or infarcted at their tip. They are characterised by a paucicellular fibrous or fibromyxoid stroma. They may contain thick-walled blood vessels, although this feature is by no means invariable and is probably dependent on the plane of the section through the polyp or the age of the polyp. The diagnosis of an endometrial polyp is not difficult as soon as these points are kept in mind.

TISSUE FRAGMENTATION AND SAMPLING ARTIFACT

Fragmentation of endometrial samples is common; however, in most cases the amount of specimen disruption is not sufficient to limit diagnosis. One of the more common sampling artifacts includes the shearing of glandular epithelium from stroma. This epithelium may then become compressed and give the false impression of true gland crowding. Careful evaluation of these foci and looking for the absence of endometrial stroma are necessary. Another common sampling artifact is glandular telescoping. This occurs when gland epithelium prolapses into itself, creating a complex, gland-in-gland structure that may mimic neoplasia (Figure 8.13). Recognition of normal background endometrium surrounding the telescoped focus is helpful.

Precursors of endometrioid carcinoma / EIN/AH 97

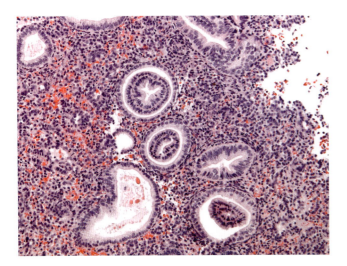

Figure 8.13 Sampling artifact. Gland-in-gland structure, also known as 'telescope' glands, is one of the classic example of sampling artifacts.

OVERSIZED EIN/AH

In these oversized cases, the precancerous process may occupy the entire specimen, so-called oversized or overrun EIN/AH. When this occurs it limits the evaluation of cytologic demarcation, which may give the false impression of a non-atypical hyperplasia, especially at low-power magnification. When this occurs, the first step is careful examination of the proliferation for single or isolated glands surrounded by the EIN/AH (Figure 8.14). These glands are typically more easily identifiable at the periphery of the lesion. If no normal background glands can be identified, then the decision must be made based on the level of architectural complexity and the more classic definition of nuclear atypia. Immunohistochemical staining with PAX2 may be helpful in this setting (see section 'Immunohistochemistry in diagnosis of EIN/AH').

ENDOMETRIAL METAPLASIA

Also called metaplastic changes or benign endometrial changes, this represents benign endometrial lesions with altered epithelial differentiation. Endometrial epithelium may undergo numerous shifts in phenotype, or metaplasias. More common types include squamous or morular, mucinous, and tubular metaplasia. Relatively rare variants include eosinophilic, secretory and hobnail metaplasia. Papillary syncytial metaplasia is a unique type that displays both eosinophilic and hobnail metaplasia, along with a papillary growth pattern, and is usually reactive. These metaplastic changes may be seen in both the benign and malignant endometrium and therefore the term 'altered differentiation' has been proposed. Interestingly, altered differentiation has numerous causes, ranging from beta-catenin mutations in morular metaplasia, inflammatory causes in eosinophilic and hobnail metaplasia, to hormonal effects in secretory changes. This problem is compounded by coexistence of epithelial metaplasias and non-atypical endometrial hyperplasia. However, metaplastic epithelium lacks epithelial disorganization, nuclear pleomorphism, excessive mitotic activity or atypical mitoses. Detailed description and representative pictures of the endometrial metaplasia are described in Chapter 7.

ATYPICAL POLYPOID ADENOMYOMA

Atypical polypoid adenomyoma is characterised by the presence of abundant fibroblastic stroma with a prominent smooth-muscle component. The glandular component shows architectural complexity and focal crowding. There may be focal cytological atypia, but the presence of fragments where architecturally complex glands without atypia are widely spaced in myofibromatous stroma helps distinguish this lesion from EIN/AH (Figure 8.15).

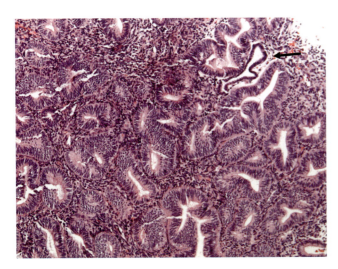

Figure 8.14 Oversized EIN/AH. Sometimes, lesion of EIN becomes larger than we typically see under the microscope. In these conditions, single or isolated glands (arrow, upper right corner) present at the periphery provide a helpful diagnostic clue.

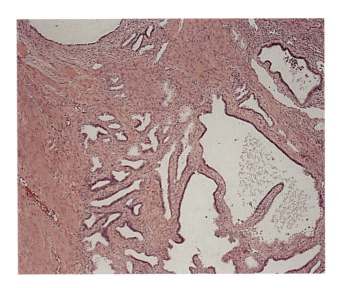

Figure 8.15 Atypical polypoid adenomyoma. The polypoid lesion shows hyperplastic glands embedded in the haphazardly arranged smooth-muscle bundles.

SECRETORY-TYPE EIN/AH

Secretory differentiation may be seen in both EIN/AH as well as low-grade endometrioid carcinomas. This state of altered differentiation is similar to that seen in normal secretory-phase endometrium, which is likely to be caused by either exogenous or endogenous progestins. The condition in the past was called as 'atypical hyperplasia superimposed by secretory changes'. Secretory endometrium may display some overlapping features with precancerous and cancerous endometrium, namely glandular crowding and perceived glandular epithelial complexity (due to the torturous nature of the endometrial glands). At low-power magnification, the secretory endometrium will display a more orderly and linear arrangement of glands than carcinoma with secretory differentiation (Figure 8.16). Fortunately, the diagnosis of secretory EIN/AH is rare, as it can be exceptionally challenging. In general, patients with secretory EIN/AH are premenopausal, with an average age in the 40s and increased levels of progestin exposure. Glands in secretory EIN/AH tend to be larger, more complex and more haphazardly arranged than the surrounding normal secretory glands (Figure 8.17). The cells will have abundant, vacuolated cytoplasm, a ruffled apical surface, and round vesicular nuclei (Figure 8.18).[34,35] Unfortunately, these cytologic features are bland and not readily recognised as atypical; therefore low-power recognition of architectural demarcation of the precancerous lesion is crucial. While the vast majority of EIN/AH arises in a background of proliferative pattern endometrium, there are rare cases that arise in a secretory background. These lesions lack the luminal complexity of secretory EIN/AH and more closely resemble proliferative glands, which allow them to be easily identified at scanning magnification.

ENDOMETRIOID CARCINOMA

The more important and common differential diagnosis in this setting is between EIN/AH and well-differentiated endometrioid carcinoma. By definition, atypical endometrial hyperplasia is a noninvasive lesion while well-differentiated endometrial adenocarcinoma is invasive into endometrial stroma and possibly also into the myometrium. In practice, the assessment of endometrial stromal invasion can be very difficult, particularly in the endometrial biopsy or curettage samples. Presence of smooth muscle in the samples with EIN/AH-like lesions is not necessarily evidence of myometrial invasion. Such findings leading to the conclusion of endometrioid carcinoma can be erroneous since the endomyometrial junction is commonly not smooth and muscle is often present.

In our experience, focal atypia and the presence of non-atypical glands admixed with atypical glands are features that support a diagnosis of EIN/AH, while

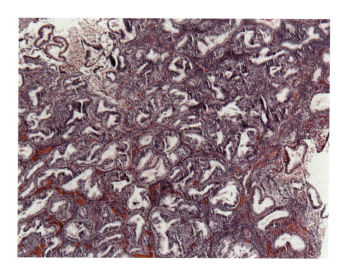

Figure 8.17 Secretory EIN/AH. The glands are larger, more complex and more haphazardly arranged than the surrounding normal secretory glands (right side of the figure).

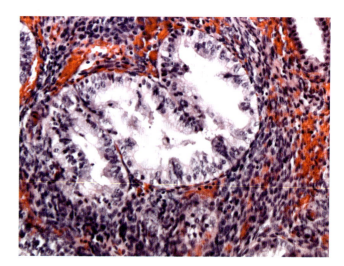

Figure 8.18 Secretory EIN/AH. In a high power, secretory EIN glands may have abundant, vacuolated cytoplasm, a ruffled apical surface and round vesicular nuclei.

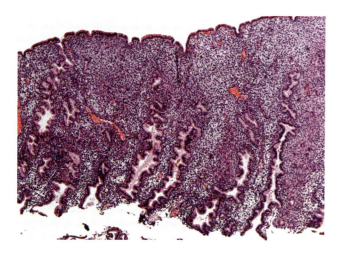

Figure 8.16 Secretory endometrium. Normal secretory endometrium is orderly arranged, which is in contrast to Figure 8.17.

conversely generalised atypia is more in keeping with endometrioid carcinoma. Features that support a diagnosis of endometrioid carcinoma rather than EIN/AH are as follows.

- Fibrotic stroma infiltrated by irregular glands
- Confluent glands with a cribriform architecture
- Excessive papillary growth pattern
- Neutrophilic inflammation is another useful pointer towards endometrioid carcinoma

It must be noted, however, that even in the absence of these features in biopsy or curettage specimens with a diagnosis of EIN/AH, up to 40% of resected uteri contained a carcinoma as discussed above. Caution is therefore advised in making a diagnosis of EIN/AH in an endometrial biopsy where cytological atypia is widespread. At the very least, surgical pathology reports should emphasise that EIN/AH cannot reliably be distinguished from well differentiated endometrioid carcinoma of the endometrium (see Chapter 9 for more details).

ENDOMETRIAL SEROUS CARCINOMA

Endometrial serous carcinoma (ESC), when present in a glandular form (nonpapillary growth pattern), can be misdiagnosed as EIN/AH due to its apparent nuclear atypia. Although it is relatively rare, it is critically important to keep this in mind since any such incident will have devastating impact for patient care. ESCs typically occur in postmenopausal women. It is difficult to be certain when ESC presents with a small amount of cancerous tissue, particularly when mainly in glandular form. The main diagnostic clue for the glandular type ESC is the striking discrepancy between architecture abnormality and nuclear grade. That being said, highly atypical cancerous cells are present in well-formed glands. As soon as this entity is kept in mind, the diagnosis can be confirmed by immunohistochemical stains with p53, p16 and ER in the majority of cases (see Chapter 9 for more details).

SUBDIAGNOSTIC LESIONS

On occasion, biopsy material may contain a focus of glands with crowding, altered cytology or both, that fails to meet the other criteria for EIN/AH. Commonly, this consists of a minute focus of crowded glands that appear different from the background endometrium, yet are not 1 mm in size, or are located at the edge of a tissue fragment (Figure 8.19). When this occurs, deeper levels should be examined. However, if the lesion continues to be subdiagnostic, then a descriptive diagnosis is appropriate. It is recommended to diagnose such lesions as 'focal gland crowding (with or without) atypia', with a comment describing the features of the lesion and recommending follow up in 2–3 (with atypia) or 6 (without atypia) months.[36] It may represent a sampling bias, but the nature of such a lesion with focal glandular crowding remains to be clarified. Clear communication with the treating

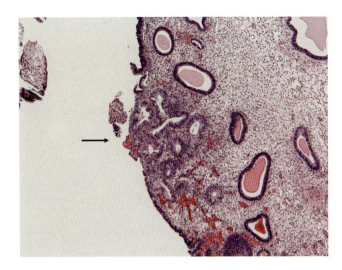

Figure 8.19 Subdiagnostic EIN/AH lesion. Typically, lesions are smaller than 1 mm in size (arrow). Otherwise, the lesion fulfils all the criteria for the EIN/AH.

physician and a recommendation of additional sampling is necessary to prevent the patient from being lost to follow-up. Sometimes, when the lesion is focal and/or the biopsy is small, which only partially fulfils criteria of an endometrioid carcinoma, then a diagnosis of 'at least EIN/AH' or 'EIN/AH bordering on endometrioid carcinoma' with a comment describing the features and their limitations is appropriate.

PROGESTIN-TREATED EIN/AH

Progestin treatment remains common for patients with a diagnosis of EIN/AH. Progestins may be given continuously, in the form of intrauterine devices or depo-provera or as interrupted therapy, that allows for progestin withdrawal endometrial shedding. Regardless of the modality, routine surveillance biopsies of the endometrium (preferably after cessation of progestins and a withdrawal bleed) necessitates familiarity with the features of progestin-treated EIN/AH. Correct interpretation of these specimens is critical to determine if the treatment is effective. The most notable effect of exogenous progestins is decidualization of the stroma, typically with a concurrent attenuated glandular component (Figure 8.20). The stromal cells appear eosinophilic and plump, while endometrial glands will decrease in size and density (Figure 8.20d). This decrease in glandular density may drive precancerous lesions below the normal threshold needed to trigger a diagnosis of EIN/AH. The background glandular epithelium may range from atrophic to hypersecretory (Arias-Stella effect). Frequently, the precancerous glands undergo metaplastic changes, most commonly consisting of eosinophilic and mucinous metaplasia. Mitotic figures may be rare to absent. Morules are typically more common after progestin administration, and may be present in otherwise unremarkable glands, serving as a histologic clue to the presence of progestin-treated EIN/AH (Figure 8.21). When evaluating biopsies from patients with known EIN/AH being treated with progestins, it is

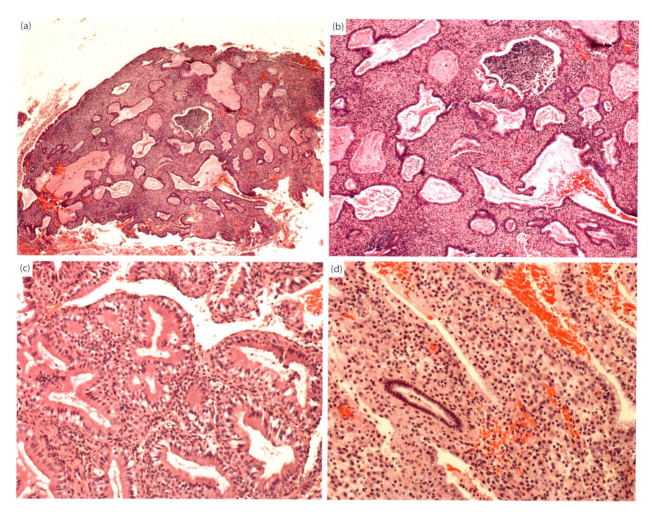

Figure 8.20 Progestin treatment effect. Endometrial hyperplasia shows various morphology after progestin treatment. **(a)** Cystically dilated glands are partially attenuated in a low-power view; **(b)** Pre-decidualized stroma is better appreciated in an intermediate power; **(c)** Focal secretory changes may be seen after progestin treatment; **(d)** Completely attenuated glands and fully decidualized stroma become apparent after a prolonged progestin therapy.

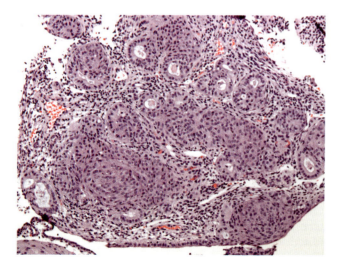

Figure 8.21 Progestin treatment effect. The patient had a history of endometrial hyperplasia and received progestin treatment afterwards. One of the common histologic changes in this scenario is squamous metaplasia.

important to compare current and previous samples. Many patients may show a spectrum of response to progestin therapy, and it is critical to relay the presence of potentially non-responsive lesions to the treating physician.[37] In cases where no lesional glands are identified, a statement stating that no EIN/AH is present in the sample is appropriate; however, if atypical glands or frank EIN/AH is present, a diagnosis of 'residual EIN/AH (with or without) progestin effect' is warranted. We have divided post progestin–treated endometrial samples into three categories in our pathology report: complete response (decidualized stroma with attenuated endometrial epithelia), non-response (residual EIN/AH) and partial response (status in between the complete and non-response). We also give an estimate of how much of the responding component is present in the endometrial evaluation sample.[38] In general, continuous progestin therapy if clinically indicated will apply if there is any portion of partial or non-responsive component identified. This practice has received positive feedback from our clinical colleagues.

Immunohistochemistry in diagnosis of EIN/AH

Searching for potential biomarkers to separate neoplastic from non-neoplastic lesions has been an active research field. Although, still in its infancy, several biomarkers have shown promising results and can be potentially useful in certain clinical settings. The two most promising biomarkers are PTEN and PAX2, which are already recommended by the European Society for Medical Oncology (ESMO) to help separate neoplastic lesions from non-neoplastic benign mimics.[39] *PTEN* is a tumor suppressor gene that is expressed in normal endometrium in both a nuclear and cytoplasmic pattern. Normal endometrium may display patchy staining, with inactivation seen in up to 49% of glands. There is an increasing trend of inactivation seen in EIN/AH (44%–63%) and adenocarcinoma (68%–83%).[5,25] The diagnostic utility of *PTEN* is hampered by its inactivation sometimes observed in normal endometrium. On the other hand, PAX2 plays a critical role in the embryogenesis of multiple organs and central nervous system. Recently PAX2 has emerged as a potential biomarker helping to separate neoplastic lesions from non-neoplastic benign endometrial lesions. Similar to PTEN, PAX2 does show loss in normal endometrium (36%), EIN/AH (71%) and carcinoma (77%).[22] As a diagnostic antibody, PAX2 is much more robust and easy to interpret due to its nuclear staining pattern. Although far from being a 'perfect' marker of EIN/AH, studies have shown that PAX2 can be used to facilitate the diagnosis of EIN/AH in certain clinical settings.[11,22,34,40] An example of PAX2 stain highlighting suspicious foci of EIN/AH is presented in Figure 8.22.

PRECURSORS OF ENDOMETRIAL SEROUS CARCINOMA

Historically, serous endometrial intraepithelial carcinoma (SEIC) is taken as the precancer of ESC.[41-44] However, it is also well recognised that SEIC is commonly associated with extrauterine disease,[45-47] and is not a precancer by all means. Thus, SEIC is better considered as a noninvasive or a morphologically unique form of ESC.[48] Therefore, SEIC is discussed in detail in Chapter 9.

Careful examination of the definition of a precancer established in the National Cancer Institute Consensus in 2006[49] resulted in the conclusion that endometrial glandular dysplasia (EmGD) fulfils most of the defined criteria as a precancer lesion of ESC. The initial diagnostic criteria of EmGD were proposed by Zheng et al. in 2004.[50] Since then, studies have established EmGD as the most likely precancerous lesion for ESC.[51-56] Lesions of EmGD display cytological and immunophenotypic features that bridge the gap between benign resting endometrium and SEIC. The dysplastic epithelium of EmGD has cytologic features that are more atypical than background benign endometrium but fall short of SEIC. The entity of EmGD, as a precancer, becomes a key step of the development of ESC.[47]

ENDOMETRIAL GLANDULAR DYSPLASIA

Studies, in the past decade mainly from Zheng's group, have established that endometrial glandular dysplasia (EmGD) is most likely the precancerous lesion for

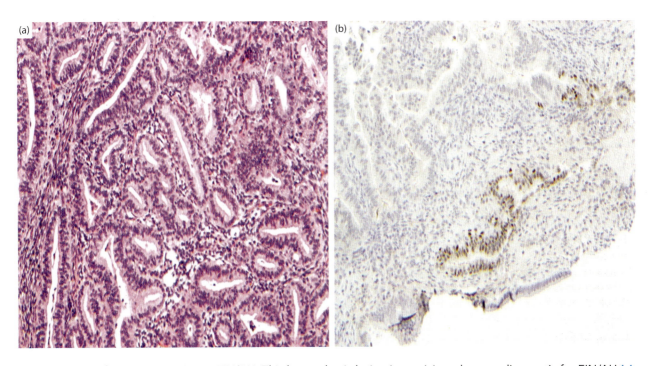

Figure 8.22 Loss of PAX2 expression in EIN/AH. This hyperplastic lesion is suspicious, but not diagnostic for EIN/AH **(a)**; loss of PAX2 stain **(b)** in the lesion supports the diagnosis as an EIN/AH.

ESC.[50–56] In the seminal report that described the entity,[50] the endometrium adjacent to a cohort of SEIC, ESC and endometrioid carcinoma cases was evaluated in detail. Among all the lesions of EmGD identified, 53% were seen in the uteri with ESC, while only 1.7% were associated with the uteri with endometrioid carcinoma.[50] The average age of the patients with an EmGD lesion was 65 years (range 57–79).[50]

Definition

EmGD is defined by those endometrial glands which show the degree of nuclear atypia falling short of SEIC, but distinct compared with the resting endometrium in the background.

Etiology and genetic profile

The etiology of EmGD is unclear, but development of EmGD is clearly linked to the *TP53* mutation. From one of our previous studies, *TP53* mutation is present in 43% of EmGD, compared with 0% in resting endometrium, 72% in SEIC, and 96% in ESC.[53] In addition, loss of heterozygosity at the chromosomal region for TP53 and 1p is noted in 31% and 18% of EmGD, respectively, compared to 78% and 47% of cancerous areas within the same uteri.[51] *TP53* gene-homologue Trp53 knockout-mice model clearly demonstrated lesions with characteristic features of EmGD, SEIC and ESC.[57]

In addition to *TP53*, other molecular changes such as IMP3, p16 and Nrf2 have been demonstrated in the lesions of EmGD.[47,55,58,59]

Prognosis and predictive factors

Compared to the lesions of EIN/AH, EmGD occurs much less frequently. The low incidence limits extensive studies. In addition, at the time EmGD is diagnosed, hysterectomies are commonly performed due to postmenopausal status and a potential risk of ESC development. Therefore, there is so far no prospective study to address its predictive and prognostic values in the clinical setting. However, in the past, we did a retrospective study to address this issue. A total of 250 ESC and 258 benign uteri were used as the initial study source. All available endometrial biopsies from a period of three months or more before hysterectomy were blindly reviewed to identify if EmGD was present prior to the development of ESC. These included an available pool of 27 biopsy specimens from the ESC group and 29 samples from the benign control group. A total of 10 EmGD cases, 9 (33%) of 27 from the ESC group and 1 (3.5%) of 29 from the benign control group, were found. The period from identifying EmGD to the presence of either a SEIC or a full-blown ESC ranged from 16 to 98 months with an average of 33 months. Patients with a diagnosis of EmGD carry a nine-fold increased risk of progression to SEIC/ESC.[52]

Compared to SEIC, which is associated with a significant number of extrauterine disease, based on our own practice, lesions of EmGD have not shown such an association so far (Zheng et al., unpublished). This provides a promise that intervention at the time of EmGD diagnosis may be an effective way to prevent the development of ESC, although confirmatory studies are needed.

Histopathology

Grossly, no visible lesions could be identified in the corresponding areas of EmGD. Microscopically, EmGD lesions are usually multifocal, with each focus usually smaller than 2 mm in size.[50,54] Occasionally, extensive involvement of an endometrial polyp can be encountered. EmGD is characterised by glands and/or surface endometrial epithelium with atypical cytologic features that clearly separate it from the benign resting endometrium, but not as severe as those of frankly malignant SEIC glands (Figures 8.23 through 8.28). These morphologic features are summarized as follows.

- Nuclei of EmGD cells are typically oval or round, enlarged, hyperchromatic or with open chromatin pattern.
- Nuclei are usually 2- to 3-fold larger as compared with those of benign resting endometrium, while the nuclei of SEIC are usually 4- to 5-fold larger.
- Degree of nuclear hyperchromasia is less than that of frankly malignant cells seen in SEIC.
- Nucleoli are usually conspicuous instead of prominent as seen in SEIC.
- Partial or complete loss of cell polarity can be seen.
- Mitotic figures and apoptotic bodies are not readily appreciable.
- Transitional area from benign resting endometrium to EmGD and from EmGD to SEIC are commonly observed if examined carefully.
- Dysplastic cells typically involve the endometrial glands within the endometrium or an endometrial polyp; less often, they involve the surface lining of endometrium or a polyp (Figure 8.26).
- Small papillary structures can be observed in EmGD glands, with thin fibrovascular cores of the EmGD papillae lined by dysplastic cells (Figure 8.27). The stroma around the EmGD glands may be fibrotic, but desmoplastic reactions are not seen.
- Unlike EIN/AH, there is no size limitation for the diagnosis of EmGD. The lesion size can range from a single gland to a hyperplastic diffuse lesion.

Of note, although background endometrium is often atrophic or weakly proliferative endometrium, it may also be proliferative, or sometimes hyperplastic, depending on the hormonal status of individual patients. Since nowadays, a considerable number of postmenopausal women are using hormonal therapy, about 40% of women with

Precursors of endometrial serous carcinoma / Endometrial glandular dysplasia 103

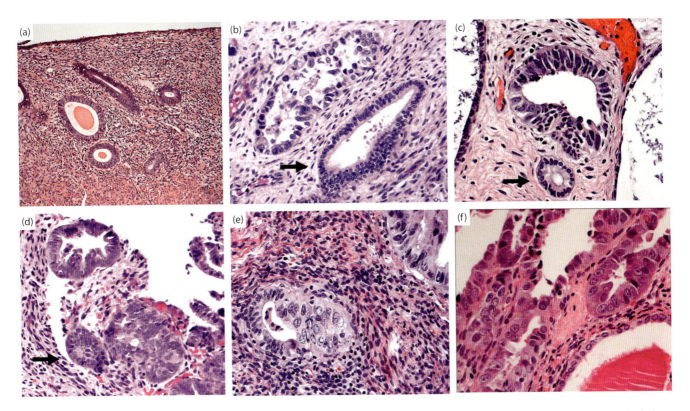

Figure 8.23 Comparison among lesions of endometrial glandular dysplasia (EmGD), serous endometrial intraepithelial carcinoma (SEIC) and the background endometrium. (a) Background resting endometrium; (b) through (d) EmGD lesions are admixed with residual normal glands (arrows); (e) A residual normal resting endometrial gland (left) abuts an EmGD (right); (f) SEIC. Severe nuclear atypia or frankly malignant cells are present in SEIC. Compared to the lesions of EmGD (b) through (e), the degree of nuclear atypia of SEIC is apparently much higher.

SEIC or ESC have a non-atrophic endometrium as a background.[50] It is not always necessary that the background of endometrium for patients with EmGD to be atrophic. This situation also applies to the diagnosis of ESC (see Chapter 9).

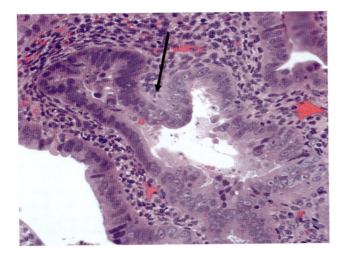

Figure 8.24 Transition from endometrial glandular dysplasia (EmGD) to serous endometrial intraepithelial carcinoma (SEIC). EmGD (upper left) transits into SEIC (lower right). Arrow indicates the lesions in between.

Immunohistochemistry in diagnosis of EmGD

As an 'intermediate' bridge between benign resting endometrium and SEIC, the diagnosis of EmGD can sometimes be problematic, especially for those pathologists who are not familiar with the lesion. Immunohistochemical studies can help to facilitate the diagnosis in these scenarios. Based on our own experience accumulated in the past decade, we have summarized the markers, which can be used in differential diagnosis.

- *p53*: The staining patterns of p53 in EmGD lesions range from patchy to diffuse. In the patchy stain pattern, it usually highlights more than half of the cells in a defined EmGD gland with strong, intense nuclear staining, which is different from reactive changes (focal weak nuclear stain). The molecular mechanism of such a staining pattern is unclear. In the diffuse stain pattern, it is usually similar to those stains in SEIC, representing the *TP53* mutation. With our own practice, we did not see a significant difference when we use different anti-p53 antibodies (1801 versus DO7). Lesions of EmGD show intermediate immunohistochemical scores of 5–6 or above (Figures 8.26 and 8.28).[50]

104 Endometrial premalignant lesions

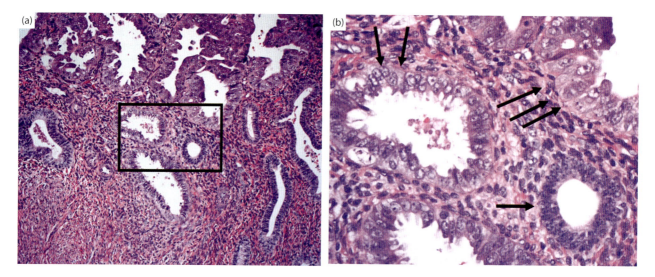

Figure 8.25 Admixture of endometrial glandular dysplasia (EmGD), serous endometrial intraepithelial carcinoma (SEIC) and resting endometrium. (a) SEIC (upper), EmGD (middle), resting endometrial glands at the center and periphery; (b) Enlarged the centered area of A shows resting background endometrial gland (lower right), EmGD (mid left) and SEIC (upper right). Please note the degree of nuclear atypia is apparently different from each other.

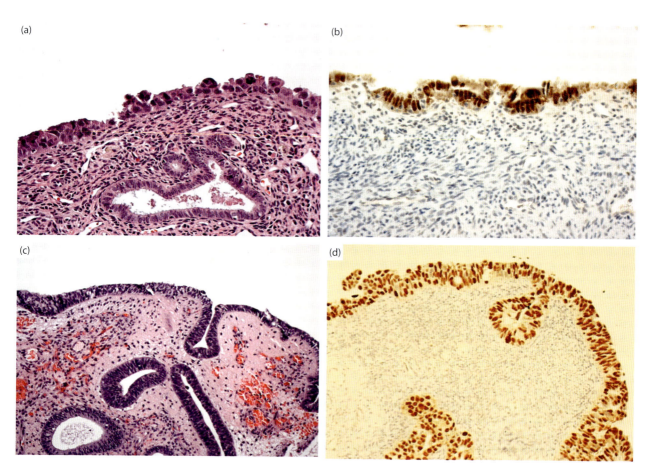

Figure 8.26 Endometrial glandular dysplasia (EmGD) with p53 stain. EmGD involves the endometrial surface epithelia (a and c) and glands (c). All show diffuse p53 nuclear stains with immunohistochemical staining score >5 (b, d).

Precursors of endometrial serous carcinoma / Endometrial glandular dysplasia

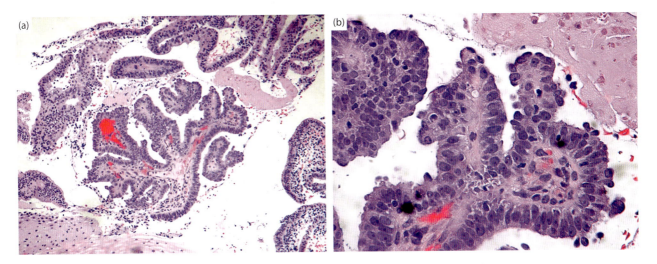

Figure 8.27 Endometrial glandular dysplasia (EmGD) with papillary architecture. (a) Low-power magnitude; (b) High-power magnitude. Note the moderate nuclear atypia.

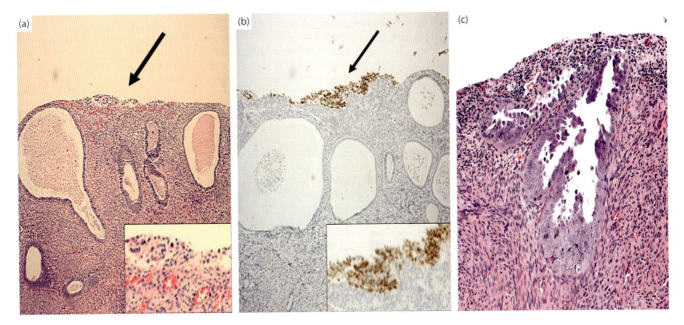

Figure 8.28 Clinical progression of endometrial glandular dysplasia (EmGD). (a) EmGD involves endometrial polyp. The arrow points the surface area, which is magnified in the lower right corner showing nuclear atypia; (b) The same area of A is stained with p53; (c) A lesion of serous endometrial intraepithelial carcinoma is found in her uterus 18 months later.

- *MIB-1 (Ki-67)*: EmGD usually demonstrates a higher proliferative index than the background resting endometrium.[50] Thus, comparison with background endometrium is important in assessing these foci. However, when the background endometrium is not resting, MIB-1 staining becomes less useful.
- *IMP3*: May highlight EmGD foci relative to the background endometrium. However, IMP3 is relatively insensitive for this purpose.[58]
- *ER/PR*: Usually reduced in EmGD, which is more prominent when compared with the background endometrium.

- *P16*: EmGD lesions are typically diffusely strong positive for p16, whereas the benign endometrial glands generally show patchy positivity. However, p16 should be used with caution and in conjunction with other markers, since tubal metaplasia is usually p16 diffusely positive.

Of note, if the diagnosis of EmGD is considered but the morphological features of lesion are ambiguous, we recommend using a panel of 6 antibodies (p53, p16, IMP3, ER, PR and MIB-1) to facilitate the diagnosis.

Differential diagnosis

EmGD can be focal or extensive. Similar to EIN/AH, prior to making the diagnosis of EmGD, benign mimics and malignant counterparts have to be excluded. The common differential diagnosis includes reactive atypia in reparative changes of the benign endometrium, endometrial metaplasia, endometrial polyp with atypical looking glands and SEIC. Correct application of the above-mentioned diagnostic criteria will be successful in the majority of cases.

REACTIVE REPARATIVE CHANGES OF THE BENIGN ENDOMETRIUM

Reactive changes are commonly seen in patients with a prior history of endometrial procedures (biopsy or curettage). Therefore, careful review of clinical notes will be helpful. The reactive changes include enlargement of nuclei, somewhat nuclear atypia and prominent nucleoli. However, nuclear-cytoplasmic ratio and nuclear polarity are usually preserved. Fine chromatin and smooth nuclear contour are common. Nuclei usually lack hyperchromasia and coarse chromatin. More importantly, unlike EmGD which is usually focal and distinct from background endometrium, the reparative changes are usually diffuse and cytologically similar to background endometrial glands. In difficult situations, immunohistochemical stains with p53, IMP-3, p16, PR and ki-67 can be very helpful.

ENDOMETRIAL METAPLASIA

Endometrial metaplasia represents benign endometrial lesions with altered epithelial differentiation. Metaplasia, such as tubular metaplasia; eosinophilic, secretory and hobnail metaplasia; papillary syncytial metaplasia and clear-cell metaplasia, may be difficult to be separated from EmGD. However, metaplastic epithelium lacks epithelial disorganization and nuclear pleomorphism. Based on our own experience, metaplasia usually lacks the level of nuclear atypia typically seen in EmGD. The background endometrium adjacent to the metaplasia usually displays bleeding or breakdown changes. Immunohistochemical stains can facilitate the diagnosis.

SEROUS ENDOMETRIAL INTRAEPITHELIAL CARCINOMA

The most important difference between SEIC and EmGD is the level of nuclear atypia. SEIC has a high-grade nuclear atypia which is similar to that of ESC. SEIC usually displays brisk mitotic activity.[41,44] On the other hand, EmGD has a moderate degree of nuclear atypia, and mitotic activity is usually conspicuous. The cytological features of EmGD and SEIC, as well as resting endometrium, are summarized in Table 8.3.

ENDOMETRIAL POLYP

Of note, EmGD can occur within an endometrial polyp either inside or at the surface. Therefore, careful evaluation of individual glands at high power is the key, especially in postmenopausal patients.

Table 8.3 The histopathological features of resting endometrium, EmGD and SEIC SEIC

	Resting endometrium[a]	EmGD	SEIC
Size	Normal	2–3 fold enlarged	4–5 fold enlarged
Polarity of cells	Intact	Partial loss	Loss
Cytoplasm	Normal	Increased	Abundant
Nuclear features			
Size	Normal	1.5–2 fold enlarged	2–4 fold enlarged
Stratification	No	Present	Present
Hyperchromasia	Mild	Mild to moderate	Moderate to severe
Chromatin	Even distributed	Fine or granular	Coarse
Shape	Low columnar	Elongated/pencil shape	Irregular
Nucleoli	Conspicuous	Inconspicuous	Prominent, like ESC
Mitotic figures	No	Occasional	Often
Apoptotic bodies	No	Often	Brisk
Growth pattern			
Surface	Nonspecific	Often	Often
Single gland	Nonspecific	Often	Often
Glandular clusters	No	Maybe present	Maybe present
Cribriforming	No	No	Maybe present
Polyp involvement	Occasional	Often	Often
Background endometrium	Resting endometrium[a]	Resting endometrium[a]	Resting endometrium[a]

Abbreviations: EmGD, endometrial glandular dysplasia; SEIC, serous endometrial intraepithelial carcinoma.
[a] Resting endometrium including: atrophic endometrium, weakly proliferative endometrium and proliferative endometrium.

PUTATIVE PRECURSOR FOR ENDOMETRIAL CLEAR-CELL CARCINOMA

Unlike EIN/AH and EmGD, which are well accepted as the precancerous lesions for endometrioid carcinoma and ESC, the precancerous lesion of endometrial clear-cell carcinoma (ECCC) is yet to be established. So far, only a few studies tried to address this issue. In 2014, Moid and Berezowski first described a distinctive lesion in a hysterectomy specimen from a 70-year-old woman which they designated endometrial intraepithelial carcinoma, clear-cell type.[60] The lesion comprised surface epithelium and glands that were lined by cells with 'clear cytoplasm, marked nuclear pleomorphism, coarse chromatin, irregular nuclear membranes, and prominent eosinophilic nucleoli' and an occasional hobnail appearance. No mitotic figures were recognised. There was no evidence of stromal or myometrial invasion. The lesions showed 'focal' staining for p53, a 'moderate to high proliferative index' and no evidence of extrauterine extension. Zheng's group further studied the characteristic clinicopathologic features of these putative precursor lesions.[61] We identified a spectrum of atypical endometrial glandular and surface changes that were distinct from both the background benign endometrium and the adjacent endometrial clear-cell carcinoma. Thus, we hypothesize that those lesions may represent the precancerous lesion of ECCC.

MORPHOLOGIC FEATURES OF CLEAR-CELL EMGD

The features of clear-cell EmGD are a spectrum of morphological changes involving a single gland, a few glandular

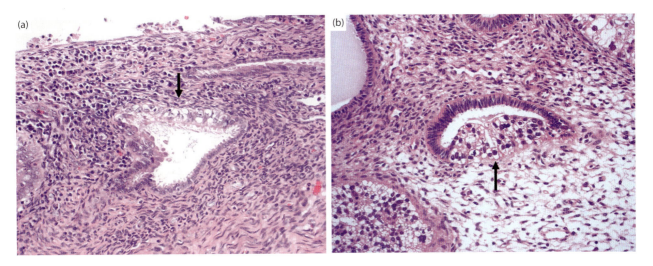

Figure 8.29 (a, b) Clear-cell endometrial glandular dysplasia (EmGD). Lesion involves only half of the gland (arrow) with atypical nuclei and clear cytoplasm.

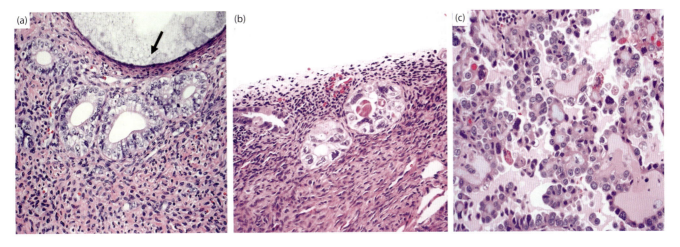

Figure 8.30 Comparison among clear cell neoplastic lesions. (a) Clear-cell endometrial glandular dysplasia: Note the clear cytoplasm and background atrophic endometrial gland (arrow); (b) Clear-cell endometrial intraepithelial carcinoma contains marked atypical nuclei, which are similar to those of clear-cell carcinoma (c).

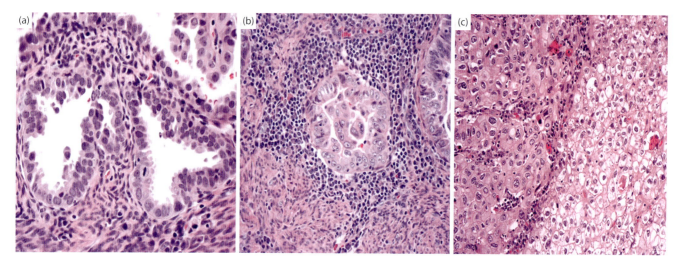

Figure 8.31 Clear-cell neoplastic lesions with eosinophilic cytoplasm. (a) Clear-cell endometrial glandular dysplasia; (b) Clear-cell endometrial intraepithelial carcinoma; and (c) Clear-cell carcinoma. All these lesions contain eosinophilic cytoplasm instead of classic clear cytoplasm.

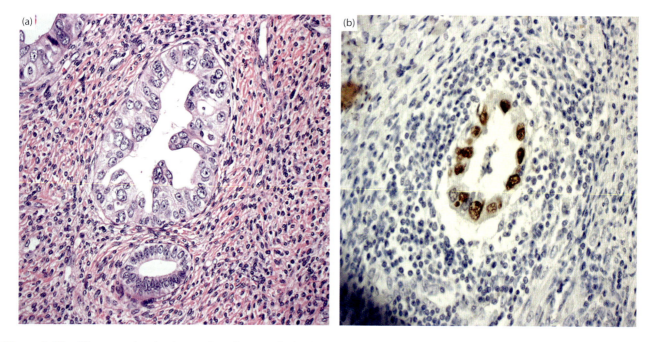

Figure 8.32 p53 expression in clear-cell endometrial glandular dysplasia. (a) The dysplastic lesion contains partial clear and partial eosinophilic cytoplasm. The nuclear atypia is apparent compared with the resting endometrial gland underneath. (b) The lesion is strongly positive for p53 immunostain with a score of 7.

clusters or surface epithelium lined by cells with cytoplasmic clearing or eosinophilia, or hobnail nuclei, and varying degrees of nuclear atypia. These changes were graded on a scale of 1 to 3,[61] primarily depending on the level of cytologic atypia of the constituent cells. A lesion is grade 1 if there is nuclear enlargement (2- to 3-fold compared with resting endometrium). Grade 3 nuclei show marked pleomorphism and prominent nucleoli comparable to frank ECCC. Grade 2 changes display intermediate features. Mitotic figures were rare in grade 1 and 2 lesions but were easily seen in grade 3 lesions. Morphologically and conceptually, grade 3 lesions were classifiable as clear-cell EIC, whereas grade 1 and 2 lesions were designated clear-cell endometrial glandular dysplasia (clear-cell EmGD). Representative images of clear-cell EmGD are illustrated in Figures 8.29 through 8.32.

FUTURE DIRECTION OF CLEAR-CELL EMGD

Of note, only a limited number of clear-cell EmGD cases have been studied. Unlike EmGD, the clinical behavior of clear-cell EmGD, such as the risk of extrauterine extension, is still unclear. In addition, the precise molecular alternation of clear-cell EmGD is yet to be elucidated. More studies are needed in the future.

REFERENCES

1. Allison KH, Reed SD, Voigt LF et al. Diagnosing endometrial hyperplasia: Why is it so difficult to agree? *Am J Surg Pathol* 2008;32:691–8.
2. Zaino RJ, Kauderer J, Trimble CL et al. Reproducibility of the diagnosis of atypical endometrial hyperplasia: A Gynecologic Oncology Group study. *Cancer* 2006; 106:804–11.
3. Hecht JL, Ince TA, Baak JP et al. Prediction of endometrial carcinoma by subjective endometrial intraepithelial neoplasia diagnosis. *Mod Pathol* 2005;18:324–30.
4. Mutter GL, Zaino RJ, Baak JP, Bentley RC, Robboy SJ. Benign endometrial hyperplasia sequence and endometrial intraepithelial neoplasia. *Int J Gynecol Pathol* 2007;26:103–14.
5. Mutter GL, Ince TA, Baak JP et al. Molecular identification of latent precancers in histologically normal endometrium. *Cancer Res* 2001;61:4311–4.
6. Purdie DM, Green AC. Epidemiology of endometrial cancer. *Best Pract Res Clin Obstet Gynaecol* 2001;15: 341–54.
7. Shapiro S, Kelly JP, Rosenberg L et al. Risk of localized and widespread endometrial cancer in relation to recent and discontinued use of conjugated estrogens. *N Engl J Med* 1985;313:969–72.
8. Kurman RJ, Kaminski PF, Norris HJ. The behavior of endometrial hyperplasia. A long-term study of 'untreated' hyperplasia in 170 patients. *Cancer* 1985;56:403–12.
9. World Health Organization. *WHO Classification of Tumors of Female Reproductive Organs.* Lyon: International Agency for Research on Cancer, 2014.
10. Mutter GL. Endometrial intraepithelial neoplasia (EIN): Will it bring order to chaos? The Endometrial Collaborative Group. *Gynecol Oncol* 2000;76:287–90.
11. Quick CM, Laury AR, Monte NM, Mutter GL. Utility of PAX2 as a marker for diagnosis of endometrial intraepithelial neoplasia. *Am J Clin Pathol* 2012;138: 678–84.
12. Parazzini F, La Vecchia C, Bocciolone L, Franceschi S. The epidemiology of endometrial cancer. *Gynecol Oncol* 1991;41:1–16.
13. Meyer LA, Broaddus RR, Lu KH. Endometrial cancer and Lynch syndrome: Clinical and pathologic considerations. *Cancer Control* 2009;16:14–22.
14. Eng C. *PTEN*: One gene, many syndromes. *Hum Mutat* 2003;22:183–98.
15. Cheng WF, Lin HH, Torng PL, Huang SC. Comparison of endometrial changes among symptomatic tamoxifen-treated and nontreated premenopausal and postmenopausal breast cancer patients. *Gynecol Oncol* 1997;66:233–7.
16. Cohen I, Perel E, Flex D et al. Endometrial pathology in postmenopausal tamoxifen treatment: Comparison between gynaecologically symptomatic and asymptomatic breast cancer patients. *J Clin Pathol* 1999;52: 278–82.
17. Esteller M, Garcia A, Martinez-Palones JM, Xercavins J, Reventos J. Detection of clonality and genetic alterations in endometrial pipelle biopsy and its surgical specimen counterpart. *Lab Invest* 1997;76:109–16.
18. Mutter GL, Chaponot ML, Fletcher JA. A polymerase chain reaction assay for non-random X chromosome inactivation identifies monoclonal endometrial cancers and precancers. *Am J Pathol* 1995;146:501–8.
19. Faquin WC, Fitzgerald JT, Boynton KA, Mutter GL. Intratumoral genetic heterogeneity and progression of endometrioid type endometrial adenocarcinomas. *Gynecol Oncol* 2000;78:152–7.
20. Vierkoetter KR, Kagami LA, Ahn HJ, Shimizu DM, Terada KY. Loss of mismatch repair protein expression in unselected endometrial adenocarcinoma precursor lesions. *Int J Gynecol Cancer* 2016;26:228–32.
21. Lucas E, Chen H, Molberg K et al. Mismatch repair protein expression in endometrioid intraepithelial neoplasia/atypical hyperplasia: Should we screen for Lynch syndrome in precancerous lesions? *Int J Gynecol Pathol.* 31 Oct 2018. doi: 10.1097/PGP.0000000000000557 [Epub ahead of print].
22. Monte NM, Webster KA, Neuberg D, Dressler GR, Mutter GL. Joint loss of PAX2 and PTEN expression in endometrial precancers and cancer. *Cancer Res* 2010;70:6225–32.
23. Levine RL, Cargile CB, Blazes MS et al. *PTEN* mutations and microsatellite instability in complex atypical hyperplasia, a precursor lesion to uterine endometrioid carcinoma. *Cancer Res* 1998;58: 3254–8.
24. Maxwell GL, Risinger JI, Gumbs C et al. Mutation of the *PTEN* tumor suppressor gene in endometrial hyperplasias. *Cancer Res* 1998;58:2500–3.
25. Mutter GL, Lin MC, Fitzgerald JT et al. Altered PTEN expression as a diagnostic marker for the earliest endometrial precancers. *J Natl Cancer Inst* 2000;92:924–30.
26. Duggan BD, Felix JC, Muderspach LI, Tsao JL, Shibata DK. Early mutational activation of the c-Ki-ras oncogene in endometrial carcinoma. *Cancer Res* 1994;54:1604–7.
27. Mutter GL, Wada H, Faquin WC, Enomoto T. K-ras mutations appear in the premalignant phase of both microsatellite stable and unstable endometrial carcinogenesis. *Mol Pathol* 1999;52:257–62.
28. Sasaki H, Nishii H, Takahashi H et al. Mutation of the Ki-ras protooncogene in human endometrial hyperplasia and carcinoma. *Cancer Res* 1993;53:1906–10.
29. Moreno-Bueno G, Hardisson D, Sarrio D et al. Abnormalities of E- and P-cadherin and catenin (beta-, gamma-catenin, and p120ctn) expression in

endometrial cancer and endometrial atypical hyperplasia. *J Pathol* 2003;199:471–8.
30. Mutter GL, Kauderer J, Baak JP, Alberts D, Gynecologic Oncology G. Biopsy histomorphometry predicts uterine myoinvasion by endometrial carcinoma: A Gynecologic Oncology Group study. *Hum Pathol* 2008;39:866–74.
31. Trimble CL, Kauderer J, Zaino R et al. Concurrent endometrial carcinoma in women with a biopsy diagnosis of atypical endometrial hyperplasia: A Gynecologic Oncology Group study. *Cancer* 2006;106:812–9.
32. Giede KC, Yen TW, Chibbar R, Pierson RA. Significance of concurrent endometrial cancer in women with a preoperative diagnosis of atypical endometrial hyperplasia. *J Obstet Gynaecol Can* 2008;30: 896–901.
33. Lacey JV, Jr., Mutter GL, Nucci MR et al. Risk of subsequent endometrial carcinoma associated with endometrial intraepithelial neoplasia classification of endometrial biopsies. *Cancer* 2008;113:2073–81.
34. Jeffus SK, Winham W, Hooper K, Quick CM. Secretory endometrial intraepithelial neoplasia. *Int J Gynecol Pathol* 2014;33:515–6.
35. Parra-Herran CE, Monte NM, Mutter GL. Endometrial intraepithelial neoplasia with secretory differentiation: Diagnostic features and underlying mechanisms. *Mod Pathol* 2013;26:868–73.
36. Huang EC, Mutter GL, Crum CP, Nucci MR. Clinical outcome in diagnostically ambiguous foci of 'gland crowding' in the endometrium. *Mod Pathol* 2010;23:1486–91.
37. Mentrikoski MJ, Shah AA, Hanley KZ, Atkins KA. Assessing endometrial hyperplasia and carcinoma treated with progestin therapy. *Am J Clin Pathol* 2012;138:524–34.
38. Guo D, Li L, Zhang H, Zheng W. Pathologic assessment and clinical impacts for endometrial cancer and precursors after progestin treatment. *Chinese J Pathol* 2015;44:216–20.
39. Colombo N, Creutzberg C, Amant F et al. ESMO-ESGO-ESTRO Consensus Conference on Endometrial Cancer: Diagnosis, treatment and follow-up. *Ann Oncol* 2016;27:16–41.
40. Allison KH, Upson K, Reed SD et al. PAX2 loss by immunohistochemistry occurs early and often in endometrial hyperplasia. *Int J Gynecol Pathol* 2012;31: 151–9.
41. Ambros RA, Sherman ME, Zahn CM, Bitterman P, Kurman RJ. Endometrial intraepithelial carcinoma: A distinctive lesion specifically associated with tumors displaying serous differentiation. *Hum Pathol* 1995;26: 1260–7.
42. Sherman ME, Bitterman P, Rosenshein NB, Delgado G, Kurman RJ. Uterine serous carcinoma. A morphologically diverse neoplasm with unifying clinicopathologic features. *Am J Surg Pathol* 1992; 16:600–10.
43. Spiegel GW. Endometrial carcinoma *in situ* in postmenopausal women. *Am J Surg Pathol* 1995;19: 417–32.
44. Zheng W, Khurana R, Farahmand S et al. p53 immunostaining as a significant adjunct diagnostic method for uterine surface carcinoma: Precursor of uterine papillary serous carcinoma. *Am J Surg Pathol* 1998;22:1463–73.
45. Hou JY, McAndrew TC, Goldberg GL, Whitney K, Shahabi S. A clinical and pathologic comparison between stage-matched endometrial intraepithelial carcinoma and uterine serous carcinoma: Is there a difference?. *Reprod Sci* 2014;21:532–7.
46. Soslow RA, Pirog E, Isacson C. Endometrial intraepithelial carcinoma with associated peritoneal carcinomatosis. *Am J Surg Pathol* 2000;24:726–32.
47. Zheng W, Xiang L, Fadare O, Kong B. A proposed model for endometrial serous carcinogenesis. *Am J Surg Pathol* 2011;35:e1–e14.
48. Zheng W, Schwartz PE. Serous EIC as an early form of uterine papillary serous carcinoma: Recent progress in understanding its pathogenesis and current opinions regarding pathologic and clinical management. *Gynecol Oncol* 2005;96:579–82.
49. Berman JJ, Albores-Saavedra J, Bostwick D et al. Precancer: A conceptual working definition – results of a Consensus Conference. *Cancer Detect Prev* 2006;30:387–94.
50. Zheng W, Liang SX, Yu H et al. Endometrial glandular dysplasia: A newly defined precursor lesion of uterine papillary serous carcinoma. Part I: Morphologic features. *Int J Surg Pathol* 2004;12:207–23.
51. Liang SX, Chambers SK, Cheng L et al. Endometrial glandular dysplasia: A putative precursor lesion of uterine papillary serous carcinoma. Part II: Molecular features. *Int J Surg Pathol* 2004;12:319–31.
52. Zheng W, Liang SX, Yi X et al. Occurrence of endometrial glandular dysplasia precedes uterine papillary serous carcinoma. *Int J Gynecol Pathol* 2007;26:38–52.
53. Jia L, Liu Y, Yi X et al. Endometrial glandular dysplasia with frequent p53 gene mutation: A genetic evidence supporting its precancer nature for endometrial serous carcinoma. *Clin Cancer Res* 2008;14: 2263–9.
54. Fadare O, Zheng W. Endometrial glandular dysplasia (EmGD): Morphologically and biologically distinctive putative precursor lesions of type II endometrial cancers. *Diagn Pathol* 2008;3:6.
55. Yi X, Zheng W. Endometrial glandular dysplasia and endometrial intraepithelial neoplasia. *Curr Opin Obstet Gynecol* 2008;20:20–5.

56. Fadare O, Zheng W. Endometrial serous carcinoma (uterine papillary serous carcinoma): Precancerous lesions and the theoretical promise of a preventive approach. *Am J Cancer Res* 2012;2:335–9.
57. Wild PJ, Ikenberg K, Fuchs TJ et al. p53 suppresses type II endometrial carcinomas in mice and governs endometrial tumour aggressiveness in humans. *EMBO Mol Med* 2012;4:808–24.
58. Zheng W, Yi X, Fadare O et al. The oncofetal protein IMP3: A novel biomarker for endometrial serous carcinoma. *Am J Surg Pathol* 2008;32:304–15.
59. Chen N, Yi X, Abushahin N et al. Nrf2 expression in endometrial serous carcinomas and its precancers. *Int J Clin Exp Pathol* 2010;4:85–96.
60. Moid F, Berezowski K. Pathologic quiz case: A 70-year-old woman with postmenopausal bleeding. Endometrial intraepithelial carcinoma, clear cell type. *Arch Pathol Lab Med* 2004 Nov;128:e157–8.
61. Fadare O, Liang SX, Ulukus EC, Chambers SK, Zheng W. Precursors of endometrial clear cell carcinoma. *Am J Surg Pathol* 2006;30:1519–30.

9

Endometrial malignant lesions

Etiology and risk factors	113	Mucinous carcinoma	130
Pathogenesis	114	Endometrial serous carcinoma	131
Clinical presentation and management	114	Clear-cell carcinoma	138
Pathologic characteristics of endometrial cancer	115	Undifferentiated and dedifferentiated carcinoma	142
Endometrioid carcinoma	123	References	144

Current concepts of endometrial cancer successfully integrate traditional histopathology with pathogenetic mechanisms. Endometrial cancers have long been classified into two major divisions (types I and II) based on light microscopic appearance, clinical behavior and epidemiology.[1] Type I, those with endometrioid histology, comprise approximately 75% of newly diagnosed endometrial cancers in North America. They are usually associated with unopposed estrogen exposure and are often preceded by precancerous lesions.[2] In contrast, type II endometrial cancers have non-endometrioid histology, typically endometrial serous carcinoma (ESC) with an aggressive clinical course. Patients with ESCs are usually not associated with unopposed estrogen stimulation, and their precancerous lesions have also been identified.[2] The morphologic and clinical differences are largely paralleled by genetic distinctions with different types of gene mutations between endometrioid and serous cancers.[3,4]

Studies by comparison of tumor subsets using genome-wide methods such as expression profiling has further broadened our understanding of relevant genetic basis for the differences between these two different histologic types of endometrial cancers.[5,6] Such a dualistic model has been popular in the last 30 years due to its reasonable separations of type I from type II cancers at the genetic and biological levels. However, both clinicians and pathologists have gradually encountered problems related to the model. Based on this model, type I or endometrioid carcinoma should have a very good prognosis, but not infrequently we have seen type I cancers behave badly,[7] just like type II endometrial cancers. In addition, patients with endometrial clear-cell carcinoma, which was classified as one of the type II cancers, do not behave as uniformly badly as patients with ESC.[8,9] There is no consensus as to the diagnostic criteria to differentiate high-grade endometrioid carcinoma and ESC,[10,11] which has caused a significant confusion in clinical practice. As we understand in general, a low-grade stage 1A endometrioid carcinoma should have almost no risk of recurrence or metastasis and, therefore, no staging procedure is necessary. However, many of us, including gynecologic oncologists and pathologists, have more or less encountered unexpected recurrence or distant metastasis from such cases. From all these perspectives, our pathology diagnosis or classification is beyond perfect. Starting from 2013, The Cancer Genome Atlas (TCGA) of endometrial cancer study has found promising data which separate the endometrial cancers into four molecular types based on their distinctive genetic characteristics.[12] More importantly, these molecular classifications of the endometrial cancers have a much better predictive value for patient survival than that of the dualistic model. This has resulted in an enhanced understanding of molecular and genetic events, reinforcement of the clinicopathologic subgroups originally defined by histologic and clinical features and development of biomarkers informative in identifying previously unknown or poorly described endometrial neoplastic lesions.

Although there is much progress made in the field, gynecologic pathology practice remain focused on morphology with the aid of immunohistochemistry to make correct diagnoses. Molecular analysis for endometrial cancer diagnosis is rarely applied in routine practice. Therefore, we will present general clinicopathologic features of the endometrial cancers followed by descriptions of individual histologic types of the cancer in this chapter.

ETIOLOGY AND RISK FACTORS

The majority of malignant endometrial neoplasms are adenocarcinomas. Factors that have been identified as causal in the development of endometrial adenocarcinoma include estrogenic stimulation (exogenous or endogenous), prolonged tamoxifen treatment, family history of endometrial cancer and pelvic radiotherapy.

UNOPPOSED ESTROGEN

Women who receive estrogens alone for peri- and postmenopausal hormone replacement are at increased risk of developing endometrial cancer. The reported relative risk for endometrial cancer in these women has ranged from 1.8 to 10 depending on the type of estrogen used and the duration of treatment.[13] Endogenous estrogenic stimulation occurs most commonly in association with obesity. The strong epidemiological link between obesity and endometrial cancer has been attributed to endometrial stimulation by endogenous estrogens derived from conversion of androgens to estrogens in the adipocytes of obese women. Although there was a positive association between body mass index and endometrial cancer risk, this was substantially reduced after adjusting for serum estrogen levels. There is also evidence suggesting a strong direct association between endometrial cancer risk and circulating estrogen and androgen levels, which can eventually convert to estrogen in peripheral fatty tissue.[14]

Endogenous estrogenic stimulation of the endometrium may also occur in association with chronic anovulation in disorders such as polycystic ovary disease and estrogen-secreting ovarian tumors such as granulosa cell tumor and thecoma. Women with these tumors are at increased risk of developing endometrial carcinoma.

Estrogen-associated endometrial malignancies have no distinctive pathological features. Most are adenocarcinomas of endometrioid type that develop on a background of endometrial hyperplasia. They tend to present at an early stage, to be well-differentiated and to have a favorable prognosis.

GENETIC FACTORS

Endometrial carcinoma risk is also informed by genetics, with several familial cancer syndromes imparting increased risk for tumors. The most common heritable risk factor for endometrial carcinoma is Lynch syndrome (LS, hereditary nonpolyposis colorectal cancer syndrome), which occurs primarily in the setting of germline mutations in the mismatch repair (MMR) genes *MSH2*, *MSH6*, *MLH1* and *PMS2*.[15,16] Rare cases of LS are attributable to mutations in the MMR-related gene *EPCAM* and to the heritable *MLH1* promoter hypermethylation.[17–19] About 2%–5% of all endometrial cancer cases are LS related and 50% of LS patients present with endometrial cancer as the sentinel symptom. Therefore, many medical centers in the world have instituted universal tumor-screening protocols to identify these patients.[20,21] Cowden syndrome, caused by germline defects in the *PTEN* gene, is associated with a far smaller proportion of endometrial cancers (well below 1%).[22,23] Even more uncommon are Cowden-like syndromes which are characterised by mutations in the succinate dehydrogenase B/C/D (*SDHB-D*) and killen (*KLLN*) genes.[24] Finally, although endometrial carcinoma has not traditionally been considered part of the *BRCA* mutation spectrum, recent evidence has challenged this notion with some studies demonstrating increased rates of uterine serous and serous-like cancers among *BRCA*-mutated patients,[25] particularly for those patients who are younger than 55 years.[26]

RADIATION

It has been suggested that radiotherapy may be a risk factor for endometrial cancer, particularly carcinosarcoma, high-grade endometrioid carcinoma and serous carcinoma. Although there are many anecdotal reports of endometrial adenocarcinoma and carcinosarcoma following radiotherapy, a definite causal link between endometrial cancer and radiotherapy has not yet been established.

PATHOGENESIS

Endometrioid carcinoma, usually a low-grade tumor that presents at an early stage, develops in a stepwise fashion from disordered proliferative endometrium → hyperplasia without atypia → atypical hyperplasia or EIN and then develops into endometrioid carcinoma. In this process of cancer development, there are multiple genes involved. These include *PTEN*, microsatellite instability, *K-ras*, etc. The detailed description about the genetic changes can be found in Chapter 8 and in the section Immunohistochemistry and Molecular Features of this chapter.

By contrast, endometrial serous carcinoma develops through the following steps: resting endometrium → p53 signature → endometrial glandular dysplasia (EmGD) → serous endometrial intraepithelial carcinoma (SEIC) → full-blown endometrial serous carcinoma. Within this process, the most important genetic change involves the *TP53* gene. The detailed description about genetic changes of *TP53* and other genes can be partly found in Chapter 8 and in the later section of this chapter as well as in the cited references.[27–29]

It is unclear how the remaining endometrial cancers develop, although development of clear cell carcinoma of the endometrium through clear cell endometrial glandular dysplasia has been briefly mentioned in the past.[30]

CLINICAL PRESENTATION AND MANAGEMENT

Endometrial cancers typically present with abnormal uterine bleeding. Diffuse pelvic pain and abdominal distention, as well as symptoms related to gastrointestinal and ureteral obstruction may occur in patients with more advanced disease. Women with symptoms concerning for endometrial carcinoma are managed with a combination of pelvic ultrasonography, endometrial biopsy and/or dilatation and curettage. Ultrasound is used to measure the endometrial stripe to assess for endometrial thickening; however, the predictive value of the endometrial thickness is relatively low. Detection rates can be increased by performing a hysteroscopic-guided biopsy, but the overall detection rate does not increase significantly compared with routine endometrial curettage.

Treatment of endometrial carcinoma is mainly surgical, including total hysterectomy and with or without bilateral salpingo-oophorectomies. Staging procedure including dissection of pelvic and sometimes para-aortic lymph nodes is also performed, although this can be avoided for low-grade, minimally invasive tumors. Adjuvant therapy is recommended in patients with advanced disease but has a less clear role in patients with low-stage tumors. Conservative management with medroxy-progesterone acetate (MPA) and megestrol acetate is sometimes offered to those patients with well-differentiated endometrioid tumors without evidence of myometrial invasion or extrauterine spread depending on clinical settings. Hormonal management can be applied for poor surgical candidates and women who strongly desire to preserve fertility.

PATHOLOGIC CHARACTERISTICS OF ENDOMETRIAL CANCER

Those pathologic parameters, which are commonly encountered in our daily practice, are described here. These include cancer grading, depth of myometrial invasion including the patterns of invasion, endocervical invasion (stromal versus mucosal), lymphovascular space invasion, peritoneal ascitic fluid status, margin status, regional lymph node metastasis and distant metastasis. The prognostic significance of micrometastasis (MM) and isolated tumor cells (ITCs) in sentinel lymph nodes is still controversial, with studies suggesting adverse influence on prognosis,[31] while some studies suggesting no effect.[32] All these parameters are required for the pathology report, and all oncologists will look for these parameters before a definitive management plan is given after the surgery. We will describe these pathologic characteristics prior to the discussion of individual histologic types of endometrial cancer as follows.

ENDOMETRIAL CARCINOMA GRADING

The main grading system for endometrial cancer is the three-tiered International Federation of Gynecology and Obstetrics (FIGO) grading system, which applies for the endometrioid carcinoma and its variants. However, this grading system does not apply to those high-grade cancers such as serous carcinomas, clear-cell carcinomas, carcinosarcomas, small/large cell neuroendocrine and undifferentiated/dedifferentiated carcinomas. When a mixed tumor is encountered, a ≥10% contribution of each histologic type of cancer is required. Endometrioid carcinomas and their variants are classified as grade 1–3 using the FIGO grading system, which is based on the proportion of nonsquamous solid growth. The Gynecologic Oncology Group (GOG) released an updated clause to the system that allows for a one-step upgrade (e.g. grade 1 → 2, grade 2 → 3) on the basis of severe cytologic atypia irrespective of the percentage of solid growth. It is important to note that severe cytologic atypia should include large pleomorphic nuclei, coarse nuclear chromatin and large irregular nucleoli in more than 50% of the tumor sample. Representative images of endometrioid carcinoma with different grades are illustrated in Figures 9.1 through 9.3.

In contrast to the 3-tiered system, a novel system proposed in 2005 combines papillary/solid growth, mitotic

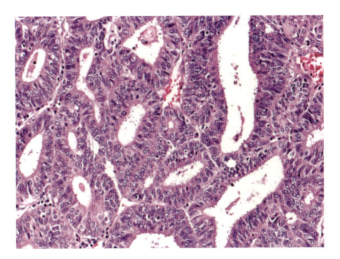

Figure 9.1 Well-differentiated endometrioid carcinoma (FIGO I) shows no or minimal solid tumor growth.

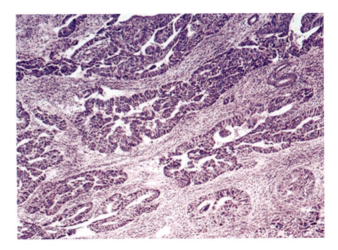

Figure 9.2 Moderately differentiated endometrioid carcinoma (FIGO II). Areas of semi-solid or solid (>5% but <50%) are present.

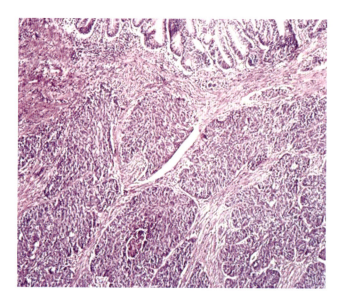

Figure 9.3 Poorly differentiated endometrioid carcinoma (FIGO III), with greater than 50% of tumor showing solid growth pattern.

activity and nuclear atypia to divide endometrioid tumors into low-grade and high-grade.[33] This two-tiered system has shown a better diagnostic reproducibility among pathologists and, in some studies, improved correlation with outcome relative to the existing FIGO system. However, prognostic power of the binary system has not been well documented.[34] Therefore, the FIGO grading system remains the most popular.

MEASUREMENT OF MYOMETRIAL INVASION

Depth of myometrial invasion measurement is a commonly encountered, clinically important question since it is one of the pivotal parameters of the cancer staging system. Invasion is estimated by measuring the deepest point of tumor infiltration from the level of the endometrial-myometrial junction. This is ideally performed on a full-thickness endomyometrial tissue section that includes the deepest point of invasion, adjacent normal endometrial-myometrial junction and the uterine serosa. When endomyometrial thickness is thicker than 3 cm, a slender bisected section is taken to fit a single cassette or two usual bisected sections are submitted in two consecutive separate cassettes.

Measurement of the depth of invasion sounds relatively simple. In reality, however, it is complex due to the following compounding factors: irregular endomyometrial junction, presence of adenomyosis and specific invasive patterns. This complexity is reflected in the relatively high interobserver variability in diagnosing endometrial cancer invasion.[35] Gynecologic pathologists typically report lower depths of invasion than nonspecialists, suggesting that overestimating invasion is a more significant problem than underestimating invasion.[35]

ENDOMETRIAL-MYOMETRIAL JUNCTION

The endomyometrial junction is typically irregular and is one of the common problems for assessing the depth of invasion accurately (Figure 9.4). This can be largely avoided by evaluating the invasion in low power. An intact endomyometrial junction should have a relatively smooth and even border. Invasion can be confirmed by finding loss of stromal cells or benign basalis endometrial glands between the cancer and myometrium interface (Figure 9.5). It is noted that endometrial stromal cells can have fibroblastic (Figure 9.6) or smooth-muscle (Figure. 9.7) metaplasia, which may cause confusion of myometrial invasion. But these metaplastic stromal cells remain positive for CD10, which can be used to aid the diagnosis. The differences between stromal metaplasia and myometrial invasion is summarized in Table 9.1.

Localizing the endometrial-myometrial junction can be problematic when the normal architecture has been distorted by tumor. In such situations, it is particularly

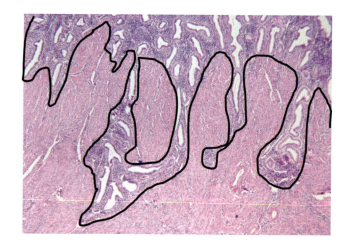

Figure 9.4 Irregular endomyometrial junction. Junction between the endometrium and the myometrium in normal uteri is usually irregular.

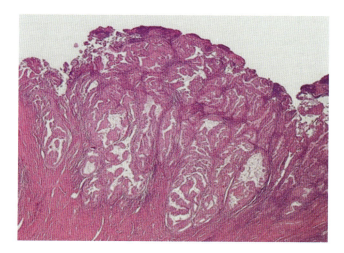

Figure 9.5 Myometrial invasion. There is loss of stroma and basal glands between the cancerous area and the myometrium.

Pathologic characteristics of endometrial cancer / Adenomyosis 117

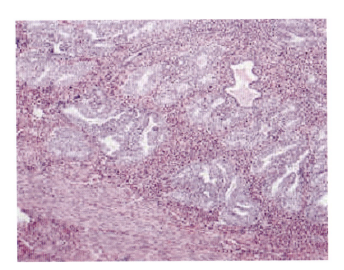

Figure 9.6 Fibroblastic metaplasia of stromal cells at endomyometrial junction. There are many stromal cells with fibroblastic metaplasia between the cancerous glands. No myometrial invasion is present in this setting.

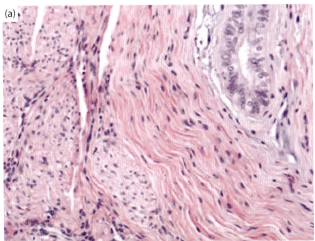

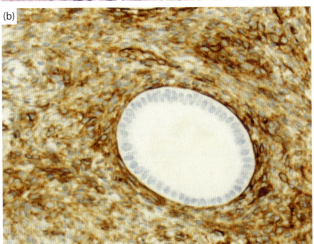

Figure 9.7 Smooth muscle metaplasia of the stromal cells in a focus of adenomyosis. Adenomyosis stroma resembles smooth muscle bundles (a, middle). The metaplastic stroma is CD10 positive (b).

Table 9.1 Evaluating stroma next to cancer near myometrium

Conditions	Myometrial invasion
Benign glands at interface of tumor and myometrium	No
Fibrous/myoid metaplasia of endometrial stroma	No
Loss of endometrial stroma	Yes
Desmoplastic stroma	Yes

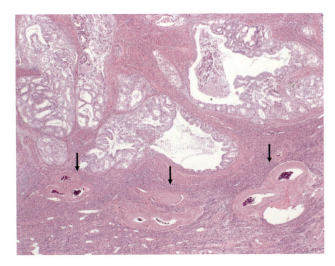

Figure 9.8 Endometrial cancer with deep myometrial invasion. The thick-walled vessels (arrows) are indicative of deep myometrial invasion. This tumor invades more than 50% of myometrium.

important not to misinterpret exophytic growth (tumor thickness) as depth of invasion. Proximity to thick-walled blood vessels can serve as a helpful clue that a tumor has invaded into the outer half of the myometrium (Figure 9.8), since such vessels are not present in the superficial myometrium. Conversely, pathologists should be cautious calling >50% invasion for tumors that are distant from thick-walled blood vessels, as this may represent an exophytic tumor with only limited myometrial invasion.

ADENOMYOSIS

Adenomyosis is easily identified when benign endometrial glands with surrounding stromal cells are seen. Endometrial cancers can arise in adenomyosis and such a situation may become problematic when that stroma is sparse or indistinct such as astromal adenomyosis. In particular, endometrial stromal cells may show smooth-muscle metaplasia, which become eosinophilic and spindled, mimicking myometrium (Figure 9.7). Differentiating adenomyosis from invasion is very challenging on frozen section and can result in errors with both over-calling and under-calling the depth of invasion. When such a situation is encountered, it is recommended to assess the sections in low power to understand the overall milieu: if extensive adenomyosis is present, caution should be exercised before calling invasion in isolated astromal glands, particularly if they are cytologically indistinguishable from neighboring adenomyosis and show a similar geographic distribution. Similarly, the presence of atypical or frankly malignant cells within a focus of adenomyosis does not qualify as invasion. This can be reinforced by identifying benign glands and apparent stromal cells within the lesion (Figure 9.9). Invasive carcinoma may arise from foci of adenomyosis. In this situation, invasive cancer grows beyond the boundaries of endometrial stroma and demonstrates true myometrial invasion. The depth of invasion is measured from the point of intact adenomyosis, rather than the endometrial-myometrial junction. A schematic chart of myometrial invasion measurement is summarized in Figure 9.10. Regarding endometrial stromal cells, many pathologists tend to stain with CD10 in order to assess the depth of invasion. It is, however, of little value since CD10 may also be positive in myometrial smooth-muscle cells surrounding invasive carcinoma. It is also worth remembering that cancer may also invade into foci of adenomyosis, which usually present as abrupt tumor masses involving foci of adenomyosis.

MYOMETRIAL INVASIVE PATTERNS

By convention, myometrial invasion can be easily identified when desmoplastic reaction or presence of irregular infiltrative glands are present (Figure 9.11). However, it can be problematic when invasive tumor presents as a bulky tumor mass with pushing borders without apparent stromal response or desmoplastic reaction. When this happens, invasion can be judged by absence of stromal cells and the benign endometrial glands or being adjacent to thick-walled blood vessels as discussed above in the last two sentences in the section, 'Endometrial-myometrial junction'. In addition to the invasive patterns (irregular infiltrative glands with a desmoplastic reaction or a bulky pushing tumor without a desmoplastic reaction), there are two recently recognized, less-common patterns specific to the endometrioid subtype that can also pose particular difficulty in the assessment of invasion. These are the microcystic elongated and fragmented (MELF) and the adenoma malignum-like patterns.

The MELF invasive pattern shows the following features, and representative pictures are presented in Figures 9.12 through 9.15.

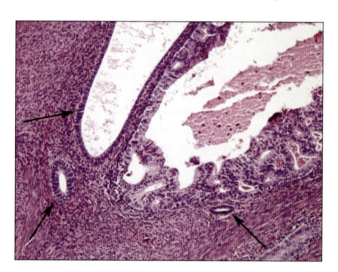

Figure 9.9 Endometrioid carcinoma arises in adenomyosis. Normal stroma and benign resting endometrial glands (arrows) are present adjacent to the cancerous glands.

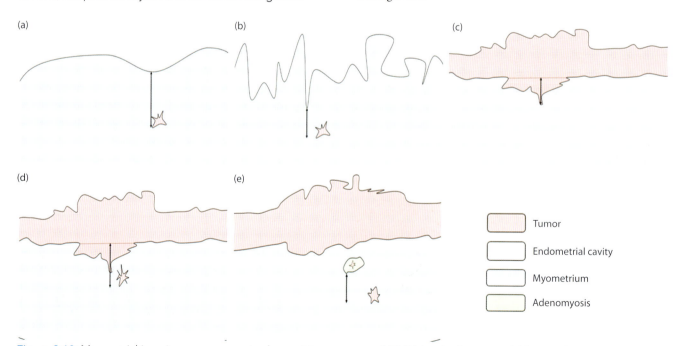

Figure 9.10 Myometrial invasion measurement scheme. Measurement of DMI (depth of myometrial invasion). (a) Measurement of DMI in an uncomplicated case. (b) Measurement of DMI in a tumor with irregular endomyometrial junctions. (c) and (d) Measurement of DMI in exophytic tumors. The depth of invasion should be measured, not the tumor thickness. (e) A proposal for measuring the DMI in cases showing deeply placed invasive carcinoma in proximity to adenomyosis colonized by carcinoma.

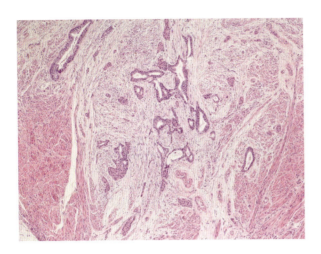

Figure 9.11 Myometrial invasion. Desmoplastic reaction surrounds the invasive cancerous glands.

- Most commonly associated with grade 1 endometrioid carcinomas
- Leading edge of tumor glands attenuate and commonly fragmented or broken, making it bland and deceivable appearance
- Glands resemble microcysts or lymphatics
- Tumor cells commonly have eosinophilic cytoplasm
- Acute inflammation commonly present in the glandular cells and lumen
- Inflammatory and fibromyxoid stroma are common

MELF is seen in 7%–45% of the endometrioid cancer cases and is associated with an increased incidence of true lymphovascular invasion, as well as increased rates of nodal metastases.[36] MELF has been postulated to represent an early phase of epithelial-mesenchymal transition, with immunohistochemical analyses demonstrating an immunophenotype more typical of mesenchymal differentiation in the infiltrating MELF

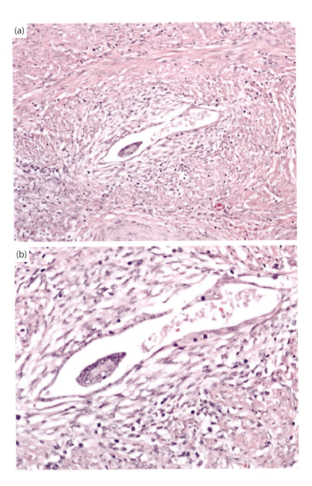

Figure 9.13 MELF myometrial invasive pattern. Intermediate-power view (a, 10x); High-power view (b, 40x). Attenuated cancerous gland is focally broken (upper right) and bland looking. A single small cancerous gland within the large glandular space simulates lymphovascular space involvement.

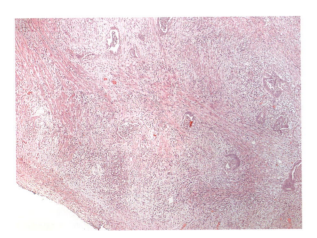

Figure 9.12 MELF myometrial invasive pattern. Invasive glands form microcysts (upper left) and clefts (lower right). Acute inflammation and edematous changes are commonly present. Uterine serosa is seen in the left lower corner.

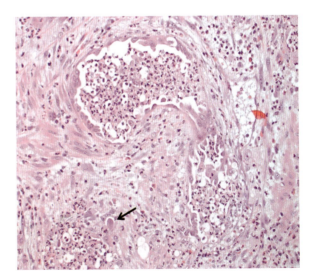

Figure 9.14 MELF myometrial invasive pattern. Invasive glands with single cancer cells containing large amount of cytoplasm (arrow), simulating macrophages. Extensive inflammation is commonly present.

120 Endometrial malignant lesions

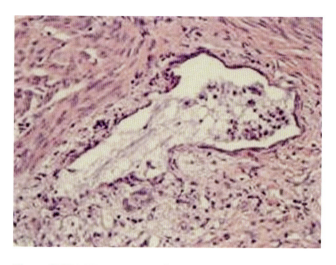

Figure 9.15 MELF myometrial invasive pattern. Microcystic gland may show incomplete glandular structure, which is surrounded by adjacent inflammatory and fibromyxoid stroma.

glands, including decreased expression of hormone receptors and e-cadherin and positive for cycling D1.[37,38]

Adenoma malignum-like infiltration is also known as 'diffusely infiltrative endometrial adenocarcinoma' (Figure 9.16). The characteristics of this invasive pattern are summarized as follows.

- Diffusely infiltrative pattern with scattered round, regular glands situated in a myometrium, simulating adenoma malignum–like invasive pattern
- No jagged contours and no desmoplastic stroma, which somehow mimics stroma-poor adenomyosis
- Tumor glands mostly arranged haphazardly

It is important to note that these endometrial cancers have no biologic or genetic relationship to adenoma malignum of the endocervix, while the name is purely described as their subtle pattern of infiltration.

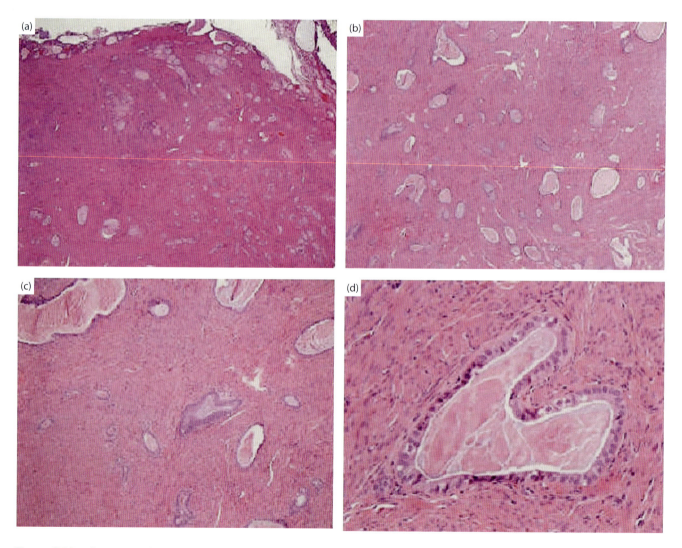

Figure 9.16 Adenoma malignum-like infiltration. Diffusely infiltrative pattern with scattered round, regular glands (a–c), and occasional angular glands (c, d). No jagged contours or desmoplastic stroma are present.

ASSESSMENT OF CERVICAL INVASION

Cervical invasion by endometrial cancer has two conditions. One is endocervical mucosa invasion and the other is cervical stromal invasion. The former has been dropped in the latest FIGO staging system, while the latter remains. Cervical stromal invasion is defined as stage II disease. Therefore, it is important to recognise it properly. However, this is not easy since the criteria for cervical stromal invasion are not well established, which is particularly true when endometrial cancer is focally localized in the junction of mucosa and cervical stroma. In general, the following clues will be helpful for the diagnosis of cervical stromal invasion. Evaluate the distribution of the background benign endocervical glands in low power. If the tumor is distributed similarly to the native endocervical glandular pattern, invasion is unlikely. This can be further confirmed by finding benign endocervical glands underneath the cancerous glands under intermediate power. However, true stromal invasion is present if tumor is seen infiltrating beyond this normal gland distribution or located deeper than normal endocervical glands, even without desmoplastic stromal reaction (Figure 9.17).

LYMPHOVASCULAR INVASION

Lymphovascular space invasion (LVSI) is seen more commonly in high-grade endometrial cancers and is relatively rare in low-grade endometrioid cancers.[39] Although LVSI is not an intrinsic component of endometrial cancer staging, it is considered as an independent negative prognostic factor for low-stage cancers and can therefore guide treatment strategies, particularly for tumors that straddle treatment algorithms based on grade and stage.[40] Deposits of cancer cells within either blood or lymphatic vessels define LVSI (Figure 9.18). Some helpful features to identify true LVSI are:

- Cancer deposits largely fit the vascular space with or without endothelial linings. This is because endothelial linings are commonly not visible under routine microscopy (Figure 9.19).

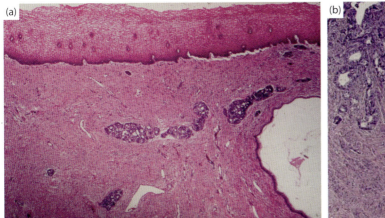
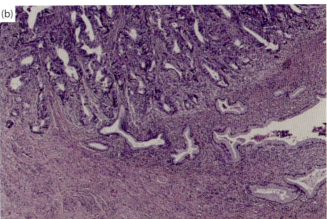

Figure 9.17 Cervical stromal invasion. Cancer glands invade below the squamous mucosa without obvious desmoplastic changes (a); There are benign endocervical glands underneath the cancer, indicative of cancer without stromal invasion (b).

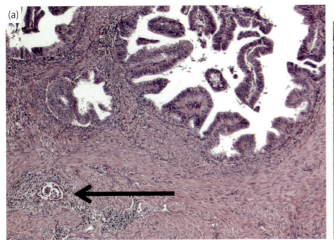
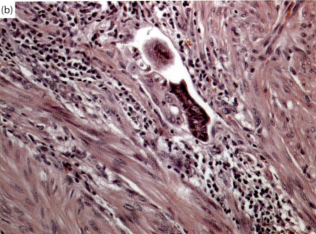

Figure 9.18 Villoglandular endometrioid carcinoma with lymphovascular invasion (a, arrow). Another area showing cancer in a lymphovascular space (b).

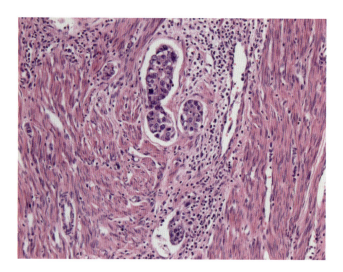

Figure 9.19 Endometrioid carcinoma with lymphovascular invasion. Clusters of tumor cells are located within the lymphovascular space of myometrium. Please note the cancer cells largely fit the shape of the lymphovascular space.

- Conformation of the tumor deposit to the vessel wall (with or without adherence to the wall)
- Proximity to thick-walled vessels or arteries

The diagnosis of LVSI can be complicated by technical artifacts (pseudoinvasion) and histologic mimics. Surgical procedures such as laparoscopic hysterectomy are a well-documented cause of vascular pseudoinvasion.[41] Detached tumor fragments (floaters) may be deposited in large vascular spaces by the grosser's knife. This pseudoinvasion typically presents as free-floating tumor fragments in large vessels. Retraction artifact around invasive nests of tumor can also mimic LVSI. Identification of an endothelial lining confirmed with immunohistochemical stains that highlight lymphatic channels (such as D2-40) can be helpful when the H&E appearance is ambiguous. However, negative D2-40 stain does not rule out LVSI. Therefore, such practice has limited value in routine practice. Localization is sometimes helpful since lymphatics travel in parallel with veins; tumor juxtaposition near a vein provides a clue of true invasion over retraction artifact.

LVSI should be differentiated from MELF invasive pattern as discussed above. In a situation like this, presence of surrounding fibromyxoid stroma helps identify MELF glands rather than vessels. Histiocytoid pattern of LVSI can lead to underestimation. This pattern is characterised by dyshesive cells with eosinophilic cytoplasm admixed with normal blood components. Because these tumor cells appear singly, rather than in obvious clusters, they can be easily overlooked on casual review. Appreciating nuclear atypia will lead to a correct diagnosis in this kind of scenario.

OTHER SITUATIONS IN ASSESSMENT OF ENDOMETRIAL CANCER

Peritoneal washing status is no longer part of endometrial cancer staging. However, positive washing is considered a poor prognostic factor for non-endometrioid and high-grade endometrioid carcinomas.[42] This situation sometimes is seen in those high-grade cancers with or without myometrial invasion. It is believed that cases like these largely metastasize through the trans-tubal route. Based on our own practice, we are able to identify free-floating cancer cells in tubal lumen in about 20% of the cases after completely examining both fallopian tubes (Figure 9.20). We therefore recommend that both fallopian tubes should be entirely submitted for microscopic examination in this situation.

Parametrial invasion has been shown to be another poor prognostic factor.[43] Parametrial tissue is not resected in the

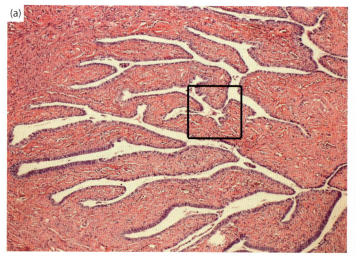
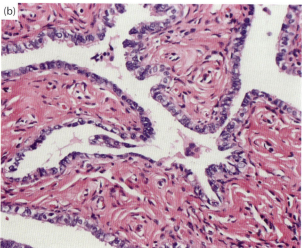

Figure 9.20 Trans-tubal metastasis: isolated serous carcinoma cells are not apparent in tubal lumen (a, boxed area, 20×) until it is magnified (b, 200×). Pictures were taken from a case of SEIC.

surgeries for the majority of endometrial cancers, except where the cancer involves the cervix when radical hysterectomy is performed. When this happens, parametria are assessed just like endocervical cancer.

In total hysterectomy specimens, the paracervical soft tissue represents the only true margin, while radical hysterectomy specimens include a vaginal and parametrial margins. Reporting on the margin status is optional.

ENDOMETRIOID CARCINOMA

CLINICAL FEATURES

Patient age ranges from 50 to 70 years in the majority of cases, with an average of 57 years old. However, it may also occur in reproductive age women with approximately 5% endometrioid carcinoma occurring at an age younger than 40 years. The most common symptom is abnormal vaginal bleeding, which is present in about 90% of the patients. Therefore, perimenopausal or postmenopausal bleeding is common. Occasional patients may have relatively normal menstrual cycles or no abnormal bleeding.

MACROSCOPY

Approximately 60% of tumors are diffusely involved the endometrial cavity, presenting as thickening of the endometrium, polypoid or exophytic lesions (Figure 9.21). Tumors can be focal, presenting as discrete nodule(s), focal undulation. A subset of tumors arises primarily from the lower uterine segment. When this pattern is present, a high suspicion of Lynch syndrome–associated endometrial carcinoma should be given. Importantly, attention should be given to the endometrium-myometrium junction. The blurring of the junction indicates possible myometrial invasion. Occasionally, no discrete tumor or mass can be identified grossly. When this happens, the entire endometrium should be submitted to look for microscopic cancer.

HISTOPATHOLOGY

Endometrioid carcinomas typically consist of back-to-back, complex, branched endometrial-type glands of varying differentiation with no or minimal intervening stroma. Cribriform structures are formed when tumor cells grow more within the glandular lumens. Occasionally, villoglandular pattern (papillary architecture) can be seen. Tumor glands are typically lined by stratified columnar epithelium. Cytoplasm of the neoplastic cells are usually eosinophilic and granular, with the lining cells sharing a common apical border which result in a glandular lumen with smooth contour. The nuclear atypia is usually mild to moderate, with inconspicuous nucleoli. However, poorly differentiated carcinoma with grade 3 nuclei is not uncommon. Tumor stroma may contain foamy cells (macrophages) due to tumor

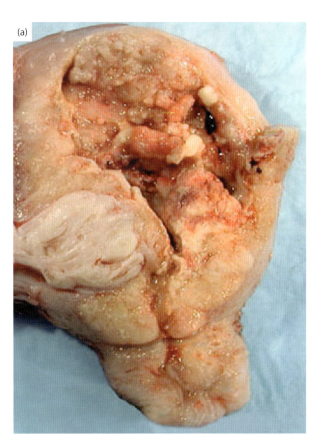

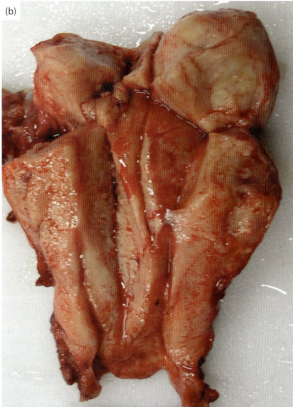

Figure 9.21 Gross presentations of endometrioid carcinoma. Tumor masses can either present as large masses (a) or form small nodules (arrow, b) in the endometrial cavity.

necrosis in approximately 15% of cases. Background of EIN/AH is more commonly seen in those endometrioid cancers with unopposed estrogen as the main etiology, while cancers caused by Lynch syndrome may not have hyperplastic background. Focal mucinous changes are very common. Representative pictures of the endometrioid carcinomas are presented in Figures 9.1 through 9.3.

IMMUNOHISTOCHEMISTRY AND MOLECULAR FEATURES

Cells of endometrioid carcinoma are typically positive for CK7, EMA, CA125, Ber EP4 and B72.3. With the exception of half of grade 3 tumors, most endometrioid carcinomas are positive for ER and PR. Vimentin is usually diffusely positive. P53 can be diffusely positive (mutational type) in some grade 3 cancers, but only rarely in grade 1 and 2 tumors. Therefore, p53 positivity alone is not enough to make the diagnosis of endometrial serous carcinoma (see section on Differential Diagnosis in Endometrial Serous Carcinoma for more details). Immunostains are commonly used for the purposes of differential diagnosis and therapeutics. For instance, it helps to distinguish between endometrial carcinomas from endocervical carcinomas. The expression of ER, PR and vimentin favor endometrial origin, while the absence of these markers, in conjunction with strong diffusely positive p16 staining, is consistent with the endocervical origin.[44,45] The details of such differential diagnosis are partially covered in Table 9.2.

TP53 mutations were found in 15% of endometrioid cancers in the TCGA study,[12] and 22% of these were frameshift or nonsense mutations.[46] Furthermore, more than one-third of grade 3 endometrioid cancers diffusely overexpress p53, which is equivalent to *TP53* mutation.[47] It also worth noticing that the *POLE*-mutated ('ultramutated') subset of cancers accounts for ~10% of endometrioid carcinomas. This molecular subset is of clinical interest because they have a very good prognosis even in the context of relatively high-grade, high-stage malignancies. It is notable that while *POLE*-mutated cancers also bear *TP53* in 35% of cases, existing data suggest that it is the underlying POLE-mutation, rather than the superimposed *TP53* mutation, that drives prognosis.[48] Therefore, it is not uncommon that endometrioid carcinomas demonstrate the mutated p53 expression pattern. From this perspective, it is not enough for a pathologist to make the diagnosis of ESC based on mutational type of p53 immunohistochemistry alone.

In addition to *TP53* changes, molecular alteration of mismatch repair (MMR) genes is also common in endometrial cancers. Complete loss of nuclear staining for one or more of the four MMR proteins MLH1, MSH2, MSH6 and PMS2 is found in approximately 30% of endometrioid carcinomas.[49] The majority of these MMR-deficient cases show dual loss of MLH1 and PMS2 attributable to epigenetic hypermethylation of the *MLH1* promoter region. A smaller subset (~5%–10%) demonstrates loss of PMS2, MSH2 and/or MSH6, *or* dual MLH1/PMS2 loss in the absence of hypermethylation, raising concern for heritable germline mutations associated with Lynch syndrome.[50] It is estimated that about 50% patients with Lynch syndrome present with endometrial cancer, mainly endometrioid type, as the sentinel symptom in the clinic.[50] Therefore, many academic institutions in the world now stain the MMR proteins for either all newly diagnosed endometrial cancers (universal) or patients under 60 years old (selective) as a screening test for Lynch syndrome.

The two most pathology diagnosis–related biomarkers are PTEN and PAX2, which have already been recommended by the European Society for Medical Oncology (ESMO) to help separate neoplastic lesions from non-neoplastic benign mimics.[51] There is an increasing trend of inactivation seen in EIN/AH (44%–63%) and adenocarcinoma (68%–83%).[52] However, loss of *PTEN* expression can also be seen in normal endometrium, which limits its clinical application in differential diagnosis. Similar to *PTEN*, *PAX2* does show loss in normal endometrium (36%), EIN/AH (71%) and carcinoma (77%).[53] Therefore, caution has to be exercised when both biomarkers are used to aid the diagnosis. In our own experience, we like to see the staining results for those areas in question rather than an overall estimation of the entire section.

Table 9.2 Differential diagnosis between endocervical adenocarcinoma and endometrioid carcinoma

	Endocervical adenocarcinoma	Endometrioid carcinoma
Clinical presentation	Cervical mass; postcoital bleeding; vaginal discharge; usually premenopausal	High estrogen level, such as obesity; irregular menses; usually perimenopausal or postmenopausal
Tumor stroma	Dense fibrous stroma, with large irregular vessels	Endometrial stroma, foamy cells
Tumor features	Adjacent adenocarcinoma in situ (AIS); often companying with squamous intraepithelial lesion (SIL); transition from AIS to adenocarcinoma can be seen; tumor cells often show high-grade atypia, apical mitosis and apoptosis	Adjacent EIN; transition from EIN to carcinoma; mitosis or apoptosis less often
Immunophenotype	p16 diffusely positive; ER/PR patchy positive or negative; vimentin negative; CEA positive	p16 patchy positive; ER/PR positive; vimentin positive; CEA negative
HPV *in situ* hybridization	Positive	Negative

ENDOMETRIOID CARCINOMA WITH SQUAMOUS DIFFERENTIATION

Approximately 20% of endometrioid carcinomas contain foci of squamous differentiation (Figure 9.22). Typical cytological and histological features of squamous epithelial, such as keratin pearl formation, intercellular bridge, dense eosinophilic cytoplasm, polygonal shaped and distinct cell border, can usually be seen in the area of squamous differentiation to aid the diagnosis. Of note, the area of squamous differentiation is not included in the estimation of solid growth for grading endometrioid carcinoma. Therefore, it is crucial to distinguish area of squamous differentiation from solid tumor growth pattern. Although usually it is easy to make the distinction by morphology, immunostaining of squamous markers such as p40, p63 and CK5/6 can be helpful in difficult cases.

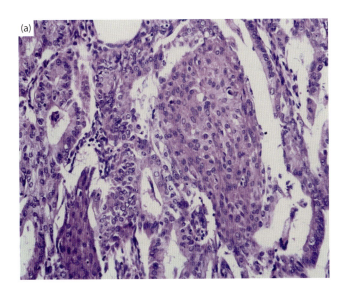

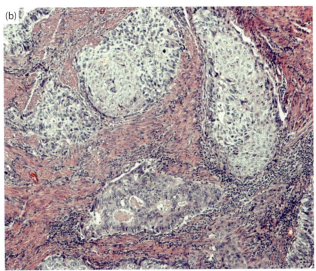

Figure 9.22 Endometrioid carcinoma with squamous differentiation. Squamous morule **(a)** and prominent squamous differentiation **(b)** are commonly present in endometrioid carcinomas.

VARIANTS OF ENDOMETRIOID CARCINOMAS

Endometrioid carcinomas have several rare variants, which behave similarly to the typical endometrioid cancers and are described below.

Villoglandular carcinoma. Villoglandular carcinoma is characterised by well-formed cancerous glands admixed with elongated papillary structures, which are lined by cells resembling those of well-differentiated endometrioid carcinoma (Figure 9.23). The papillary structures are typically thin, slender and lack broad, fibrovascular cores. Both squamous differentiation and psammoma bodies may be present, but the latter is much less frequent. Cytologically, it is typically bland looking with mild nuclear atypia. Villoglandular carcinomas usually have a good prognosis and typically without deep myometrial invasion. However, when myometrial invasion is present, it may show LVSI and behave aggressively.

Secretory carcinoma. Typically, secretory carcinoma consists of confluent villoglandular voluminous glands with glycogen-enriched subnuclear vacuoles (resembles secretory endometrium) and almost always well differentiated (Figure 9.24). This is different from endometrioid carcinoma with focal secretory changes, which is likely related to the progestin usage. In contrast, the secretory glands in secretory carcinoma are diffuse, which is not related to progestin application, although the detailed molecular mechanisms are unknown. Most secretory carcinomas occur in postmenopausal women without hormone therapy.

Other rare variants of the endometrioid carcinoma include ciliated cell carcinoma (Figure 9.25), spindle cell variant (Figure 9.26), corded and hyalinized variant (Figure 9.27), endometrioid carcinoma mimic ovarian sex-cord stromal tumor (Figure 9.28). Correct recognition of these variants should not be difficult as long as their growth patterns are kept in mind. Biomarker expression is similar to the typical endometrioid carcinoma.

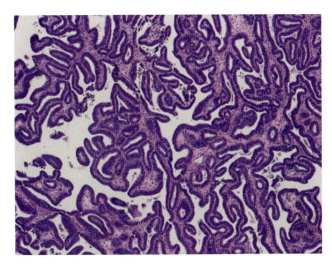

Figure 9.23 Endometrioid carcinoma, villoglandular variant.

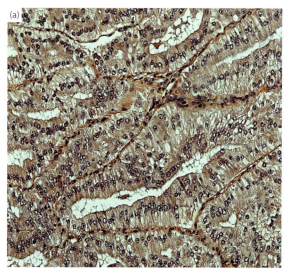
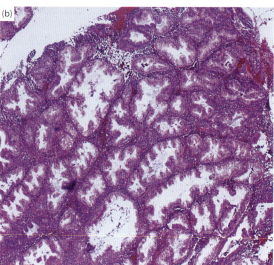

Figure 9.24 Comparison between secretory carcinoma and crowded glands of secretory endometrium. Secretory carcinoma with crowded back-to-back glands containing subnuclear vacuoles **(a)**. The normal secretory endometrium with crowded yet well-organized glands **(b)**.

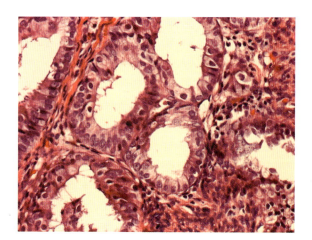

Figure 9.25 Ciliated-cell carcinoma. The tumor glands resemble tubal epithelium, lined by epithelia bearing cilia.

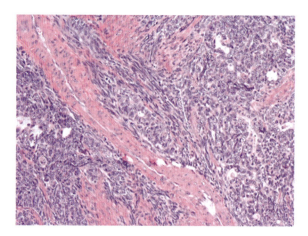

Figure 9.26 Endometrioid carcinoma, spindle-cell variant. The spindle-shaped cancer cells with minimal nuclear atypia simulate stromal cells.

DIFFERENTIAL DIAGNOSIS

Atypical hyperplasia (AH)/endometrial intraepithelial neoplasia (EIN). Well-differentiated endometrioid carcinoma versus EIN/AH is a commonly encountered diagnostic dilemma in daily practice. This is mainly because these two entities represent a spectrum of endometrial glandular proliferations without a clear-cut line separating them. Diagnostic criteria described by all major textbooks for these entities lack a quantitative definition and there are many overlap points in between. Although there is a significant degree of interobserver variability to separate these two entities, the majority of gynecologic pathologists use the following points for the diagnosis of well-differentiated endometrioid carcinoma over EIN/AH. In general, presence of stromal invasion is a definition of cancer. In this particular setting, glandular fusion of at least 2 mm in linear extent matches to the criteria of 'stromal invasion' (Figure 9.29). It is worthwhile to emphasise that in this situation, invasion into the stroma need not be seen directly as infiltrative glands percolating through stroma; rather, it is inferred by the loss of stroma between glands. This requirement derives from rigorous work done about 40 years ago.[54] The study investigated nuclear atypia, mitotic activity, necrosis, cellular stratification and stromal invasion in 204 endometrial curetting specimens and determined that stromal invasion was the most predictive factor of endometrial carcinoma on subsequent hysterectomy. Basically, presence of florid, expansile and/or cribriform growth patterns in low power is an indication of stromal invasion or cancer diagnosis. However, it becomes difficult in cases of small biopsies with closely-packed individual glands showing minimal intervening stroma. Furthermore, the requirement for absolutely no intervening stroma may result in undercalling certain cancer cases since many endometrioid cancers commonly maintain small amount of intervening stroma. That being said endometrial glandular growth patterns are more reliable than lack of intervening stroma in those proliferating

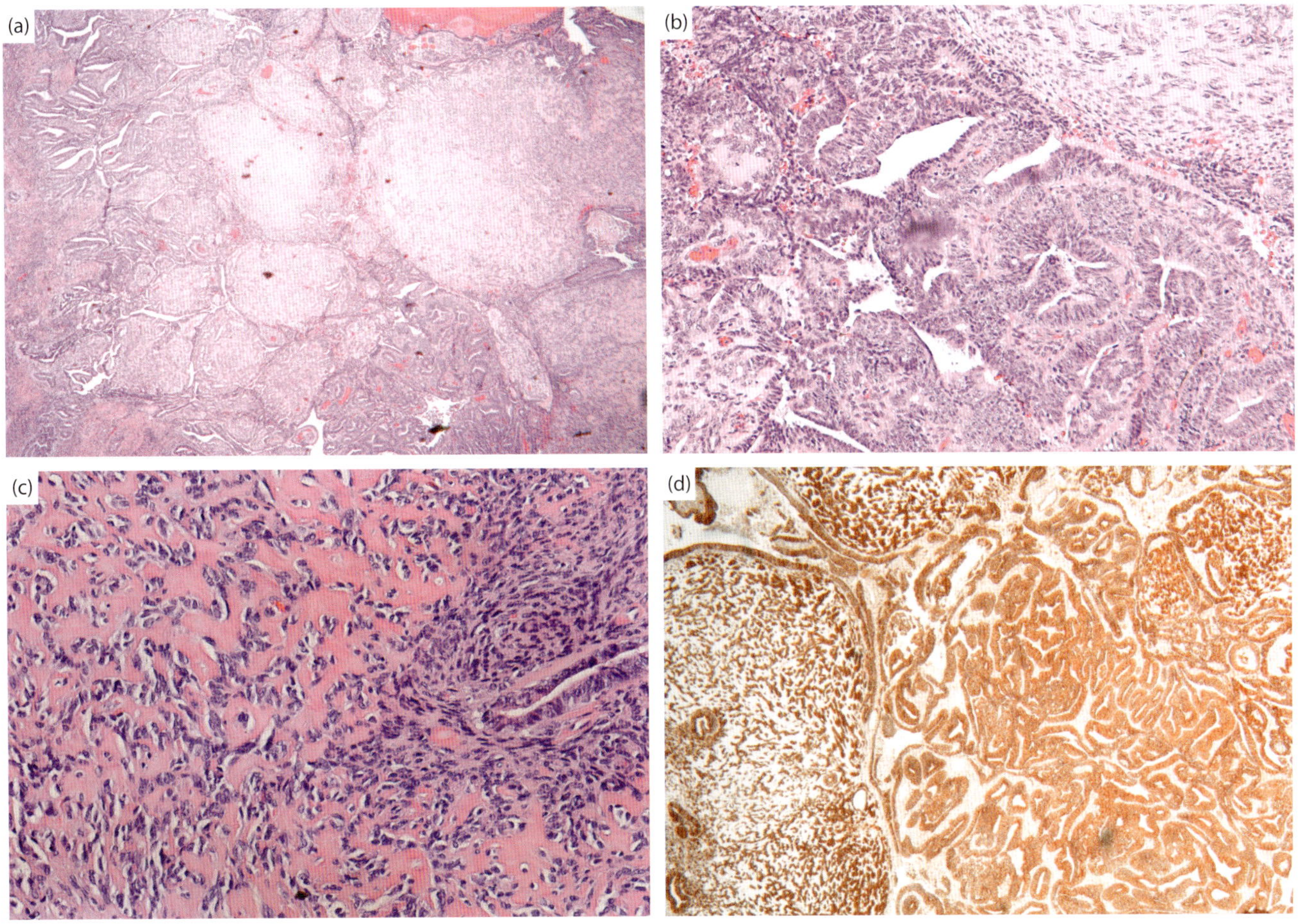

Figure 9.27 Endometrioid carcinoma, corded and hyalinized variant. Regular endometrioid carcinoma is present in the periphery, while several nodules containing corded glands within the hyalinized stroma is seen mainly in the center (a, low power). A higher-power view shows both typical endometrioid area and corded and hyalinized component (b, upper right corner). Further magnified corded and hyalinized component (c). Both components are diffusely positive for beta-catenin (d).

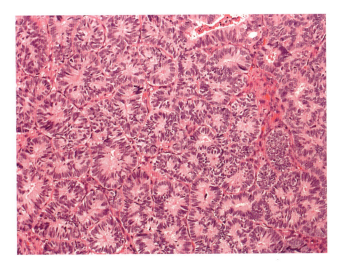

Figure 9.28 Endometrioid carcinoma mimicking ovarian sex-cord tumor. Tumor consists of compact anastomosing cords and tubule-like structures simulating an ovarian sex-cord stromal tumor.

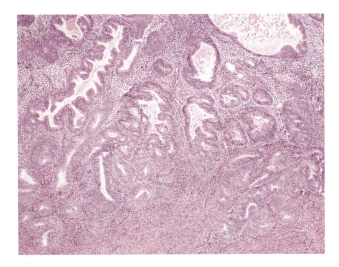

Figure 9.29 Endometrioid carcinoma. Cancerous area, measuring about 3 mm, is apparent in the endometrial–myometrial interface.

glands. Gynecologic oncologist, the colleague in the clinical side, will actually manage the patient not much differently in terms of pathologic diagnosis of EIN versus well-differentiated endometrioid carcinoma. This is because they understand there is significant overlap in these two entities with EIN as a precancerous lesion bearing a significant risk for cancer. Hysterectomy with or without staging remains a choice for both entities.

Endometrial serous carcinoma. The glandular variant of endometrial serous carcinoma (ESC) can demonstrate endometrioid architecture, while the solid variant of serous carcinoma can be confused with high-grade endometrioid carcinoma. On the other hand, endometrioid carcinoma can demonstrate intraluminal papillary structures (Figure 9.30), which can be mistaken as ESC. The main difference between these two entities is the degree of nuclear atypia. Usually, ESC shows severe nuclear atypia or grade 3 nuclei, while endometrioid carcinoma has lower grade nuclear atypia or grade 1–2 nuclei. A panel of immunostains can facilitate the diagnosis in difficult settings. ESC typically demonstrates strong diffuse p53 positivity or completely negative staining (all or none staining pattern or mutational type), diffuse p16 positivity, reduced ER and PR positivity. In contrast, wild p53 staining pattern, patchy p16, presence of ER and only partial loss of PR are typical of endometrioid carcinoma. However, it is worth noting that mutational type p53 staining pattern can be commonly seen in cases of endometrioid carcinoma irrespective of grading. Therefore, p53 positivity (mutational type) alone does not warrant the diagnosis of ESC. More information about immunohistochemical stains to aid the diagnosis of endometrial carcinoma histologic types is described in the differential diagnosis of ESC below in this chapter.

Endocervical adenocarcinoma. When adenocarcinoma is found in both endometrial and/or endocervical biopsy/curettage specimens, the following possibilities should be considered: (1) cervical involvement by endometrial carcinoma, (2) endometrial extension by endocervical adenocarcinoma, and (3) two primary tumors. It is important to clarify the primary site of the tumor, since the clinical management will be different. The most helpful features and tools to differentiate the entities from each other are summarized in Table 9.2. Basically, dense fibrous stroma suggests endocervical adenocarcinoma, while endometrial stroma with foamy cells is suggestive of endometrial origin (Figure 9.31). The usual type (HPV related) of endocervical adenocarcinoma usually has a high-grade nuclear atypia, more apical mitotic figures and apoptotic bodies (Figure 9.32). Adjacent adenocarcinoma in situ or squamous intraepithelial lesion (SIL) is more suggestive of endocervical primary, while presence of EIN/AH is consistent with endometrial primary. A panel of immunostains can help to facilitate the diagnosis (Figure 9.33). The biomarkers within this table including p16, ER/PR, vimentin and CEA

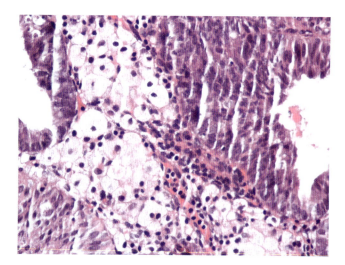

Figure 9.31 Endometrioid carcinoma. Foamy cells are present in the stroma, indicating endometrial location.

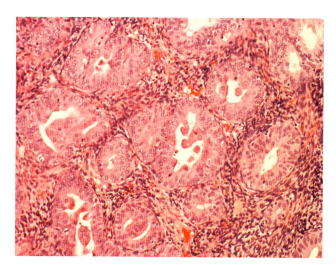

Figure 9.30 Intra-luminal papillae in endometrioid carcinoma.

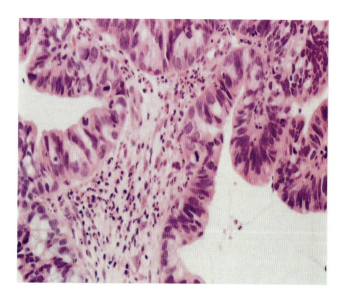

Figure 9.32 Endocervical carcinoma. There are frequent apoptotic bodies and apical mitotic figures, strongly suggestive endocervical origin.

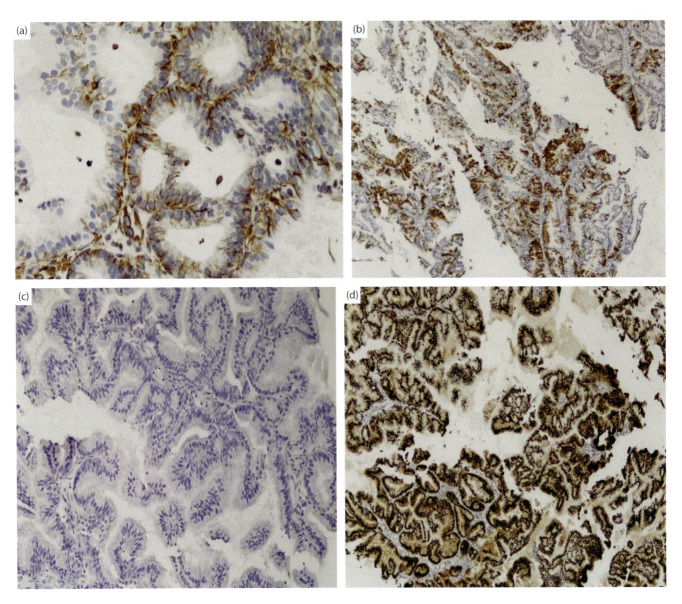

Figure 9.33 Endometrial mucinous carcinoma. Vimentin positive (a), p16 patchy positive (b), CEA negative (c), ER diffusely positive (d). Such immune phenotypes are supportive of endometrial origin rather than endocervical origin.

are commonly applied by surgical pathologists in their routine practice. Typically, endocervical adenocarcinoma is positive for p16 and CEA and negative or less positive for ER/PR and vimentin. On the other hand, endometrial carcinoma shows a reverse pattern in a typical scenario. We would like to provide the following tips, which can improve the diagnostic accuracy significantly. Among all the biomarkers listed above, the most useful markers are p16 and ER. P16 should be diffusely and strongly positive in the usual-type endocervical carcinoma and only patchy positive or negative in endometrial carcinoma. Here we should emphasise that the diffuse positive means that more than 99% of the cancerous cells are strongly positive both in cytoplasm and nuclei. This is because some endometrioid carcinomas, particularly FIGO grade 2 or higher cases, may show 'diffuse' staining, say 90% positivity of the cancer cells. However, this remains different from the staining pattern for an endocervical carcinoma. Similarly, ER is typically strongly and diffusely positive in a well-differentiated endometrial endometrioid carcinoma, but it may also be positive in endocervical carcinoma. In this scenario, the degree of positivity and the intensity of the staining is less in endocervical cancer than that of endometrial endometrioid cancer. Appropriate interpretation of these two biomarkers can lead to accurate diagnosis in more than 90% of the cases in this setting. In contrast to p16 and ER, the rest of the markers are somewhat less specific. PR expression may be lost or reduced in both cancers. Vimentin and CEA only work properly in up to 70% of the cases. In rare difficult situations, HPV in situ hybridization can be used. It is almost 100% positive in usual-type endocervical carcinoma, while negative in endometrial endometrioid carcinoma. However, the method is not readily available in most pathology laboratories.

PROGNOSIS AND PREDICTIVE FACTORS

FIGO stage, age, histological grade, depth of myometrial invasion and lymphovascular invasion are the most important predictors of lymph-node involvement and outcome. The risk of nodal spread and recurrence is related to depth of myometrial invasion. Overall, stage remains the most dominant predictive factor for patient outcome. At the molecular level, copy number high genotype obtained by molecular sequencing analysis remains as the most reliable predictive factor of poor survival for patients with endometrial cancer.[12]

MUCINOUS CARCINOMA

CLINICAL FEATURES AND GENETIC PROFILE

Mucinous carcinoma is a rare variant of endometrioid carcinoma, accounting for 1%–9% of endometrial carcinoma.[55] Tumors are almost always stage I disease, with myometrial invasion typically limited to the inner half. Mucinous carcinoma including endometrioid carcinoma with mucinous differentiation is commonly associated with hormone therapy, particularly progestin dominant hormones. The genetic feature of this type of endometrial cancer is mainly KRAS mutation.[56]

PATHOLOGIC FEATURES AND DIFFERENTIAL DIAGNOSIS

Grossly, endometrial mucinous carcinoma locates mainly within the endometrial cavity and rarely involving the cervix. For those cancers within the endometrial cavity, there are no gross differences from endometrioid cancers.

Microscopically, mucinous carcinoma usually shows glandular or villoglandular architecture and consists of at least 50% columnar or pseudostratified epithelial cells containing intracytoplasmic mucin.[57] It is the intracellular, not intraluminal, mucin, which is required for the diagnosis since many endometrioid carcinomas may contain mucin components in the glandular lumen. Mucin stains such as mucicarmine can help to demonstrate the presence of intracellular mucin. Histologically, cancerous glands resemble endocervical glands (Figure 9.34). Nuclear atypia is mild to moderate and mitotic activity is usually low. Other malignant features include architectural complexity and epithelial stratification. Frank tumor necrosis is rarely seen but presence of inflammatory cells within the cancer is common, similar to mucinous carcinoma elsewhere.

Of note, focal mucinous differentiation is very common and can be seen in approximately half of endometrioid carcinomas. In practice, the diagnosis of endometrioid carcinoma with mucinous differentiation is appropriate if the malignant mucinous epithelia consist of less than 50% of total tumor volume.

Rare cases of intestinal type of endometrial mucinous carcinoma have been reported.[58] It is known that intestinal type mucinous carcinomas are more frequently seen in the endocervix. Therefore, if an intestinal type adenocarcinoma is encountered in the endocervical and endometrial biopsy specimens, the likelihood of endocervical primary is much higher than endometrial primary. In addition, when the mucinous carcinoma is poorly differentiated, the intracytoplasmic mucin is often depleted or less prominent, commonly leading to a misdiagnosis of non-mucinous carcinoma (Figure 9.35). This can be avoided by finding cancer cells with relatively better intracellular mucin. It should not be difficult since a better mucinous differentiated area is commonly present even in poorly differentiated cancer

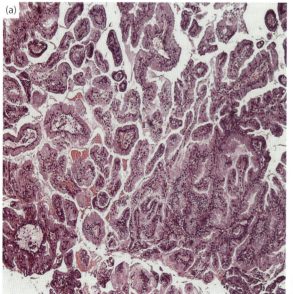
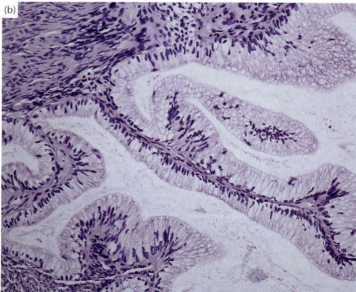

Figure 9.34 Mucinous carcinoma, endocervical type (a); Intracytoplasmic mucin and intraluminal mucin (b).

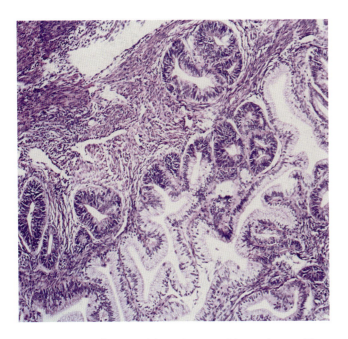

Figure 9.35 Endometrioid carcinoma with mucinous differentiation. Typical endometrioid carcinoma is on the top, while apparent endocervical like mucinous differentiation is seen in the bottom and the right of the picture.

cases. Furthermore, mucinous differentiation is also frequently encountered when patients are using progestin or progestin dominant oral contraceptives, which is a common medical practice to prescribe such medicine to those patients experiencing abnormal bleeding prior to hysterectomy.

It also worth noting that mucinous carcinoma is common elsewhere in addition to the endometrium and cervix. This includes ovary and organs outside of the female reproductive tract. Therefore, appropriate differential diagnosis should always apply when a different primary or metastasis is considered.

ENDOMETRIAL SEROUS CARCINOMA

CLINICAL FEATURES

Although endometrial serous carcinomas (ESC) represent only 10% of endometrial carcinomas, they are estimated to account for approximately 40% of endometrial-associated mortality.[59,60] ESC is less often associated with excessive prolonged estrogen exposure than endometrioid carcinoma. It occurs more frequently in black, multiparous and non-obese women. Other risk factors include current smoker, post tubal ligation, and history of breast carcinoma and/or tamoxifen usage.[26,61] ESCs most often occur in postmenopausal elderly women, with a mean age in the late 60s.

Although the etiology is unclear, we now understand that *TP53* mutation is the most important single event, which can cause the development of ESC from benign endometrium. This was supported by the model of endometrial serous carcinogenesis we developed during last decade[28] and p53 knockout mouse model produced afterwards.[62] It is believed that there are multiple genetic changes (copy number high) within the cancer cells induced by genomic instability because of *TP53* mutation.[46,63]

MACROSCOPY

The tumor may form a large, necrotic mass, which may fill up the entire endometrial cavity and often accompanied by deep myometrial invasion (Figure 9.36). Of note, the tumor can be microscopic only, with no appreciable mass or only conspicuous induration. Therefore, in cases with no obvious mass but biopsy-proven endometrial cancer, one or two random sections during the frozen section evaluation are needed to search for probable myometrial invasion (Figure 9.37). Sometimes, SEIC or ESC may arise on the surface of an endometrial polyp.

HISTOPATHOLOGY

Serous endometrial intraepithelial carcinoma (SEIC). SEIC is typically seen in glands and surface epithelia and often multifocal without myometrial invasion. The glands are typically well separated and do not display crowding or confluence. The lining epithelia show severe nuclear atypia and are morphologically identical to those of conventional invasive ESC (Figure 9.38). SEIC has a tendency to involve an endometrial polyp,[64–67] although it also occurs in non-polypoid endometrium. Therefore, close examination of polyps, especially in the postmenopausal population, may help to identify the lesions in a subtle condition.

Historically, SEIC represents a unique entity without myometrial invasion but with a high amount of extrauterine disease. However, the diagnosis of SEIC has caused much undertreatment resulting in recurrence within 2 years after hysterectomy. Nowadays, pathologists and clinicians have realized that SEIC represents an ESC without myometrial

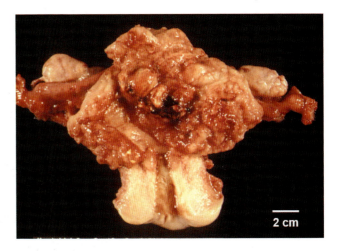

Figure 9.36 Endometrial serous carcinoma. Massive tumor masses are present in the endometrial cavity and extensive myometrial invasion is present in the side of myometrial wall.

132 Endometrial malignant lesions

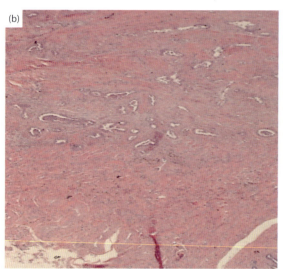

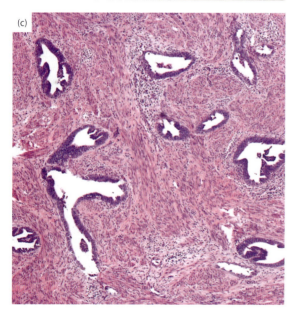

Figure 9.37 Endometrial serous carcinoma. Tumor only forms a small induration in the fundal area of the uterus (a), but with extensive myometrial invasion (b) and the invasive cancer is mainly glandular (c).

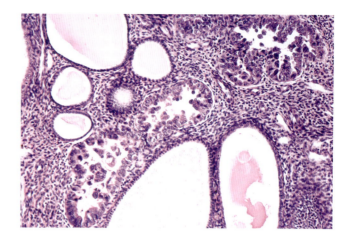

Figure 9.38 Serous endometrial intraepithelial carcinoma. A few serous cancerous glands are present in the background of atrophic endometrium.

invasion and management for SEIC should be identical to that of ESC. Therefore, the nomenclature (diagnosis) of SEIC should be avoided, particularly in the biopsy specimens, to avoid potential confusion.

Endometrial serous carcinoma (ESC). The cytological features of ESC variably display features such as severe pleomorphism, hobnail nuclei, hyperchromasia with coarse chromatin pattern, large prominent nucleoli, and abundant mitotic figures. ESC mainly has three morphologic structures including papillary, glandular and solid growth patterns.

- Papillary growth pattern. This is the conventional type of ESC, which used to be named as uterine papillary serous carcinoma (UPSC) because of the papillary structure. ESC with papillary structures typically show either thick or thin papillae and small detached buds and tufts within the cancerous glands (Figure 9.39). As we know these days, the papillary structure is not specific for serous carcinoma. This is why the term UPSC is no longer popular.
- Glandular growth pattern. This growth pattern resembles endometrioid or sometimes villoglandular carcinoma significantly (Figures 9.40 through 9.42). It is particularly true when it is viewed in low power. The feature of the glandular type ESC is well-differentiated or low-grade architecture with high-grade nuclei.
- Solid growth pattern. Sheets of cancer cells, which are similar to those high-grade poorly or undifferentiated carcinomas (Figure 9.43), compose this pattern.

In addition to the high nuclear grade, ESC cells have more eosinophilic cytoplasm, except in the solid growth pattern. Myometrial invasion, mitosis and tumor necrosis are commonly present. Psammoma bodies are occasionally present. Abrupt transitions from normal to ESC or from SEIC to ESC are common. Lesions of EmGD can be identified in about half of the uteri with ESC if multiple sections from noncancerous areas are taken (see Chapter 8 for more details). Regarding benign background endometrium, we would like to emphasise that it is not always atrophic. It can

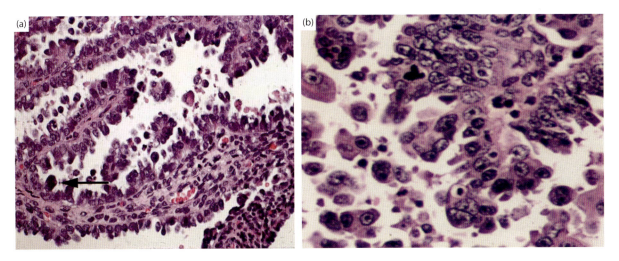

Figure 9.39 Endometrial serous carcinoma. Large papillae lined by high-grade cancer cells with large amount of eosinophilic cytoplasm. Occasional psammoma body is seen (a, arrow). There are many small detached clusters or single cancer cells (b).

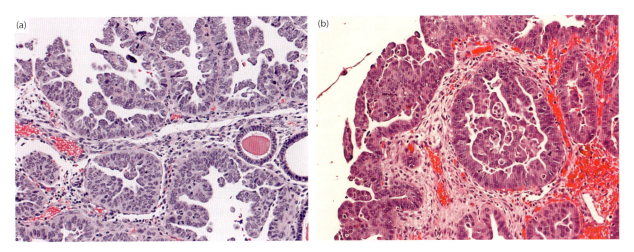

Figure 9.40 Endometrial serous carcinoma with villoglandular architecture (a) and intraluminal papillae (b). Apparently, these cancer cells have high-grade nuclei.

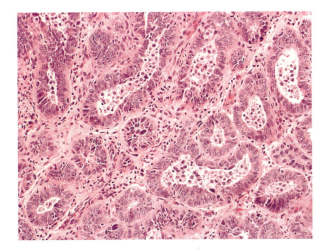

Figure 9.41 Endometrial serous carcinoma with glandular growth pattern. High-grade serous cancer cells form glandular architecture without papillary formation. Intraluminal tumor necrosis or dying cancer cells are present.

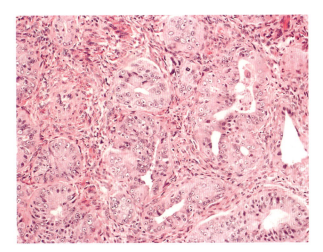

Figure 9.42 Endometrial serous carcinoma with glandular growth pattern. Cancer cells have eosinophilic cytoplasm and prominent nucleoli, the histologic features are characteristic of endometrial serous carcinoma.

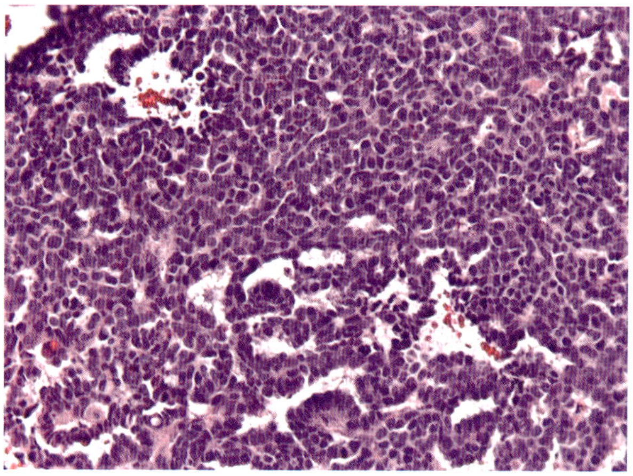

Figure 9.43 Endometrial serous carcinoma with solid growth pattern. The serous carcinoma only shows focal glandular formation.

be weakly proliferative, or proliferative or even hyperplastic depending on the hormone levels of individual patients. We want to emphasise this because the association between ESC and atrophic endometrium is so strong in pathologists' minds that many of them are hesitant to call ESC when non-atrophic endometrium is present.

Mixed ESC and endometrioid carcinoma. It is not uncommon that ESC is found along with endometrioid carcinoma. As shown in Figure 9.44, well-differentiated endometrioid carcinoma can abruptly transition into typical ESC. A mixed tumor is defined by each component constituting more than 10% of the tumor volume. When endometrioid carcinoma is less than 10%, it is not necessary to diagnose a mixed tumor. But if the serous component is present in less than 10% of the tumor volume, a diagnosis of endometrioid carcinoma with serous differentiation is recommended.

Of note, the mixed tumors including those with serous differentiation still carry a worse prognosis than those pure endometrioid carcinomas.[68] Ample sampling is always a good practice when a minor mixed component is encountered. The pathology report should clearly state the amount of ESC in a mixed cancer.

IMMUNOHISTOCHEMISTRY

Mutational type of p53 expression pattern remains a feature of ESC. This is defined by all (diffuse) or none staining pattern of p53 immunohistochemistry. Diffuse staining pattern requires more than 75% of the cancer nuclei stain strongly. None staining pattern equals to a null p53 expression. There are no strongly stained cancer cells.

- P16 is typically diffusely positive in both cytoplasm and nuclei in every ESC cell.
- Ki-67 is high, commonly more than 70%.
- IMP3 is more positive in ESCs than that in endometrioid cancers.
- ER is either reduced significantly or completely lost, while PR is commonly lost.
- MMR proteins (MLH1, PMS2, MSH2 and MSH6) are usually negative.
- PTEN and PAX2 are usually negative.

Careful evaluation of the internal controls and noncancerous areas will lead to correct interpretation of the staining results.

MOLECULAR FEATURES

ESCs correlate well with the copy-number high group in the TCGA molecular classification of the endometrial cancer, and have extensive copy-number alterations, few DNA methylation changes and more than 90% *TP53* mutations.[46,63] In addition, ESC shares genomic features with ovarian serous

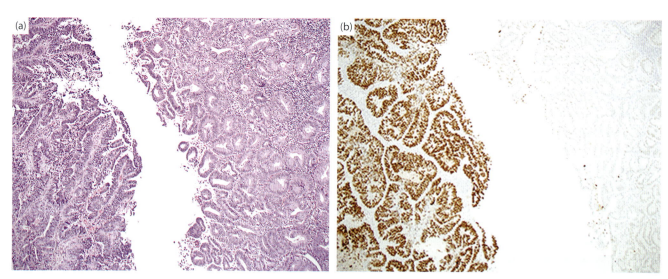

Figure 9.44 Mixed endometrioid carcinoma and serous carcinoma. Endometrioid carcinoma is present in the right, while serous carcinoma is on the left (a). Subsequent staining with p53 shows wild type in the endometrioid area, while mutational type (diffusely positive) in the serous component (b).

and basal-like breast carcinomas. The clonal relationship between serous endometrial intraepithelial carcinoma (SEIC) and associated ESC has been well established, with the same somatic mutations in multiple genes.[69]

Other genetic changes include PIK3CA (24%–40%), FBXW7 (20%–30%) and PPP2R1A (18%–28%).

DIFFERENTIAL DIAGNOSIS

The major differential diagnosis of ESC is from endometrioid carcinoma. This is the most common and the most difficult in daily practice. The main difficulty occurs between glandular type ESC and endometrioid carcinoma. We provide the following clues to help the diagnosis.

- Clinical history may be helpful. Patients with ESC tend to be 60 years or older. History of breast cancer and known BRCA mutation increases the likelihood of ESC.
- Discrepancy between architecture and nuclear grading is suggestive of glandular-type ESC. As illustrated in Figures 9.42 and 9.43, glandular ESC presents with well-formed 'endometrioid'-looking glandular architecture, while possessing grade 3 nuclei. In contrast, the architecture and nuclear grading of typical endometrioid carcinomas are usually consistent. However, there is a subset of high-grade glandular endometrial adenocarcinomas with ambiguous features that could reflect either serous or endometrioid differentiation.[70] In this situation, a panel of immunohistochemical stains may facilitate the diagnosis (see below bullet points).
- Background endometrium provides a useful clue to aid the diagnosis. Endometrioid carcinoma usually accompanies hyperplastic endometrium, while ESC is generally associated with atrophic or resting endometrium. However, this feature is not always consistent since hormone therapy is common nowadays. In our practice, ESC is not uncommonly associated with proliferative or even hyperplastic background endometrium.
- A panel of immunostains (Table 9.3) may be useful to lead to the accurate diagnosis. As mentioned in the section of endometrioid carcinoma, TP53 mutations can be found in a significant portion of endometrioid carcinomas. Therefore, mutational-type p53 stain results alone are no longer sufficient as a diagnostic marker for ESC. Additional markers need to be included in order to make the correct diagnosis. We divide the differential diagnosis into two scenarios. One is morphologically more likely or unlikely to ESC and the other is ambiguous. In the former situation, combination of p53 and p16 are essential and IMP3 or ER/PR are optional. When p53 is mutational type and p16 is diffusely positive in almost 100% of cancer cells, it is diagnostic for ESC (Figure 9.45). When only one or neither is matched, it is diagnostic of an endometrioid carcinoma (Figure 9.46). In the latter condition, morphologically ambiguous endometrial adenocarcinomas require more comprehensive biomarker stains. In addition to p53 and p16, we apply MMR protein panel PTEN, as well as PAX2, in the differential diagnosis. The expanded panel of the biomarkers increases the likelihood of accurate diagnosis in the pathology practice without genomic sequencing. As discussed above in the molecular features of endometrial cancer, alteration of MMR genes, PTEN and PAX2, is unlikely in ESC cases. Loss of any PTEN or PAX2, or MMR protein expression, is consistent with endometrioid carcinoma. One such example is presented in Figure 9.47.
- Rely more on morphology. We would like to reiterate that we should rely on morphology over immunophenotype to make the diagnosis when discrepancy occurs. When morphology of tumor is clearly not ESC, we should not order the immunostains.

With the points illustrated above, the majority ESC cases can be accurately diagnosed.

PROGNOSTIC AND PREDICTIVE FACTORS

It is well established that SEIC is likely to be associated with extrauterine disease in the absence of myometrial invasion or presence of any other serous neoplasm outside of the uterus.[71–74] That is to say that histologic type of endometrial serous carcinoma, no matter with or without myometrial invasion, bears a poor prognosis. However, ESC with earlier stage has a better survival than cases with advanced stage.[75,76] The overall 5-year survival rate for ESC is 36% and 10-year survival is only 18%.

Table 9.3 Immunophenotypes of endometrial clear-cell carcinoma, ESC and endometrioid carcinoma

Biomarkers	Clear-cell carcinoma	ESC	Endometrioid carcinoma
ER and/or PR	Low level or negative	Negative	Strong positive
P53	Mostly wild type, occasional mutated type	Mutated type	Mostly wild type, rarely mutated type
Napsin A	>85% positive	<8% positive	Negative
p504S (AMCAR)	75% positive	15% positive	22% positive
HNF-1β	Positive	Negative	Negative
Squamous cell markers (p40, p63 and CK5/6)	Negative	Negative	Positive in area of squamous metaplasia

Abbreviation: ESC, endometrial serous carcinoma.

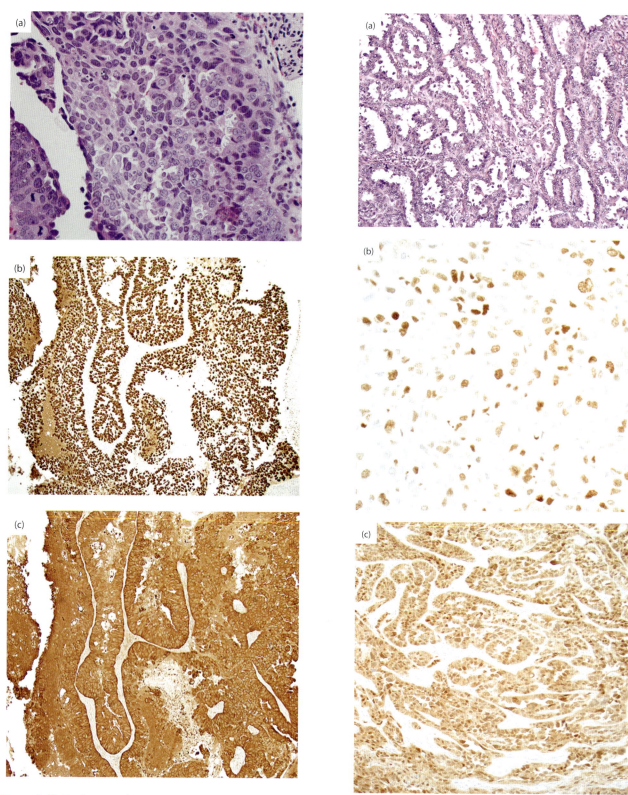

Figure 9.45 Endometrial serous carcinoma with p53 and p16 stains. Morphologically, this cancer is compatible with endometrial serous carcinoma (H&E, a). It is supported by mutational type p53 stain (b) and diffusely positive for p16 (c).

Figure 9.46 Endometrial carcinoma with ambiguous morphology. This endometrial adenocarcinoma shows intermediate nuclear grade and focal hobnail nuclei. It is not typical of endometrioid or serous carcinoma (a). Immunohistochemical stain with p53 shows patchy positive or wild type staining pattern (b); but p16 is intermediate to strong and diffuse (c). A diagnosis of FIGO grade 2 endometrioid carcinoma is rendered in this scenario.

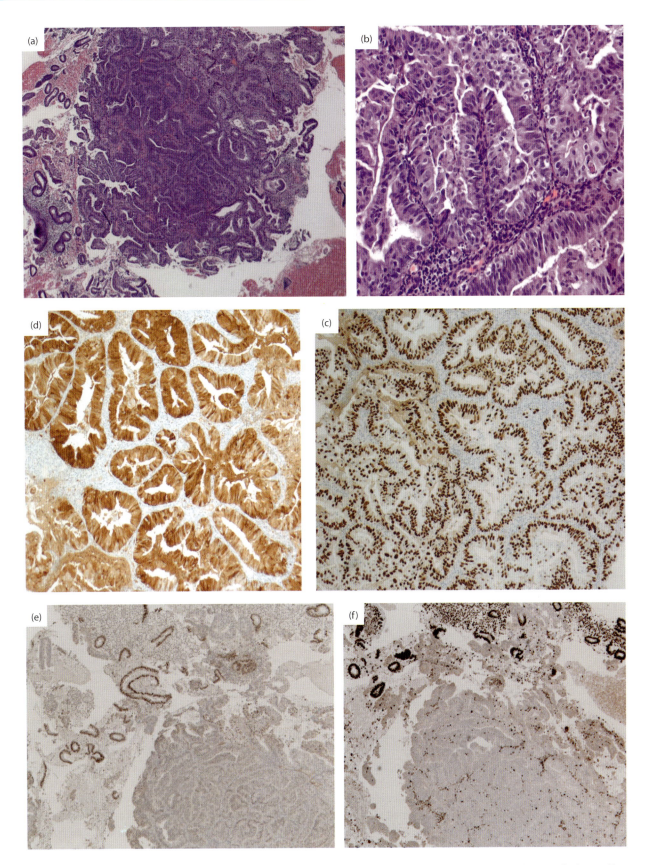

Figure 9.47 Endometrial carcinoma with ambiguous morphology. This endometrial adenocarcinoma morphologically is also ambiguous with a concern for endometrial serous carcinoma (a and b, H&E). Immunohistochemical stains initially show mutational type of p53 (c) and diffuse stain of p16 (d). Because of relatively low nuclear grade, additional stains show loss of Pax2 (e) and loss of MSH6 (f). The final diagnosis for this case is FIGO grade 2 endometrioid carcinoma.

Although *TP53* is commonly mutated in ESC, it is not an ideal marker demonstrated by p53 immunostain alone since many endometrioid carcinomas also have mutational staining pattern as discussed above. Copy-number high genotype obtained by molecular sequencing analysis represents the most reliable predictive factor of poor survival for patients with endometrial cancer.[12]

CLEAR-CELL CARCINOMA

CLINICAL FEATURES

Endometrial clear-cell carcinoma (ECCC) occurs mostly in postmenopausal women, with an average age of 65 years. Similar to ESC, it is more common in Africa and America than in Asia. Classic clinical presentation is abnormal bleeding. Some patients with ECCC may have a history of pelvic radiation, tamoxifen treatment and synthetic progestin usage.

It used to be considered as a cancer with a poor prognosis similar to patients with ESCs. However, recent molecular sequencing studies demonstrate that ECCCs constitute a histologically and genetically heterogeneous group of tumors with varying outcomes.[77]

PROGNOSTIC AND PREDICTIVE FACTORS

The overall survival varies greatly, from 21% to 75%, probably reflecting the heterogenicity of the disease.[78–80] According to the FIGO Annual Report 2006, 5-year overall survival was 62.5% for patients with this histological type compared with 83.2% for those with endometrioid carcinoma of the endometrium.[81]

PATHOLOGIC FINDINGS

Similar to other endometrial cancers, ECCC may present with variable size of tumor masses ranging from grossly barely visible to large masses with irregular infiltrative borders and frank tumor necrosis. It may also occur in an endometrial polyp.

Microscopically, ECCCs may display papillary (Figure 9.48), tubular/ tubulocystic (Figure 9.49) or solid architectures (Figure 9.50). Nuclear atypia is prominent, with marked nuclear pleomorphism and irregular nucleoli. The papillae are often short and branching, with broad-based hyalinized stoma. Large, polygonal tumor cells have clear to eosinophilic cytoplasm with glycogen and distinct margins (Figure 9.51). Occasionally, tumor cells can be small, flat or low columnar or hobnail shaped (Figure 9.52). Densely eosinophilic extracellular globules or hyaline bodies may be present. Putative precursor lesions with isolated glands or endometrial surface epithelia (within an otherwise normal endometrial region) that display cytoplasmic clarity or eosinophilia with varying degrees of nuclear atypia[82] may be present in the noncancerous area. Benign endometrium is usually atrophic, not hyperplastic.

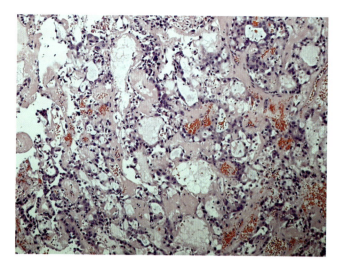

Figure 9.48 Clear-cell carcinoma. Cancer cells with clear cytoplasm are sitting in the hyaline stroma.

IMMUNOHISTOCHEMISTRY

ECCCs are typically negative for both ER and PR. Expression of p53 and p16 are usually less than that of ESC (Figure 9.53), but sometimes can be diffusely positive.

There are several relatively specific biomarkers developed recently for ECCCs. Napsin A is positive in 85% of ECCCs (Figure 9.54), only 8% in ESCs and 0% in endometrioid carcinoma.[30] Therefore, positive expression of Napsin A is supportive of ECCC diagnosis.

AMCAR (p504S) also demonstrates relative specificity for ECCC (Figure 9.55), with positivity in 75% of the cases and about 15% in ESC and 22% in endometrioid carcinoma cases.[30] Therefore, it is less sensitive and specific than Napsin A.

HNF-1β is another biomarker used to aid the diagnosis of ECCC.[83] However, the frequent expression in secretory endometrium, endometriosis and endometrioid carcinoma with secretory changes limits its clinical utility.

MOLECULAR FEATURES

There are limited data showing genetic or molecular features of ECCC due to its low incidence. However, a TCGA study revealing the molecular features of ECCC has been done recently. It shows that all molecular subgroups, including POLE mutation, MMR-deficient, copy-number low and copy-number high, are basically evenly distributed within the ECCC cases analyzed.[77] From this perspective, ECCC represents a heterogenous group of endometrial cancer with previously defined morphology. Future studies with molecular approach will be more informative in diagnosis as well as in clinical management.

DIFFERENTIAL DIAGNOSIS

By convention, differential diagnosis for ECCCs covers the following aspects.

Clear-cell carcinoma / Differential diagnosis 139

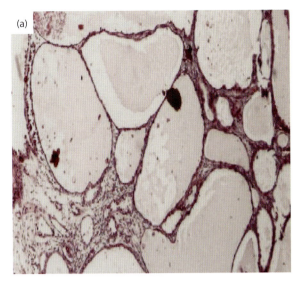

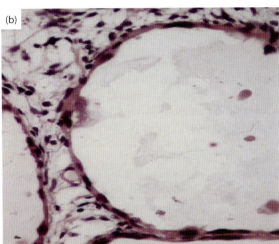

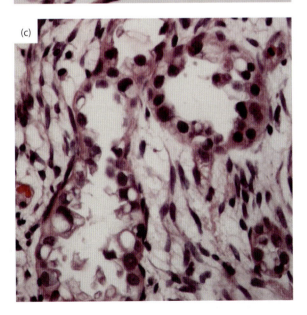

Figure 9.49 Clear-cell carcinoma with cystic tubular growth pattern. A dominant cystic growth pattern is seen in low power (a). Cancer cells in this growth pattern may show flat single layer of atypical cells (b) or cells with highly atypical nuclei with hobnail features (c).

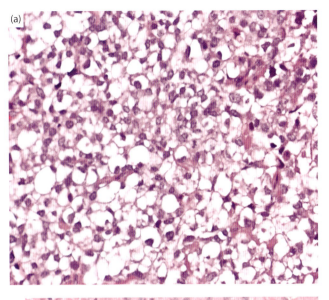

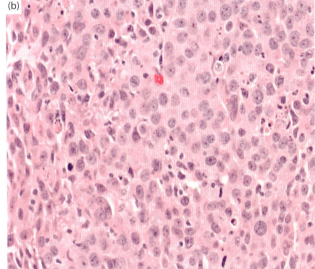

Figure 9.50 Clear-cell carcinoma with solid-growth pattern. Clear-cell carcinoma of the endometrium shows many cancer cells with abundant clear cytoplasm (a). Clear-cell carcinoma sometimes may have eosinophilic cytoplasm (b).

Arias-Stella (A-S) reaction. A-S reaction is caused by increased gonadotropin stimulation during pregnancy. Affected endometrial glands can show marked nuclear atypia. Smudgy nuclei are often present. Epithelial cells are usually enlarged with abundant eosinophilic to vacuolated cytoplasm. Cells often protrude into lumen imparting hobnail appearance. It can be confused with clear-cell carcinoma. However, unlike clear-cell carcinoma, the mitotic activity in A-S reaction is typically absent (Figure 9.56), while clear cell carcinoma usually lack smudgy nuclei. In addition, decidualized stroma, young age and cessation of menstruation are useful clues for the A-S reaction.

ESC. Cases of ESC may show focal clear cytoplasm. Cancer cells of ECCC may lack cytoplasm clearing. In those situations, the distinction between these two entities can

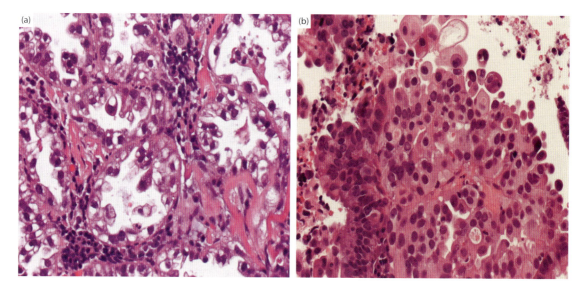

Figure 9.51 Clear-cell carcinoma. Intraluminal papillae (a) and partial solid-growth pattern with individual detached cancer cells (b) are other morphologic features of an endometrial clear-cell carcinoma.

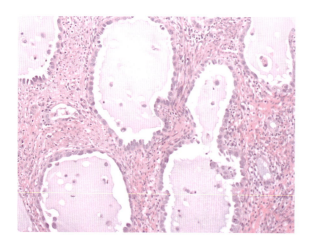

Figure 9.52 Clear-cell carcinoma. In the cystic growth pattern, cancer cells of the clear-cell carcinoma can be small, flat or low columnar or hobnail shaped.

be problematic. Microscopically, nucleoli of ECCC are less prominent than those of ESC. Characteristically, ECCCs commonly have hyalinized stroma, which is not present in ESC. In addition, hobnailing nuclei are more prominent in ECCC than in ESC. In difficult cases, the panel of immunostains, including p53, p16, ER, Napsin A and p504S, is useful to facilitate the diagnosis.

Endometrioid carcinoma. One of the diagnostic pitfalls surrounding endometrioid carcinomas with prominent squamous differentiation is the confusion with clear-cell carcinoma when the squamous component has extensive cytoplasmic clearing. This is caused by abundant glycogenation of squamous cytoplasm and should not be mistaken for true clear-cell differentiation or solid component of ECCC. In this situation, absence of significant cytologic atypia, as well as lack of hobnail appearance, is a clue of squamous differentiation, as is the absence of architectural features (fibrous and

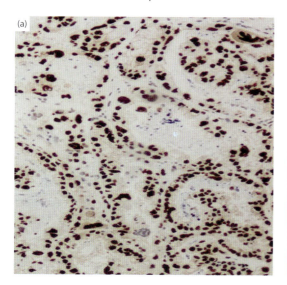
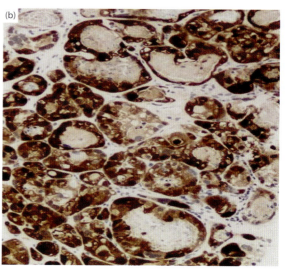

Figure 9.53 Clear-cell carcinoma with p53 staining. The expression of p53 (a) and p16 (b) are usually less than that of ESC.

Clear-cell carcinoma / Differential diagnosis 141

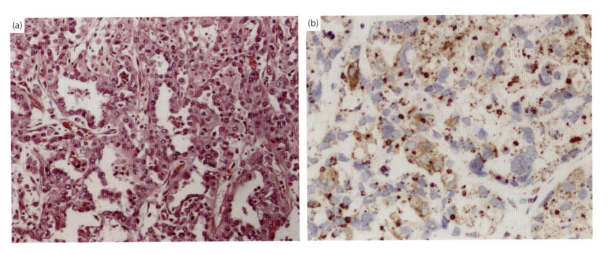

Figure 9.54 Clear cell carcinoma with Napsin A stain. Clear-cell carcinoma (a) shows chunky and granular staining pattern of Napsin A (b).

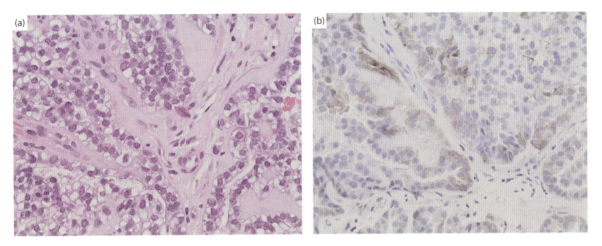

Figure 9.55 Clear cell carcinoma with AMCAR (p504S) stain. Clear-cell carcinoma (a) shows focal granular stains of AMCAR (p504S) in cytoplasm (b).

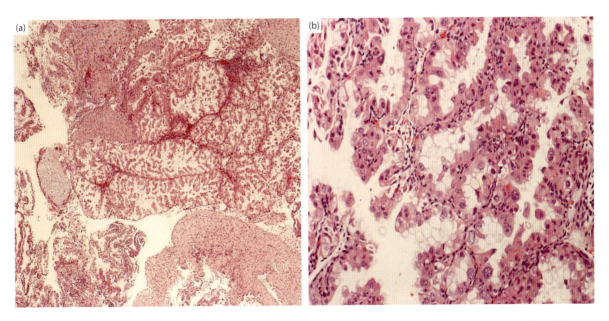

Figure 9.56 Endometrium with A-S reaction. Many hypersecretory endometrial glands are present (a). These hypersecretory glands have hobnail features, but lack of mitosis (b).

hyalinized stroma, tubulocystic growth) indicative of ECCC. Finally, the clear-cell changes in squamous differentiation often merge with areas of more conventional endometrioid carcinoma, further supporting squamous-like clear cytoplasmic changes rather than a true ECCC. Again, immunohistochemical stains with squamous cell markers as well as markers of ECCC will facilitate the diagnosis (Table 9.3).

UNDIFFERENTIATED AND DEDIFFERENTIATED CARCINOMA

By definition, endometrial undifferentiated carcinoma is a highly malignant carcinoma without specific lineage differentiation. Dedifferentiated carcinoma is composed of two dramatically different cancer components with one as undifferentiated carcinoma and the other as low-grade (FIGO 1 or 2) endometrial carcinoma.

CLINICAL FEATURES

The age of onset is about a decade younger than that of serous or clear-cell carcinoma, with a median age of approximately 50 years.[84] The behavior of these cancers is highly aggressive, with recurrence or death from tumor in 55%–95% of affected women.[84,85] However, it is recently found that such cancers may have a very good prognosis if POLE mutation is present.[86]

PATHOLOGIC FINDINGS

Undifferentiated carcinoma is characterised by a patternless, solid, sheet-like growth of tumor cells (Figure 9.57).

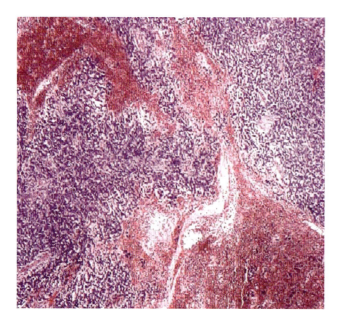

Figure 9.57 Undifferentiated carcinoma. Sheets of cancer cells without any clue of histologic differentiation are seen. Frank tumor necrosis is present.

There are no nests, papillae, glands, trabeculae or spindled patterns. The tumor is composed of small to intermediate sized, discohesive round to ovoid shaped cells, resembling large-cell lymphoma, high-grade endometrial stromal sarcoma or small-cell carcinoma. The tumor nuclei may show vesicular chromatin pattern and prominent nucleoli. Focal squamous differentiation, myxoid changes, rhabdoid differentiation, neuroendocrine differentiation (less than 10%) and spindle cells may be present. Frequent mitoses, apoptosis and frank tumor necrosis are commonly present.

Dedifferentiated carcinoma is composed of otherwise typical undifferentiated carcinoma and a secondary low-grade (FIGO 1 or 2) endometrioid carcinoma (Figure 9.58). These two components are typically present adjacent to rather than admixed with each other.

IMMUNOHISTOCHEMISTRY

The majority of undifferentiated carcinomas show patchy strong positivity to cytokeratin, with some cases showing diffuse positivity or throughout negativity. Even in cases of patchy positivity, the positive tumor cells demonstrate strong reactivity to cytokeratin. In our own experience, CK 7 is the most useful in this setting. This is an important feature to distinguish it from mesenchymal malignancy. Tumors are generally negative for both ER and PR. Focal neuroendocrine differentiation (less than 10% of tumor volume) is common, with some of tumor cells reactive to neuroendocrine markers such as chromogranin A, synaptophysin, and CD56. About half of the cases show loss of MMR protein expression. In dedifferentiated carcinomas, the low-grade endometrioid carcinoma components have the identical immunophenotypical profile as in endometrioid carcinoma.

MOLECULAR FEATURES

Approximately 50% of tumors display high microsatellite instability (MSI), with most of the cases due to hypermethylation of MLH1 promotor. A subset of cases arises in individuals with Lynch syndrome which is due to the mutation of MMR genes,[70,84] and approximately 11% of cases contain POLE mutations.[86]

DIFFERENTIAL DIAGNOSIS

The main differential diagnoses for undifferentiated carcinoma include poorly differentiated or FIGO grade 3 endometrioid carcinoma, neuroendocrine carcinoma and mesenchymal malignancy. As described above, undifferentiated carcinoma shows a patternless feature without any clue of histologic differentiation. In contrast, poorly differentiated or FIGO grade 3 endometrioid carcinoma often shows focal areas of glandular differentiation, which is haphazardly admixed with the solid components. Immunohistochemically, partial maintenance of

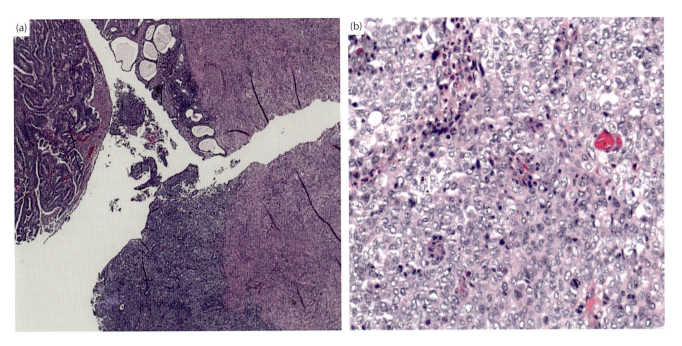

Figure 9.58 Dedifferentiated carcinoma of the endometrium. Well-differentiated adenocarcinoma is present in the left upper left corner, while undifferentiated component is present in the mid-low part (a). Magnified undifferentiated carcinoma shows sheets of malignant cells without any recognisable histological pattern (b).

ER expression is common in FIGO grade 3 cancers, while it is commonly absent in undifferentiated carcinoma. Cytokeratin (CK7) is likely diffusely positive in FIGO grade 3 cancers but only patchy or focally positive in undifferentiated carcinoma. Regarding neuroendocrine carcinoma and poorly differentiated carcinoma with neuroendocrine differentiation, we arbitrarily use 10% neuroendocrine differentiation as a dividing line. The diagnosis of undifferentiated carcinoma is made when neuroendocrine differentiation is less than 10% of the tumor volume. In contrast, if neuroendocrine markers, typically more than 2, are positive in more than 10% of the tumor volume, the diagnosis of neuroendocrine carcinoma is appropriate. Mesenchymal malignancies such as undifferentiated endometrial sarcoma or leiomyosarcoma are other entities in the differential diagnosis list. At close examination at both low and high magnitudes, we should find at least focally spindled pleomorphic cells, which are suggestive of sarcomas. In addition to CK7, multiple cytokeratin markers are negative, which will be important clues separating undifferentiated carcinoma from other mesenchymal malignancy. Other markers such as smooth muscle markers and cyclin D1 may also help to confirm sarcoma. Leiomyosarcomas are positive for smooth-muscle markers such as desmin and H-caldesmon. It is known that approximately 50% of undifferentiated endometrial sarcomas show overexpression of cyclin D1 but featured uniform nuclei.[87] Therefore, positive cyclin D1 expression is supportive for an undifferentiated endometrial sarcoma. Although leiomyosarcoma or undifferentiated endometrial sarcoma can be focally positive for cytokeratin, positive expression of the smooth-muscle markers or cyclin D1 is sufficient for leimyosarcoma or undifferentiated endometrial sarcoma. When all the markers including cytokeratins are negative and the tumor is morphologically ambiguous, a diagnosis of undifferentiated neoplasm should be considered.

The differential diagnosis for dedifferentiated carcinoma typically include mixed carcinoma and FIGO grade 3 endometrioid carcinoma. By definition, a mixed endometrial carcinoma is composed of two or more different histological types of endometrial carcinoma, at least one of which is of serous or clear cell.[88] The key is to identify the undifferentiated carcinoma component of the tumor, which should lack cytological or histological features of serous or clear-cell carcinoma. When still in doubt based on morphology, serous carcinoma markers (such as p53, p16, ER, PR, et al.), or clear-cell carcinoma markers (such as Napsin A and p504S) can be helpful. Most importantly, serous carcinoma and clear cell carcinoma are usually strongly positive for cytokeratin, while undifferentiated carcinoma should only be focal patchy positivity. High-grade or FIGO grade 3 endometrioid carcinomas also contain solid components as well as areas of well-differentiated carcinoma. However, the two dramatically different components in these cancers are typically admixed with each other, and areas of intermediate grade or semi-solid components are commonly present. Occasionally, collision tumors or poorly differentiated squamous cell carcinoma metastasizing into a uterus with a well-differentiated endometrioid carcinoma may happen. The second component of a collision tumor is likely to be of a different histology than an undifferentiated component in dedifferentiated carcinoma. A history of cervical squamous cell carcinoma will facilitate the diagnosis of cancer involvement in the endometrium.

REFERENCES

1. Bokhman JV. Two pathogenetic types of endometrial carcinoma. *Gynecol Oncol* 1983;15:10–7.
2. Fadare O, Zheng W. Insights into endometrial serous carcinogenesis and progression. *Int J Clin Exp Pathol* 2009;2:411–32.
3. Sherman ME, Bur ME, Kurman RJ. p53 in endometrial cancer and its putative precursors: Evidence for diverse pathways of tumorigenesis. *Hum Pathol* 1995;26:1268–74.
4. Coller HA, Grandori C, Tamayo P et al. Expression analysis with oligonucleotide microarrays reveals that MYC regulates genes involved in growth, cell cycle, signaling, and adhesion. *Proc Natl Acad Sci U S A* 2000;97:3260–5.
5. Risinger JI, Maxwell GL, Chandramouli GV et al. Microarray analysis reveals distinct gene expression profiles among different histologic types of endometrial cancer. *Cancer Res* 2003;63:6–11.
6. Zorn KK, Bonome T, Gangi L et al. Gene expression profiles of serous, endometrioid, and clear cell subtypes of ovarian and endometrial cancer. *Clin Cancer Res* 2005;11:6422–30.
7. Clarke BA, Gilks CB. Endometrial carcinoma: Controversies in histopathological assessment of grade and tumour cell type. *J Clin Pathol* 2010;63: 410–5.
8. Fadare O, Zheng W, Crispens MA et al. Morphologic and other clinicopathologic features of endometrial clear cell carcinoma: A comprehensive analysis of 50 rigorously classified cases. *Am J Cancer Res* 2013;3:70–95.
9. Han G, Soslow RA, Wethington S et al. Endometrial carcinomas with clear cells: A study of a heterogeneous group of tumors including interobserver variability, mutation analysis, and immunohistochemistry with HNF-1beta. *Int J Gynecol Pathol* 2015;34: 323–33.
10. Felix AS, Brasky TM, Cohn DE et al. Endometrial carcinoma recurrence according to race and ethnicity: An NRG Oncology/Gynecologic Oncology Group 210 Study. *Int J Cancer* 2017.
11. Gilks CB, Oliva E, Soslow RA. Poor interobserver reproducibility in the diagnosis of high-grade endometrial carcinoma. *Am J Surg Pathol* 2013;37: 874–81.
12. Cancer Genome Atlas Research Network, Kandoth C, Schultz N, Cherniack AD et al. Integrated genomic characterization of endometrial carcinoma. *Nature* 2013;497:67–73.
13. Rose PG. Endometrial carcinoma. *N Engl J Med* 1996;335:640–9.
14. Lukanova A, Lundin E, Micheli A et al. Circulating levels of sex steroid hormones and risk of endometrial cancer in postmenopausal women. *Int J Cancer* 2004;108:425–32.
15. Hampel H, Frankel W, Panescu J et al. Screening for Lynch syndrome (hereditary nonpolyposis colorectal cancer) among endometrial cancer patients. *Cancer Res* 2006;66:7810–7.
16. Lynch HT, Lynch P, Lanspa S et al. Review of the Lynch syndrome: History, molecular genetics, screening, differential diagnosis, and medicolegal ramifications. *Clin Genet* 2009;76:1–8.
17. Hitchins MP, Ward RL. Constitutional (germline) MLH1 epimutation as an aetiological mechanism for hereditary non-polyposis colorectal cancer. *J Med Genet* 2009;46:793–802.
18. Huth C, Kloor M, Voigt AY et al. The molecular basis of EPCAM expression loss in Lynch syndrome-associated tumors. *Mod Pathol* 2012;25:911–6.
19. Tutlewska K, Lubinski J, Kurzawski G. Germline deletions in the EPCAM gene as a cause of Lynch syndrome–literature review. *Hered Cancer Clin Pr* 2013;11:9.
20. Clarke BA, Cooper K. Identifying Lynch syndrome in patients with endometrial carcinoma: Shortcomings of morphologic and clinical schemas. *Adv Anat Pathol* 2012;19:231–8.
21. Mills AM, Liou S, Ford JM et al. Lynch syndrome screening should be considered for all patients with newly diagnosed endometrial cancer. *Am J Surg Pathol* 2014;38:1501.
22. Folkins AK, Longacre TA. Hereditary gynaecological malignancies: Advances in screening and treatment. *Histopathology* 2013;62:2–30.
23. Mahdi H, Mester JL, Nizialek EA et al. Germline PTEN, SDHB-D, and KLLN alterations in endometrial cancer patients with Cowden and Cowden-like syndromes: An international, multicenter, prospective study. *Cancer* 2015;121:688–96.
24. Ni Y, Zbuk KM, Sadler T et al. Germline mutations and variants in the succinate dehydrogenase genes in Cowden and Cowden-like syndromes. *Am J Hum Genet* 2008;83:261–8.
25. Shu CA, Pike MC, Jotwani AR et al. Uterine cancer after risk-reducing salpingo-oophorectomy without hysterectomy in women with *BRCA* mutations. *JAMA Oncol* 2016;2:1434–40.
26. Liang SX, Pearl M, Liang S et al. Personal history of breast cancer as a significant risk factor for endometrial serous carcinoma in women aged 55 years old or younger. *Int J Cancer* 2011;128:763–70.
27. Zheng W, Schwartz PE. Serous EIC as an early form of uterine papillary serous carcinoma: Recent progress in understanding its pathogenesis and current opinions regarding pathologic and clinical management. *Gynecol Oncol* 2005;96:579–82.
28. Zheng W, Xiang L, Fadare O, Kong B. A proposed model for endometrial serous carcinogenesis. *Am J Surg Pathol* 2011;35:e1–4.
29. Jia L, Liu Y, Yi X et al. Endometrial glandular dysplasia with frequent p53 gene mutation: A genetic

evidence supporting its precancer nature for endometrial serous carcinoma. *Clin Cancer Res* 2008;14:2263–9.
30. Fadare O, Desouki MM, Gwin K et al. Frequent expression of napsin A in clear cell carcinoma of the endometrium: Potential diagnostic utility. *Am J Surg Pathol* 2014;38:189–96.
31. Frimer M, Khoury-Collado F, Murray MP, Barakat RR, Abu-Rustum NR. Micrometastasis of endometrial cancer to sentinel lymph nodes: Is it an artifact of uterine manipulation? *Gynecol Oncol* 2010;119:496–9.
32. Todo Y, Kato H, Okamoto K et al. Isolated tumor cells and micrometastases in regional lymph nodes in stage I to II endometrial cancer. *J Gynecol Oncol* 2016;27:e1.
33. Alkushi A, Abdul-Rahman ZH, Lim P et al. Description of a novel system for grading of endometrial carcinoma and comparison with existing grading systems. *Am J Surg Pathol* 2005;29:295–304.
34. Guan H, Semaan A, Bandyopadhyay S et al. Prognosis and reproducibility of new and existing binary grading systems for endometrial carcinoma compared to FIGO grading in hysterectomy specimens. *Int J Gynecol Cancer* 2011;21:654–60.
35. Ali A, Black D, Soslow RA. Difficulties in assessing the depth of myometrial invasion in endometrial carcinoma. *Int J Gynecol Pathol* 2007;26:115–23.
36. Quick CM, Laury AR, Monte NM, Mutter GL. Utility of PAX2 as a marker for diagnosis of endometrial intraepithelial neoplasia. *Am J Clin Pathol* 2012;138:678–84.
37. Stewart C, Brennan B, Leung Y, Little L. MELF pattern invasion in endometrial carcinoma: Association with low grade, myoinvasive endometrioid tumours, focal mucinous differentiation and vascular invasion. *Pathology* 2009;41:454–9.
38. Zaino RJ. Unusual patterns of endometrial carcinoma including MELF and its relation to epithelial mesenchymal transition. *Int J Gynecol Pathol* 2014;33:357–64.
39. Nofech-Mozes S, Ackerman I, Ghorab Z et al. Lymphovascular invasion is a significant predictor for distant recurrence in patients with early-stage endometrial endometrioid adenocarcinoma. *Am J Clin Pathol* 2008;129:912–7.
40. Prat J. Prognostic parameters of endometrial carcinoma. *Hum Pathol* 2004;35:649–62.
41. Krizova A, Clarke BA, Bernardini MQ et al. Histologic artifacts in abdominal, vaginal, laparoscopic, and robotic hysterectomy specimens: A blinded, retrospective review. *Am J Surg Pathol* 2011;35:115–26.
42. Haltia UM, Butzow R, Leminen A, Loukovaara M. FIGO 1988 versus 2009 staging for endometrial carcinoma: A comparative study on prediction of survival and stage distribution according to histologic subtype. *J Gynecol Oncol* 2014;25:30–5.
43. Watanabe Y, Satou T, Nakai H et al. Evaluation of parametrial spread in endometrial carcinoma. *Obstet Gynecol* 2010;116:1027–34.
44. Dabbs DJ, Sturtz K, Zaino RJ. The immunohistochemical discrimination of endometrioid adenocarcinomas. *Hum Pathol* 1996;27:172–7.
45. Ansari-Lari MA, Staebler A, Zaino RJ, Shah KV, Ronnett BM. Distinction of endocervical and endometrial adenocarcinomas: Immunohistochemical p16 expression correlated with human papillomavirus (HPV) DNA detection. *Am J Surg Pathol* 2004;28:160–7.
46. Schultheis AM, Martelotto LG, De Filippo MR et al. TP53 Mutational Spectrum in Endometrioid and Serous Endometrial Cancers. *Int J Gynecol Pathol* 2016;35:289–300.
47. Alvarez T, Miller E, Duska L, Oliva E. Molecular profile of grade 3 endometrioid endometrial carcinoma: Is it a type I or type II endometrial carcinoma? *Am J Surg Pathol* 2012;36:753–61.
48. Hussein YR, Weigelt B, Levine DA et al. Clinicopathological analysis of endometrial carcinomas harboring somatic POLE exonuclease domain mutations. *Mod Pathol* 2015;28:505–14.
49. Long Q, Peng Y, Tang Z, Wu C. Role of endometrial cancer abnormal MMR protein in screening Lynch-syndrome families. *Int J Clin Exp Pathol* 2014;7:7297–303.
50. Wang Y, Wang Y, Li J et al. Lynch syndrome related endometrial cancer: Clinical significance beyond the endometrium. *J Hematol Oncol* 2013;6:22.
51. Colombo N, Creutzberg C, Amant F et al. ESMO-ESGO-ESTRO Consensus Conference on Endometrial Cancer: Diagnosis, treatment and follow-up. *Ann Oncol* 2016;27:16–41.
52. Mutter GL, Ince TA, Baak JP et al. Molecular identification of latent precancers in histologically normal endometrium. *Cancer Res* 2001;61:4311–4.
53. Monte NM, Webster KA, Neuberg D, Dressler GR, Mutter GL. Joint loss of PAX2 and PTEN expression in endometrial precancers and cancer. *Cancer Res* 2010;70:6225–32.
54. Kurman RJ, Norris HJ. Evaluation of criteria for distinguishing atypical endometrial hyperplasia from well-differentiated carcinoma. *Cancer* 1982;49:2547–59.
55. Ross JC, Eifel PJ, Cox RS, Kempson RL, Hendrickson MR. Primary mucinous adenocarcinoma of the endometrium: A clinicopathologic and histochemical study*. *Am J Surg Pathol* 1983;7:715–29.
56. Yoo SH, Park BH, Choi J et al. Papillary mucinous metaplasia of the endometrium as a possible precursor of endometrial mucinous adenocarcinoma. *Mod Pathol* 2012;25:1496–507.
57. Kurman RJ, Carcangiu ML, Herrington CS, Young RH. *WHO Classification of Tumours of Female Reproductive Organs*. Vol. 6. ISBN - 9789283224358, 2014.
58. Zheng W, Yang GC, Godwin TA, Caputo TA, Zuna RE. Mucinous adenocarcinoma of the endometrium with intestinal differentiation: A case report. *Hum Pathol* 1995;26:1385–8.

59. Hendrickson M, Ross J, Eifel P, Martinez A, Kempson R. Uterine papillary serous carcinoma: A highly malignant form of endometrial adenocarcinoma. *Am J Surg Pathol* 1982;6:93–108.
60. Berman JJ, Albores-Saavedra J, Bostwick D et al. Precancer: A conceptual working definition – results of a Consensus Conference. *Cancer Detect Prev* 2006;30:387–94.
61. Brinton LA, Felix AS, McMeekin DS et al. Etiologic heterogeneity in endometrial cancer: Evidence from a Gynecologic Oncology Group trial. *Gynecol Oncol* 2013;129:277–84.
62. Wild PJ, Ikenberg K, Fuchs TJ et al. p53 suppresses type II endometrial carcinomas in mice and governs endometrial tumour aggressiveness in humans. *EMBO Mol Med* 2012;4:808–24.
63. Network CGAR. Integrated genomic characterization of endometrial carcinoma. *Nature* 2013;497:67–73.
64. Haley SL, Malhotra RK, Qiu S, Eltorky ME. The immunohistochemical profile of atypical eosinophilic syncytial changes vs serous carcinoma. *Ann Diagn Pathol* 2011;15:402–6.
65. Silva EG, Jenkins R. Serous carcinoma in endometrial polyps. *Mod Pathol* 1990;3:120–8.
66. Yasuda M, Katoh T, Hori S et al. Endometrial intraepithelial carcinoma in association with polyp: Review of eight cases. *Diagn Pathol* 2013;8:25.
67. McCluggage WG, Sumathi VP, McManus DT. Uterine serous carcinoma and endometrial intraepithelial carcinoma arising in endometrial polyps: Report of 5 cases, including 2 associated with tamoxifen therapy. *Hum Pathol* 2003;34:939–43.
68. Carcangiu ML, Chambers JT. Uterine papillary serous carcinoma: A study on 108 cases with emphasis on the prognostic significance of associated endometrioid carcinoma, absence of invasion, and concomitant ovarian carcinoma. *Gynecol Oncol* 1992;47:298–305.
69. Kuhn E, Kurman RJ, Vang R et al. TP53 mutations in serous tubal intraepithelial carcinoma and concurrent pelvic high-grade serous carcinoma--evidence supporting the clonal relationship of the two lesions. *J Pathol* 2012;226:421–6.
70. Garg K, Leitao MM, Jr., Wynveen CA et al. p53 overexpression in morphologically ambiguous endometrial carcinomas correlates with adverse clinical outcomes. *Mod Pathol* 2010;23:80–92.
71. Carcangiu ML, Tan LK, Chambers JT. Stage IA uterine serous carcinoma: A study of 13 cases. *Am J Surg Pathol* 1997;21:1507–14.
72. Hui P, Kelly M, O'Malley DM, Tavassoli F, Schwartz PE. Minimal uterine serous carcinoma: A clinicopathological study of 40 cases. *Mod Pathol* 2005;18: 75–82.
73. Semaan A, Mert I, Munkarah AR et al. Clinical and pathologic characteristics of serous carcinoma confined to the endometrium: A multi-institutional study. *Int J Gynecol Pathol* 2013;32:181–7.
74. Wheeler DT, Bell KA, Kurman RJ, Sherman ME. Minimal uterine serous carcinoma: Diagnosis and clinicopathologic correlation. *Am J Surg Pathol* 2000;24:797–806.
75. Giuntoli RL, 2nd, Gerardi MA, Yemelyanova AV et al. Stage I noninvasive and minimally invasive uterine serous carcinoma: Comprehensive staging associated with improved survival. *Int J Gynecol Cancer* 2012;22:273–9.
76. Seward S, Ali-Fehmi R, Munkarah AR et al. Outcomes of patients with uterine serous carcinoma using the revised FIGO staging system. *Int J Gynecol Cancer* 2012;22:452–6.
77. DeLair DF, Burke KA, Selenica P et al. The genetic landscape of endometrial clear cell carcinomas. *J Pathol* 2017;243:230–41.
78. Abeler VM, Kjorstad KE. Clear cell carcinoma of the endometrium: A histopathological and clinical study of 97 cases. *Gynecol Oncol* 1991;40:207–17.
79. Ryu SY, Park SI, Nam BH et al. Prognostic significance of histological grade in clear-cell carcinoma of the ovary: A retrospective study of Korean Gynecologic Oncology Group. *Ann Oncol* 2009;20:1032–6.
80. Gadducci A, Cosio S, Spirito N, Cionini L. Clear cell carcinoma of the endometrium: A biological and clinical enigma. *Anticancer Res* 2010;30: 1327–34.
81. Creasman WT, Odicino F, Maisonneuve P et al. Carcinoma of the corpus uteri. FIGO 26th Annual Report on the Results of Treatment in Gynecological Cancer. *Int J Gynaecol Obstet* 2006;95(Suppl 1):S105–43.
82. Fadare O, Liang SX, Ulukus EC, Chambers SK, Zheng W. Precursors of endometrial clear cell carcinoma. *Am J Surg Pathol* 2006;30:1519–30.
83. Fadare O, Parkash V, Gwin K et al. Utility of alpha-methylacyl-coenzyme-A racemase (p504s) immunohistochemistry in distinguishing endometrial clear cell carcinomas from serous and endometrioid carcinomas. *Hum Pathol* 2013;44:2814–21.
84. Tafe LJ, Garg K, Chew I, Tornos C, Soslow RA. Endometrial and ovarian carcinomas with undifferentiated components: Clinically aggressive and frequently underrecognized neoplasms. *Mod Pathol* 2010;23:781–9.
85. Altrabulsi B, Malpica A, Deavers MT et al. Undifferentiated carcinoma of the endometrium. *Am J Surg Pathol* 2005;29:1316–21.
86. Rosa-Rosa JM, Leskela S, Cristobal-Lana E et al. Molecular genetic heterogeneity in undifferentiated endometrial carcinomas. *Mod Pathol* 2016;29: 1390–8.
87. Kurihara S, Oda Y, Ohishi Y et al. Coincident expression of beta-catenin and cyclin D1 in endometrial stromal tumors and related high-grade sarcomas. *Mod Pathol* 2010;23:225–34.
88. World Health Organization. *WHO Classification of Tumors of Female Reproductive Organs.* International Agency for Research on Cancer. Lyon, 2014.

10

Gestational trophoblastic disease

Normal histology and immunohistochemistry of trophoblasts	147
Hydatidiform mole	149
Androgenetic/biparental mosaic/chimeric conceptions	157
Abnormal (non-molar) villous lesion	160
Choriocarcinoma	161
Placental site trophoblastic tumor	164
Epithelioid trophoblastic tumor	166
Exaggerated placental site	168
Placental site nodule	169
Other unclassified trophoblastic lesions	170
References	171

The diagnosis of gestational trophoblastic disease (GTD) has witnessed revolutionary changes in recent years with improved availability of immunohistochemistry and genotyping as valuable adjuncts. These tools have enabled pathologists to precisely delineate the genomic aberrations in morphologically abnormal conceptions, but they also expose the shortcomings of pure histomorphologic analysis and uncover complex pathologic conditions that were previously unrecognised. Immunohistochemistry is playing an increasing role in the diagnosis of hydatidiform mole and trophoblastic tumors, but the pitfalls of interpretation have also been better recognised. Surgical pathologists now require a much more sophisticated understanding of the pathology of gestational trophoblastic disease in order to identify cases that require additional investigations and interpret the ancillary studies within the clinical context.

The term 'gestational trophoblastic disease' can be viewed as comprising three groups of conditions. The first group is made up of gestations with morphologic abnormalities in the chorionic villi and variable extent of trophoblastic proliferations, mostly related to the underlying genomic constitutions. This includes hydatidiform mole and androgenetic/biparental mosaic/chimeric conceptions, as well as several types of abnormal (non-molar) villous lesions. The second group is trophoblastic tumors, which include choriocarcinoma, placental site trophoblastic tumor and epithelioid trophoblastic tumor. The third group is non-neoplastic trophoblastic lesions, mainly comprising exaggerated placental site and placental site nodule, together with some rare lesions that are being characterised.

NORMAL HISTOLOGY AND IMMUNOHISTOCHEMISTRY OF TROPHOBLASTS

The three types of trophoblasts are cytotrophoblasts, syncytiotrophoblasts and intermediate trophoblasts. Their functions and morphologic characteristics are listed in Table 10.1.[1,2]

IMMUNOHISTOCHEMICAL MARKERS FOR VARIOUS TYPES OF TROPHOBLASTS

The following antibodies are most commonly applied as trophoblastic markers in daily practice:

Table 10.1 Types of trophoblasts

	Function	Histologic morphology
Cytotrophoblasts	Proliferative 'stem cells' that differentiate into syncytiotrophoblasts or intermediate trophoblasts	Small uniform round nuclei with scant cytoplasm
Syncytiotrophoblasts	Mature differentiated cells that synthesize hormones and regulate gas/nutrient exchange	Multinucleated with abundant amphophilic cytoplasm

(*Continued*)

Table 10.1 (Continued) Types of trophoblasts

	Function	Histologic morphology
Intermediate trophoblasts (IT)		
1. Villous intermediate trophoblasts	Anchor villi to implantation site	Polygonal cells with clear to eosinophilic cytoplasm (Figure 10.1)
2. Implantation site intermediate trophoblasts	Infiltrate the decidua, myometrium and spiral arteries	Large pleomorphic hyperchromatic nuclei with abundant eosinophilic cytoplasm, occasionally multinucleated (Figure 10.2)
3. Chorionic-type intermediate trophoblasts	Form the chorionic laeve of fetal membranes	Polygonal cells with clear to eosinophilic cytoplasm, occasionally multinucleated (Figure 10.3)

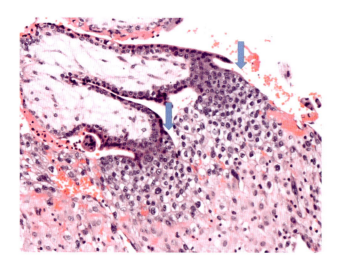

Figure 10.1 Normal histology of trophoblasts at implantation site. Note the polar proliferation of villous intermediate trophoblasts (arrows).

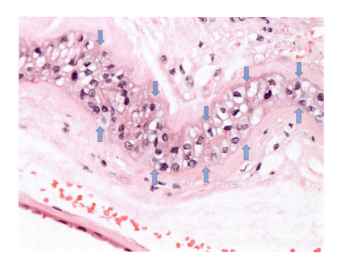

Figure 10.3 Normal histology of chorionic-type intermediate trophoblasts. Chorionic-type intermediate trophoblasts are typically polygonal with clear to pale eosinophilic cytoplasm (arrows).

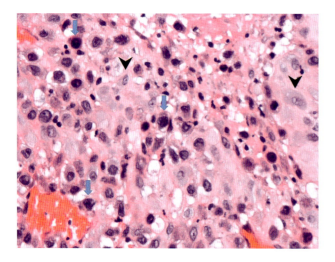

Figure 10.2 Normal histology of implantation-site intermediate trophoblasts. The intermediate trophoblasts are recognised by their enlarged hyperchromatic nuclei (arrows), in contrast with the pale nuclei of the intervening decidua (arrow heads).

- *Cytokeratin (such as AE1/AE3 or Cam5.2)*: Positive in all types of trophoblasts.[3]
- *Human chorionic gonadotropin (β-hCG)*: Positive in syncytiotrophoblasts, negative in cytotrophoblasts, variable in intermediate trophoblasts (mostly staining multinucleated intermediate trophoblasts).[4]
- *Human placental lactogen (hPL)*: Positive in intermediate trophoblasts and syncytiotrophoblasts, negative in cytotrophoblasts.[4]
- *α-inhibin*: Positive in syncytiotrophoblasts, negative in cytotrophoblasts, variable in intermediate trophoblasts (mainly staining implantation site intermediate trophoblasts).[5,6]
- *p63*: Positive in chorionic-type intermediate trophoblasts and cytotrophoblasts, negative in villous/implantation site intermediate trophoblasts and syncytiotrophoblasts.[7]
- *Other markers*: Mel-CAM (CD146) and HLA-G were proposed as markers of intermediate trophoblasts.[8,9] Placental alkaline phosphatase (PLAP) was reported to be mostly positive in chorionic-type intermediate trophoblasts.[1]

Apart from the above trophoblastic markers, other immunohistochemical markers relevant to diagnosing trophoblastic diseases include p57, Ki67 and SALL4.

HYDATIDIFORM MOLE

Hydatidiform moles (HM) are genetically abnormal conceptions with excessive paternal contribution to the fetal genomes. Although traditionally they are classified into complete or partial moles by morphologic features, the genomic constitutions have now superseded morphology as the defining criteria for typing of hydatidiform mole. This has also been endorsed by the 2014 WHO Classification of Tumours of Female Reproductive Organs.[10]

MOLECULAR PATHOLOGY OF HYDATIDIFORM MOLE

The genetic findings and etiology of complete and partial hydatidiform moles are compared in Table 10.2.[11,12]

CLINICAL SIGNIFICANCE OF HYDATIDIFORM MOLE

The risk of persistent gestational trophoblastic neoplasia (GTN) for hydatidiform mole is quoted as follows, mostly based on earlier studies:[12]

- Complete hydatidiform mole (CHM) – 15%–20% risk of persistent GTN; 2%–3% risk of choriocarcinoma
- Partial hydatidiform mole (PHM) – 0.5%–5% risk of persistent GTN; <0.5% risk of choriocarcinoma

More recent studies with genotypic verification of the histologic diagnosis appear to suggest a much lower risk of persistent GTN for hydatidiform mole, with a study suggesting 5% risk of CHM[13] and several suggesting minimal risk for PHM.[13,14]

CLINICAL AND MACROSCOPIC FEATURES OF HYDATIDIFORM MOLE

In the past, well-developed CHM typically presented with vaginal bleeding in the second trimester, large uterine size, hyperemesis and toxemia, associated with 'snowstorm' appearance without fetal development on ultrasound scan.[12,15] Macroscopically, these cases could have a large volume of specimen containing grape-like vesicles (Figure 10.4). Currently, most cases of CHM are detected earlier and present as missed miscarriage in the first trimester.[15] PHM typically

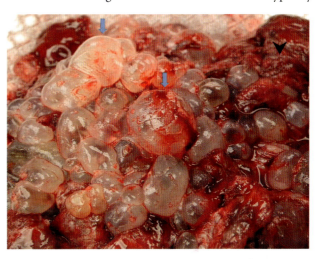

Figure 10.4 Macroscopic appearance of well-developed complete hydatidiform mole. The florid vesicle formation observed here (arrows) is uncommonly observed nowadays. This case features CHM coexisting with a normal twin delivered at term, with normal-appearing placental tissue (arrow head) in the background. (Courtesy of Dr. So Chun Hong, Department of Obstetrics and Gynaecology, Princess Margaret Hospital, Hong Kong.)

Table 10.2 Molecular pathology of hydatidiform mole

	Complete hydatidiform mole (CHM)	Partial hydatidiform mole (PHM)
Key genetic feature	Purely androgenetic (paternal only) fetal genome	Excessive paternal contribution to fetal genome, with maternal genome present
Pathogenesis	Fertilization of an ovum with absent or loss of maternal haploid genome, by a single sperm with chromosomal reduplication (monospermic/homozygous; 80%–90%), or two sperms (dispermic/heterozygous; 10%–20%)	Fertilization of an ovum with normal maternal haploid genome, by two sperms (dispermic/heterozygous PHM; >90%), or a single sperm (monospermic/homozygous PHM; <10%) with reduplication of paternal genome or diploid paternal genome
Typical genomic composition	Androgenetic diploidy (46, XX/46, XY)	Diandric-monogynic triploidy (69, XXY/69, XXX/69, XYY)
Possible variations of genomic compositions	• Tetraploid CHM • CHM with gain or loss of chromosomes • Biparental CHM (familial biparental CHM associated with maternal *NLRP7/KHDC3L* mutation)	• Tetraploid PHM • PHM with gain or loss of chromosomes

present slightly later in the first trimester or second trimester with vaginal bleeding or as missed or incomplete miscarriage. Macroscopically, CHM in the first trimester and PHM may have no gross abnormality or only mild hydropic change.

HISTOLOGIC FEATURES OF HYDATIDIFORM MOLE

The histologic features of complete hydatidiform mole vary with the gestational age. Classical morphologic features are generally seen in well-developed CHM evacuated in the second trimester, whereas the morphology of very early CHM (VECHM) evacuated in the first trimester is usually quite different. The morphologic features of partial hydatidiform mole are now recognised as being more variable than previously believed, with significant overlap with those of various abnormal (non-molar) villous lesions (see separate section Abnormal [non-molar] villous lesion). The overall morphologic characteristics are presented in Table 10.3.[12]

Issues relating to the differential diagnosis between various molar and non-molar conditions are presented in Table 10.4.

IMMUNOHISTOCHEMISTRY FOR P57

p57 is a protein encoded by a strongly paternally imprinted gene (*CDKN1C* on chromosome 11), such that its expression

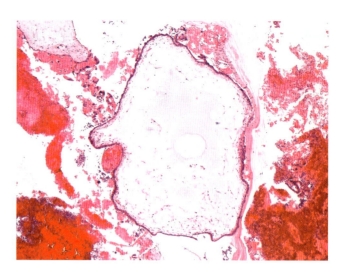

Figure 10.5 Complete hydatidiform mole with cistern formation in the villi, characterised by an empty space containing fluid and devoid of villous stromal cells.

in cytotrophoblasts and villous stromal cells requires the presence of the maternal allele of the gene.[17] This implies that p57 would not be expressed in these cells for CHM (due to absence of maternal genome), with preserved expression for PHM or non-molar conceptions.

Before assessing the staining in the chorionic villi, it is useful to assess the internal controls. No matter in CHM,

Table 10.3 Histologic features of hydatidiform mole

	CHM (well-developed)	**VECHM (very early CHM in first trimester)**	**PHM**
Chorionic villi	Diffusely enlarged villi with marked villous hydrops and cistern formation (Figures 10.5 and 10.6)	Villous size usually normal, often polypoid and 'cauliflower-shaped'	Typically two populations of villi, one enlarged with villous hydrops and the other normal-sized fibrotic (Figure 10.11), but sometimes forming a spectrum
Trophoblastic proliferation	Circumferential trophoblastic proliferation (Figure 10.7)	Mild trophoblastic proliferation, usually random and non-polar (Figure 10.9)	Mild trophoblastic proliferation (Figure 10.12)
Trophoblastic atypia	Prominent cytologic atypia in implantation site trophoblasts (Figure 10.8)	Moderate trophoblastic atypia	No or mild trophoblastic atypia (Figure 10.13)
Villous stroma	Usually hypocellular with absence of vessels	Usually hypercellular and myxoid with stellate fibroblasts and prominent karyorrhexis (Figure 10.10)	Variable villous hydrops (Figure 10.14) with occasional cistern formation
Villous contour	Typically round and smooth but trophoblastic pseudo-inclusions are common	Trophoblastic pseudo-inclusions are less frequent	Irregular scalloped borders with syncytiotrophoblast knuckles and trophoblastic pseudo-inclusions (Figure 10.15)
Fetal development	Fetal (nucleated) red blood cells, although typically absent, could be present in CHM[16]	Fetal (nucleated) red blood cells, although typically absent, could be present in CHM[16]	Fetal (nucleated) red blood cells (Figure 10.16) and fetal development may be present

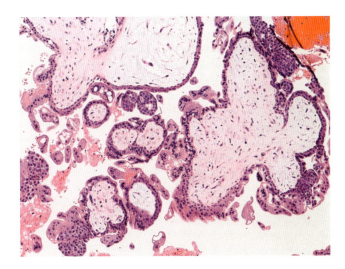

Figure 10.6 Complete hydatidiform mole. The smaller chorionic villi also display variable degree of villous hydrops and irregular villous contour.

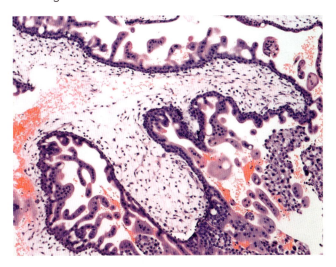

Figure 10.7 Complete hydatidiform mole. Note the circumferential trophoblastic proliferation.

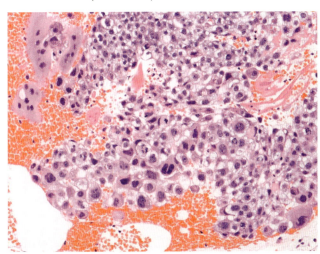

Figure 10.8 Complete hydatidiform mole. Trophoblastic atypia is typically seen in the intermediate trophoblasts. Mitotic activity may be observed.

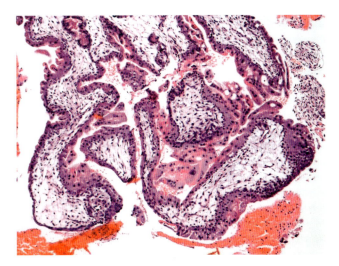

Figure 10.9 Very early complete hydatidiform mole. Note the typical myxoid hypercellular villous stroma with rich vasculature. Trophoblastic proliferation is relatively mild with random distribution.

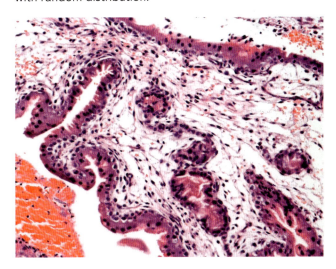

Figure 10.10 Very early complete hydatidiform mole. Note the irregular villous outline and karyorrhectic debris.

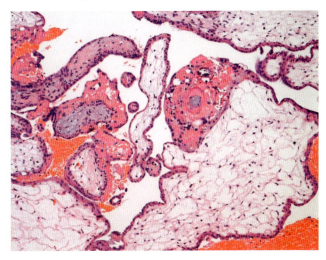

Figure 10.11 Partial hydatidiform mole. Note the coexistence of hydropic villi and fibrotic villi.

152 Gestational trophoblastic disease

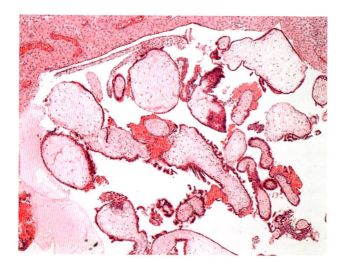

Figure 10.12 Partial hydatidiform mole. Mild trophoblastic proliferation may be observed.

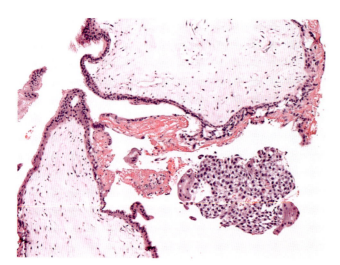

Figure 10.13 Partial hydatidiform mole. The absence of trophoblastic atypia is a helpful clue to distinguish from CHM.

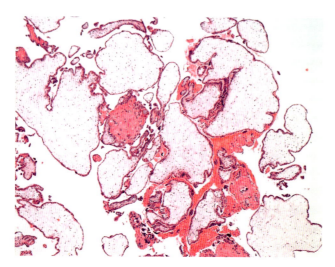

Figure 10.14 Partial hydatidiform mole. Hydropic villi with irregular scalloped borders are characteristic.

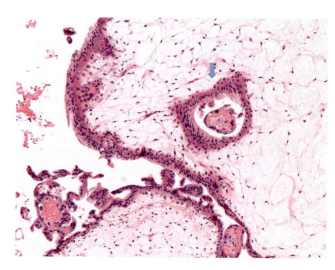

Figure 10.15 Partial hydatidiform mole with trophoblastic pseudo-inclusion (arrow).

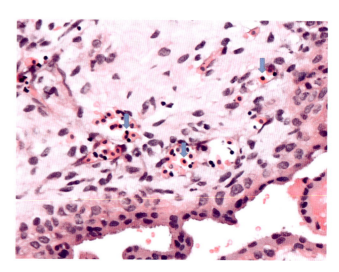

Figure 10.16 Partial hydatidiform mole. Fetal (nucleated) red blood cells (arrows) could be present in the villous vasculature.

PHM or non-molar conceptions, p57 is consistently negative in syncytiotrophoblasts but positive in intermediate trophoblasts and/or maternal decidua, irrespective of the genetic constitution.

Typical results and interpretation of p57 staining are listed in Box 10.1.[17]

However, a number of possible pitfalls and other abnormal staining patterns in the interpretation of p57 immunohistochemistry have now been recognised in the literature.[17] These important exceptions are listed in Table 10.5.[17]

GENOTYPING BY SHORT TANDEM REPEAT (STR) POLYMORPHISM ANALYSIS

Studies have found that the diagnostic reproducibility of hydatidiform moles, even combining morphology with p57 immunostaining, is still suboptimal when compared

Table 10.4 Common differential diagnostic difficulties in hydatidiform mole

Differential diagnosis	Key points for distinction and reporting
1. CHM or PHM?	• Trophoblastic atypia is usually helpful for recognising CHM. • Negative p57 staining would confirm CHM (Figure 10.17).
2. VECHM or non-molar (hydropic or early) gestation?	• Early non-molar gestation could have cellular myxoid villous stroma that mimics VECHM. • Hydropic abortion could have significant villous enlargement and edema with rare cisterns. • The pattern of trophoblastic proliferation is usually helpful, as non-molar gestations generally have polar trophoblastic proliferation instead of randomly distributed proliferation for VECHM. • Negative p57 staining would confirm CHM (Figure 10.18).
3. PHM or non-molar gestation?	• Hydropic abortion, chromosomal trisomy syndromes and digynic triploid gestations are possible mimics of PHM (see section on 'Abnormal (non-molar) villous lesion'). • Immunostaining for p57 is not helpful as both will be positive (Figure 10.19). • STR genotyping, if available, is able to distinguish PHM from the non-molar mimics. • In case of indeterminate cases based on histology and p57 result, the report could be signed out as 'products of gestation with hydropic change' or 'products of gestation with atypical features', with a comment describing the differential diagnosis and recommending serial hCG monitoring.
4. PHM or androgenetic/biparental mosaic/chimeric conception?	• Androgenetic/biparental mosaic/chimeric conceptions may display hydropic irregular villi without trophoblastic hyperplasia, with or without a second component resembling CHM (see section on 'Androgenetic/biparental mosaic/chimeric conceptions'). • Immunostaining for p57 may be helpful, but careful correlation with morphology is needed in view of possible heterogeneity of villi. STR genotyping could differentiate the two possibilities although the allelic profiles of mosaic/chimeric gestations may be difficult to interpret. • If there is a component with morphology compatible with CHM and negative p57 staining, the case could be reported as CHM, with a comment on the possibility of a mosaic/chimeric component. • If there is no definite CHM component, but the villi show discordant pattern for p57, the case may be reported as 'products of gestation with features suspicious of androgenetic/biparental mosaic/chimeric conception', with a comment that definitive differential diagnosis from PHM requires genotyping analysis and serial hCG monitoring is recommended. • If the p57 result is inconclusive or equivocal, the case may be reported as 'products of gestation with atypical features' with a comment indicating that PHM could not be excluded and serial hCG monitoring is recommended.

Abbreviation: STR, short tandem repeat.

to genotypic data as the gold standard.[23,24] With the availability of short tandem repeat (STR) genotyping using commercial kits, this valuable method is increasingly adopted by clinical laboratories for definitive diagnosis of hydatidiform moles and other genetically abnormal conceptions.

Principles and technical aspects of STR genotyping

Short tandem repeats (STRs) are repetitive sequences of DNA that show high degrees of polymorphism among individuals, each allele characterised by a specific number of repeats. At each STR locus, an individual inherits one paternal allele and one maternal allele. Commercially available kits for STR genotyping generally cover a number of STR loci from different chromosomes (including the amelogenin locus for sex chromosomes). Using DNA extracted from the maternal decidua and the chorionic villi, the allelic profiles can be compared to delineate the genetic composition of the gestation.

Murphy et al. outlined the detailed methodology for performing and interpreting STR analysis, with the key points summarized below.[25]

- H&E section of formalin-fixed paraffin-embedded (FFPE) tissue is reviewed to identify well-separated areas of maternal decidua and chorionic villi for microdissection. Care must be taken to avoid contamination of chorionic villi by maternal blood or decidua. Usually a smaller area with pure villi is preferable, excluding even a tiny fragment of maternal tissue.

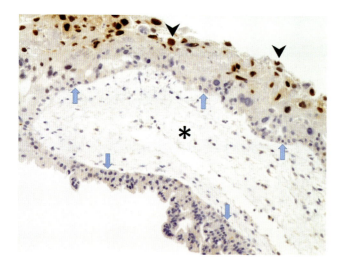

Figure 10.17 Complete hydatidiform mole. p57 immunohistochemistry demonstrates negative staining in the cytotrophoblasts (arrows) and villous stromal cells (asterisk), whereas the intermediate trophoblasts (arrow heads) serve as internal positive control.

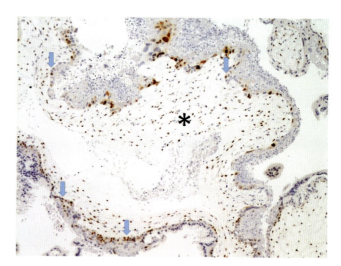

Figure 10.19 Partial hydatidiform mole. Positive p57 staining in the cytotrophoblasts (arrows) and villous stroma (asterisk) of this hydropic villus would help to exclude CHM.

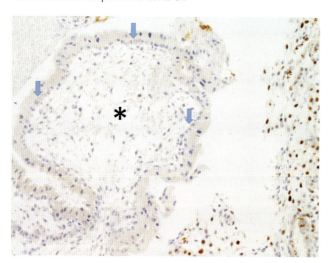

Figure 10.18 Very early complete hydatidiform mole. Negative staining for p57 in cytotrophoblasts (arrows) and villous stroma (asterisk) is a valuable diagnostic adjunct in difficult cases.

> **BOX 10.1: Typical results and interpretation of p57 immunohistochemistry**
>
> **p57 positive**
>
> - Defined as diffuse or extensive (>50%) staining of cytotrophoblasts and villous stromal cells[17]
> - Interpretation – consistent with non-molar specimen or PHM
>
> **p57 negative**
>
> - Defined as absent or limited (<10%) staining of cytotrophoblasts and villous stromal cells[17]
> - Interpretation – consistent with CHM

- Microdissection will be performed on unstained sections guided by annotated areas, followed by DNA extraction from the FFPE tissue.
- PCR amplification of the STR loci should be performed in duplicate. Analysis of the PCR product by capillary electrophoresis would identify the alleles (in the form of peaks) for maternal and villous tissue, respectively.
- For each allele identified in the villous tissue, it may be classified as paternal (non-maternal) or likely maternal (possibly paternal due to shared allele).
- For each locus with two alleles identified in the villous tissue, the allelic ratio can be calculated by dividing the peak height of the longer allele by the peak height of the shorter allele. The expected allelic ratio for diploidy is 1.0, but in practice a ratio between 0.61 and 1.17 would be considered consistent with diploidy. The expected allelic ratio for triploidy is either 0.5 or 2.0, but in practice a ratio of 0.33–0.60 or 1.5–2.0 would be considered consistent with triploidy.

Interpretation of STR genotyping data

Typical profiles of STR genotyping data for chorionic villous tissue include the following:[12,17,25]

- Non-molar gestation – one maternal allele and one non-maternal allele of similar peak height
- Complete hydatidiform mole – exclusively non-maternal alleles (one or two at each locus) with absence of maternal allele (Figure 10.20)
- Partial hydatidiform mole – one maternal allele, in combination with either (a) one non-maternal allele of approximately double the peak height or (b) two non-maternal alleles of similar peak height

Table 10.5 Pitfalls in interpretation of p57 immunohistochemistry

1. **Equivocal pattern** (staining in 10%–50% of the cytotrophoblasts and villous stromal cells)	• PHM is a possibility, as found in a prospective study.[18] • Technical factors in staining performance and antigen degradation related to improper fixation might be implicated. • Consider genotyping for definitive diagnosis.
2. **Staining pattern conflicting with morphology or genotyping** (so-called 'aberrant' staining)	• For morphologically typical CHM with diffuse positive p57 staining, the possibility of CHM with retained maternal chromosome 11 should be considered.[19,20] The presence of maternal allele on chromosome 11 would lead to p57 expression. Genotyping should be considered if available. • Similarly, PHM with loss of maternal chromosome 11 has been found to have negative p57 staining.[21] • Before undertaking genotyping for cases with unexpected staining pattern, careful evaluation of the morphology and immunostaining should be undertaken to look for any heterogeneity. Additional histologic sampling should be considered.
3. **Discordant pattern** (combination of positive/negative staining in cytotrophoblasts and villous stroma within individual villi, i.e. positive cytotrophoblasts and negative villous stroma, or vice versa)	• Androgenetic/biparental mosaic/chimeric conception has been found to be associated with discordant pattern of staining for p57.[17,22] • However, it has not been fully evaluated whether this staining pattern is sufficiently sensitive or specific for this particular group of lesions,[12] so the diagnosis of androgenetic/biparental mosaic/chimeric conception still requires genotyping to confirm and should not be solely made by p57 immunostaining.
4. **Divergent pattern** (two populations of villi with 2 different morphologies and 2 different staining patterns)	• For one population being negative and the other positive, consider the possibility of CHM coexisting with a non-molar twin gestation • For one population being positive and the other discordant, consider the possibility of androgenetic/biparental mosaic/chimeric conception • For one population being negative and the other discordant, consider the possibility of androgenetic/biparental mosaic/chimeric conception with CHM component • In any case showing divergent pattern, careful correlation of the villous morphology with the staining pattern is crucial to guide microdissection for genotyping analysis

Other possible conditions that may be detected by STR genotyping include digynic triploidy and chromosomal trisomies, as well as androgenetic/biparental mosaic/chimeric conceptions. Their respective genotyping profiles will be discussed in subsequent sections.

Pitfalls and problems with STR genotyping

Proper implementation of STR genotyping for clinical diagnosis requires a thorough awareness of its potential pitfalls. Certain common problems have been raised by Murphy et al. as listed below.[25]

- *Poor amplification* (usually related to suboptimal DNA quality in archived specimens) could lead to skewed peak heights that may be misinterpreted as triploidy.
- *Contamination of villous tissue with maternal tissue* could lead to falsely high maternal allele content, which may be misinterpreted as trisomy or triploidy. The presence of 20% of maternal tissue is sufficient to confound interpretation.
- *Not all loci are informative* in the entire panel, which may be related to the DNA quality (with difficulty amplifying the longer amplicons) or shared alleles.

Villous tissue showing allele(s) common to one or both maternal alleles would be difficult to ascertain the source of the allele(s).

Other rare scenarios of interpretation difficulties include familial biparental complete mole or egg donor pregnancy.[12]

UNUSUAL GENOTYPIC FINDINGS OR PRESENTATIONS IN HYDATIDIFORM MOLE

The foregoing discussion has focused on typical findings in complete and partial moles, which account for the majority of cases. However, there are uncommon cases with peculiar genotypic findings or clinical presentations that may be infrequently encountered.

Tetraploid hydatidiform mole

There are reported cases of tetraploid CHM[26,27] which usually show histologic features of CHM with p57 negative staining[28] and also carry risk of persistent GTN.[26] Rare cases of tetraploid PHM (with 3 paternal and 1 maternal chromosome complements) have also been recognised, with

156 Gestational trophoblastic disease

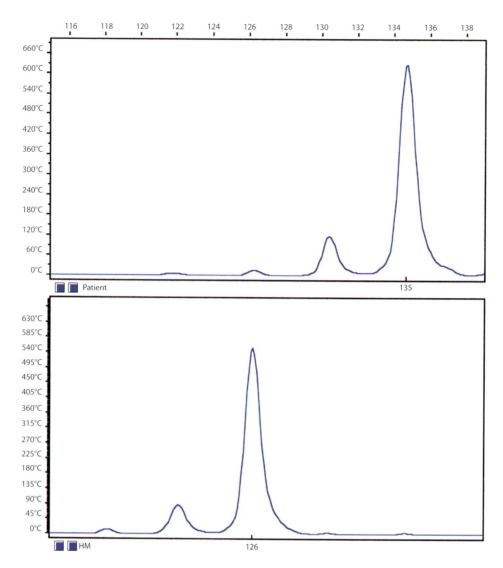

Figure 10.20 Microsatellite polymorphisms of the decidua (upper panel) and villi (lower panel) of a case of CHM. The patient is homozygous for the allele with amplification product 135 bp. The hydatidiform mole is homozygous giving rise to amplification product of 126 bp.

morphology compatible with PHM and p57 exhibiting positive but often diminished expression.[29]

Hydatidiform mole with gain or loss of chromosomes

As mentioned previously, rare cases of CHM could harbor additional chromosome(s) of maternal origin[19,20] which might lead to unexpected positive p57 staining results when involving chromosome 11. Conversely, loss of maternal chromosome 11 has been reported in PHM,[21] which could give rise to negative p57 staining.

Twin gestation with hydatidiform mole coexisting with non-molar gestation

There are many reported cases of twin pregnancy comprising CHM with normal fetus.[30–33] Histologic findings in these cases may display two distinct populations of villi, one resembling CHM and the other normal appearing, with divergent patterns of p57 staining.[17,31] Chorionic villi with morphologic features of placental mesenchymal dysplasia (PMD) may also be seen,[32] which might exhibit discordant p57 staining.[17,33,34] Current data suggest that these cases could be derived from a single oocyte fertilized by one or more spermatozoa.[30]

In contrast, twin gestations with PHM coexisting with non-molar gestation are even rarer.[35,36] It has been suggested that some earlier reported cases with diploid karyotype or no karyotypic data might represent CHM in twin pregnancy based on contemporary criteria.[35]

Recurrent hydatidiform mole

Patients with multiple molar pregnancies have been the subject of intense scientific interest.[37–39] Studies of these cases have revealed the underlying mechanisms in a subset of these patients, who have familial predilection for biparental complete hydatidiform moles related to germline mutation in the *NLRP7* or *KHDC3L* genes.[39] The current understanding of this intriguing condition is provided in Box 10.2. Nonetheless, there are patients with recurrent hydatidiform moles but genetically proven to be androgenetic (instead of biparental) without detectable germline mutation,[40,41] suggesting the presence of other unrecognised factors for this phenomenon.

BOX 10.2: Familial biparental hydatidiform mole (FBHM) and *NLRP7/KHDC3L* gene mutations

- Familial biparental hydatidiform mole (FBHM) is a rare, autosomal recessive condition characterised by inherited predisposition to develop complete hydatidiform mole of biparental diploid constitution.[37]
- Initially identified as an abnormal locus on chromosome 19q13.4,[38] germline mutation in the *NLRP7* gene (homozygous or compound heterozygous) has been identified as the underlying cause in many patients with FBHM.[42]
- *KHDC3L* gene mutation is another possible etiology in a smaller number of FBHM cases.[43]
- Histologically, biparental complete hydatidiform moles (BiCHM) share similar morphologic features as the conventional androgenetic CHM, although a minority of cases may exhibit a lesser degree of trophoblastic hyperplasia.[44]
- BiCHM shows negative staining for p57 in the cytotrophoblasts and villous stromal cells,[44] similar to usual CHM. However, STR genotyping would reveal the biparental diploid allelic profiles resembling non-molar pregnancy.
- In daily practice, when cases with negative p57 and apparently biparental diploid genotype (without family history or recurrent molar pregnancy) are encountered, the differential diagnosis of androgenetic/biparental mosaic/chimeric conception should also be carefully considered.[45]
- The discovery of the underlying biology of BiCHM has provided clues to the pathogenetic mechanisms for development of hydatidiform mole, which is believed to be a manifestation of defective genomic imprinting.[11]
- Studies have shown abnormal hypomethylation of paternally expressed genes (leading to overexpression) and hypermethylation of maternally expressed genes (leading to silencing) in BiCHM,[46,47] which suggest that abnormal genomic imprinting is the likely mechanism for trophoblastic hyperplasia and failure of fetal development in CHM.[11]

INVASIVE HYDATIDIFORM MOLE (INCLUDING METASTATIC MOLE)

Invasive mole is a form of persistent GTN that is defined by the presence of molar villi invading the myometrium, myometrial vessels or extrauterine sites.[10,48] Both CHM and PHM have been implicated in invasive mole. As cases of persistent GTN are generally managed without surgery, invasive mole is now seldom encountered in pathology specimens, mostly restricted to uncommon cases that require hysterectomy. In hysterectomy specimens, invasive mole is diagnosed by presence of molar villi directly invading myometrium without intervening decidua, or presence of molar villi within myometrial vessels. Lymphovascular invasion by atypical trophoblastic cells may be observed.[48] For some cases, trophoblastic proliferation with significant cytologic atypia that raises suspicion of an emerging choriocarcinoma could be present.[48] A diagnosis of choriocarcinoma arising from CHM (which is a controversial entity not recognized by some authorities) requires very stringent criteria, which should only be rendered in the presence of an infiltrative, cytologically malignant trophoblastic proliferation, morphologically indistinguishable from choriocarcinoma, which is separate from molar villi.[48]

Invasive mole involving extrauterine sites (usually lungs) may be referred to as metastatic mole, which requires presence of molar villi in the extrauterine site for diagnosis. Clinical or radiological evidence of extrauterine lesion alone might represent either metastatic mole or choriocarcinoma.

ANDROGENETIC/BIPARENTAL MOSAIC/CHIMERIC CONCEPTIONS

The concept of androgenetic/biparental mosaic/chimeric conception as a pathologic entity has only been recently characterised.[22,49] These conceptions are composed of two different cell lines, one with purely androgenetic genome (paternal only) and the other biparental.[22] The two cell lines may arise through mosaicism (due to mitotic error in a single zygote) or chimerism (due to fusion of two zygotes),[22] but it is believed that possible mechanisms include monospermic and dispermic fertilizations, endoreduplications and abnormal cell divisions.[22,45] The previously discussed scenario of twin gestation with CHM coexisting with non-molar gestation could be regarded as a form of chimerism at the placental level, thus sharing some features as described below.

MORPHOLOGIC FEATURES

Based on the study of 11 androgenetic/biparental mosaic/chimeric conceptions by Lewis et al., all cases contain villi of variable size and shape with hydropic enlargement but lacking trophoblastic hyperplasia (Figure 10.21), while six of these cases harbor an additional component of villi with trophoblastic hyperplasia equivalent to CHM (Figure 10.22).[22]

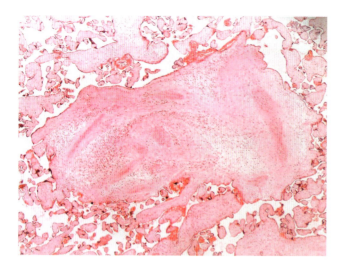

Figure 10.21 Androgenetic/biparental mosaic/chimeric conception (same case as Figure 10.4). Enlarged chorionic villi with stromal hypercellularity but without trophoblastic hyperplasia could be seen in such cases. The stem villus shown here also displays some morphologic resemblance to placental mesenchymal dysplasia (see Box 10.3).

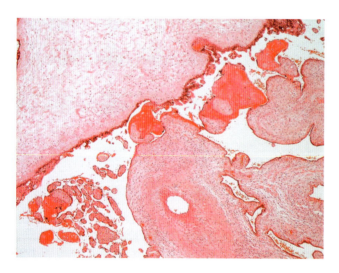

Figure 10.22 Androgenetic/biparental mosaic/chimeric conception (same case as Figure 10.4). Some of these cases may contain two populations of villi, including hydropic villi with trophoblastic hyperplasia comparable to CHM (upper left), as well as variably enlarged villi without trophoblastic hyperplasia.

In the villi without trophoblastic hyperplasia, cistern formation, trophoblastic inclusions and stromal hypercellularity were occasionally present.[22]

IMMUNOHISTOCHEMICAL AND GENOTYPING STUDIES

As reported in this study, a characteristic discordant pattern of p57 staining is commonly observed in the population of villi without trophoblastic hyperplasia, usually with positive staining in cytotrophoblasts and negative staining in villous stromal cells (Figure 10.23).[22] The component of

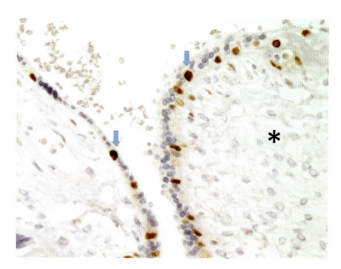

Figure 10.23 Androgenetic/biparental mosaic/chimeric conception (same case as Figure 10.4). Discordant pattern of p57 immunohistochemistry is typically seen in these cases, as reflected here by positive staining in cytotrophoblasts (arrows) and negative staining in villous stromal cells (asterisk).

villi with trophoblastic hyperplasia is generally negative for p57 as expected in CHM (Figure 10.24).[22] The presence of discordant p57 staining in androgenetic/biparental mosaic/chimeric conceptions has also been observed in other studies,[34] although the specificity of this pattern has not been adequately evaluated.[12]

STR genotyping studies performed on villi without trophoblastic hyperplasia could give complex allelic profiles with excess of paternal alleles (paternal:maternal allelic ratio usually >2:1), while the profile for villi with trophoblastic hyperplasia would demonstrate androgenetic diploidy (Figures 10.25 and 10.26).[22]

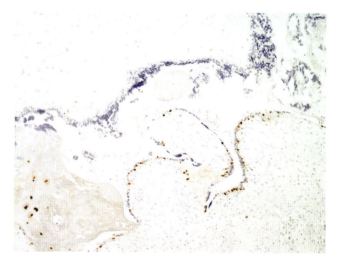

Figure 10.24 Androgenetic/biparental mosaic/chimeric conception (same case as Figure 10.4). Note the divergent pattern for p57 immunohistochemistry, featuring negative staining in the villi resembling CHM (upper) and discordant pattern for the villi without trophoblastic hyperplasia (lower).

Androgenetic/biparental mosaic/chimeric conceptions / Immunohistochemical and genotyping studies 159

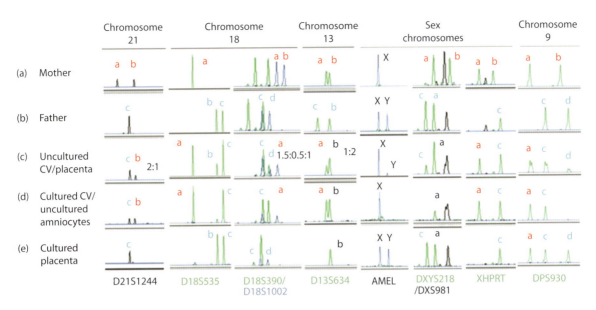

Figure 10.25 Quantitative fluorescent polymerase chain reaction (QF-PCR) study in a case of fetus coexisting with complete hydatidiform mole with trisomy 9 (same case as Figure 10.4). QF-PCR was performed on parental blood (a,b) and various tissues of the pregnancy (c–e) using short tandem repeat (STR) markers on chromosomes 21, 18, 13, 9, X and Y. The small panels showed the capillary electrophoresis data of 10 of the STR markers used. Small letter above the allelic peak represents maternal allele (red); paternal allele (blue) or shared maternal or paternal allele (black). The bottom panel indicates the name of the STR markers used. Results from cultured CV, same as uncultured amniocytes (d), showed normal 13, 18, 21, XX. Results from cultured placenta (e) showed paternally derived 13, 18, 21, XY and trisomy 9. Results of uncultured CV, same as uncultured placenta (c) showed a mosaic pattern of (d) and (e). CV, chorionic villi. (Reprinted with permission from Kan ASY et al. *J Obstet Gynaecol Res* 2018;44:955–9.)

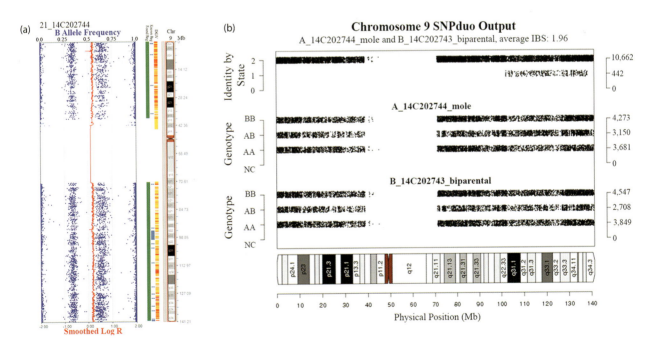

Figure 10.26 Single nucleotide polymorphism (SNP) studies performed on a case of fetus coexisting with complete hydatidiform mole (CHM) with trisomy 9 (same case as Figures 10.4 and 10.25). (a) Illumina HumanCytoSNP-12 microarray on cultured placental tissue (CHM) showing trisomy 9. (b) SNPduo analysis comparing SNP microarray genotyping data generated from CHM in the middle panel and cultured chorionic villi (fetus) in the lower panel. The data are consistent with the biparental fetal cell line containing one paternal and one maternal chromosome 9 that is identical to that carried by the CHM. The dispermic CHM also carries a segment of chromosome 9 (paternal) that is not present in the fetal cell line (identity by state = 1). (Reprinted with permission from Kan ASY et al. *J Obstet Gynaecol Res* 2018;44:955–9.)

> **BOX 10.3: Placental mesenchymal dysplasia – a morphologic entity with new genetic meanings**
>
> - Placental mesenchymal dysplasia (PMD) is the term used to describe the placental condition characterised by cystic structures in a large placenta, histologically demonstrating aneurysmal dilatation of chorionic plate and stem villous thick-walled vessels, hydropic stem villi with cisterns and absent trophoblastic proliferation.[50] Earlier studies have demonstrated diploid karyotype and thus distinguished them from PHM.[51]
> - While the fetus in PMD may be completely normal or growth-restricted, there is a well-known association with Beckwith-Wiedemann syndrome (BWS) in a subset of PMD cases.[50] BWS is associated with abnormal gene expression from an imprinted region of chromosome 11p15.5, which harbors the *CDKN1C* gene encoding the p57 protein.[50]
> - Genetic studies on cases of PMD have demonstrated the presence of androgenetic cell lines in the villi with morphologic features of PMD,[34,51] suggesting that androgenetic/biparental mosaicism is the underlying etiology of PMD, at least for some cases.
> - Discordant pattern for p57 staining has also been reported in cases of PMD.[34]
> - It has been postulated that the villi without trophoblastic hyperplasia in androgenetic/biparental mosaic/chimeric conceptions may represent an early form of placental mesenchymal dysplasia.[22]
> - With the current understanding of PMD, it appears that a substantial proportion of these cases could represent a morphologic manifestation of androgenetic/biparental mosaic/chimeric conception.

CLINICAL SIGNIFICANCE

Cases of persistent GTN have been seen associated with androgenetic/biparental mosaic/chimeric conceptions,[22,45] although the exact risk is difficult to ascertain with the small number of reported cases. It is believed that in view of the androgenetic cell lines and associated risk of persistent GTN in these conceptions, follow-up and management as for molar pregnancy would be recommended.[22]

ABNORMAL (NON-MOLAR) VILLOUS LESION

The term 'abnormal (non-molar) villous lesion' was introduced in the 2014 WHO Classification to describe a diverse group of gestations that may display histologic features mimicking partial hydatidiform mole, but are non-molar by genotype.[10] Examples of these conditions include hydropic abortions, chromosomal trisomy syndromes and digynic triploid conceptions. In these conditions, p57 immunohistochemistry would demonstrate preserved positivity in cytotrophoblasts and villous stromal cells, similar to PHM.[34]

HYDROPIC ABORTIONS

Hydropic abortions refer to any non-molar gestations with hydropic change in the villi. They usually show milder hydropic change than molar pregnancy, with smooth villous contour and absence of circumferential trophoblastic hyperplasia (Figure 10.27).[12] Polar trophoblastic proliferation at the anchoring villi can be seen. Trophoblastic atypia is absent. Rare cistern formation (Figure 10.28) or trophoblastic pseudo-inclusion might be occasionally encountered. The major differential diagnosis is PHM, which requires STR genotyping for definitive distinction in morphologically indeterminate cases.

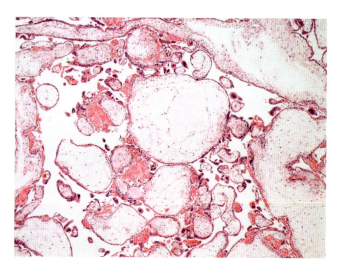

Figure 10.27 Hydropic abortion. Chorionic villi typically exhibit a spectrum of hydropic change without trophoblastic hyperplasia.

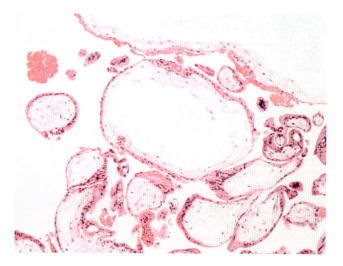

Figure 10.28 Hydropic abortion. Cistern may be rarely observed in the chorionic villi.

CHROMOSOMAL TRISOMY SYNDROMES

Gestations with trisomy in different chromosomes have been reported to display variable degrees of abnormal villous morphology, resembling PHM.[52,53] Possible findings include focal villous hydrops, trophoblastic hyperplasia, irregular villous outlines and trophoblastic pseudo-inclusions.[52,53] The degree of trophoblastic hyperplasia may be comparable to that in molar pregnancy, especially for trisomy involving chromosomes 7, 15, 21 and 22.[52] Differential diagnosis from PHM requires STR genotyping, which might also reveal the actual chromosome involved based on the allelic profile.[54]

DIGYNIC TRIPLOID CONCEPTIONS

Digynic triploid conceptions, which contain two sets of maternal chromosomes and one set of paternal chromosomes, are estimated to account for about one-third of triploid gestations, with no documented increased risk of persistent GTN.[55] These cases have been found to show irregular villous contours, trophoblastic pseudo-inclusions and mild trophoblastic hyperplasia, but usually no villous hydrops.[56] STR genotyping is able to differentiate these cases from PHM.

CHORIOCARCINOMA

Choriocarcinoma is a malignant trophoblastic neoplasm characterised by tumor cells resembling all three types of trophoblastic cells (cytotrophoblasts, syncytiotrophoblasts and intermediate trophoblasts),[57] which display overtly malignant nuclear features. Choriocarcinoma may be gestational or non-gestational, depending on whether the tumor develops from pregnancy. Non-gestational choriocarcinoma is rare and generally of germ cell origin, which is much less chemosensitive and has a poorer prognosis.[58] Gestational choriocarcinoma, in contrast, has a favorable response to chemotherapy.[58] The following description will focus on gestational choriocarcinoma only.

CLINICAL FEATURES

Gestational choriocarcinoma may present with vaginal bleeding, commonly coupled with features suggesting missed abortion or ectopic pregnancy, or fetal distress/demise in cases with concurrent pregnancy.[58] Over 50% of cases are preceded by complete hydatidiform mole, while the remaining cases may follow abortion (spontaneous or induced), normal pregnancy (term or preterm) or ectopic pregnancy.[58] Patients are usually within reproductive age, with the interval from previous pregnancy (if not concurrent) ranging from weeks to several years.[58]

MACROSCOPIC FEATURES

Gestational choriocarcinoma grossly manifests as a bulky mass in the uterine corpus with hemorrhage and necrosis on its cut surface. The intraplacental variant of choriocarcinoma may mimic an area of infarct within the placental disc.[59]

DIAGNOSTIC FEATURES

Typical histologic findings of choriocarcinoma include the following:

- Intimate admixture of mononucleate and multinucleated tumor cells resembling all three types of trophoblasts (Figure 10.29)
  - The mononucleate cells comprise smaller uniform cells with less cytoplasm, resembling cytotrophoblasts, and larger cells with more pleomorphic nuclei and amphophilic or eosinophilic cytoplasm, resembling intermediate trophoblasts.[57] Multinucleated cells resemble syncytiotrophoblasts. (Figures 10.30 and 10.31)
- Malignant nuclear features with marked nuclear pleomorphism and prominent nucleoli, with frequent mitotic figures including atypical forms (Figures 10.32 and 10.33)
- Hemorrhage and necrosis usually present in the background (a useful clue) (Figures 10.34 and 10.35)
- Chorionic villi usually absent
  - Traditionally, the presence of chorionic villi used to be considered incompatible with the diagnosis of choriocarcinoma. However, it has been increasingly recognised that choriocarcinoma could be diagnosed coexisting with complete hydatidiform mole or within placenta,[58] as elaborated below.

In rare circumstances, choriocarcinoma arising from complete hydatidiform mole may be diagnosed (with extreme caution and very stringent criteria) based on the presence of cytologically malignant trophoblastic proliferation

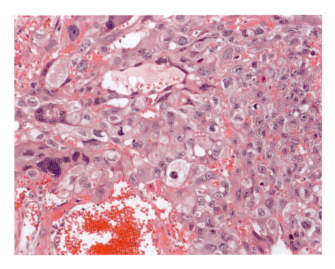

Figure 10.29 Choriocarcinoma. Typical admixture of overtly malignant cells, including mononucleate cells most of which resembling intermediate trophoblasts, as well as multinucleate cells that resemble syncytiotrophoblasts.

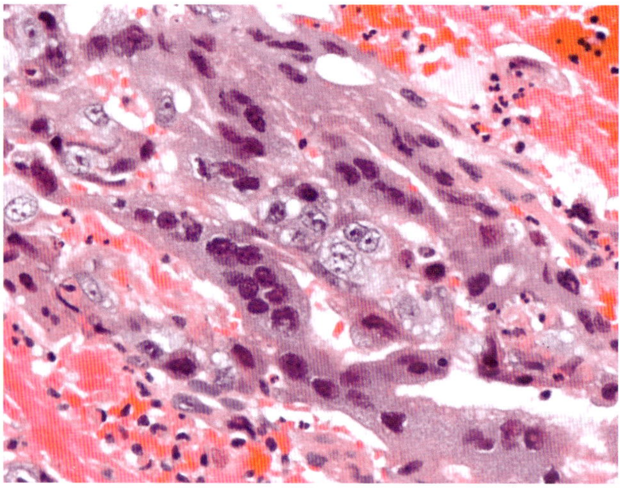

Figure 10.30 Choriocarcinoma. Note the intimate admixture of multinucleate and mononucleate tumor cells.

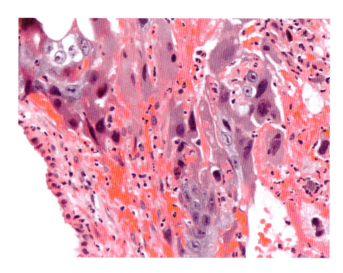

Figure 10.33 Choriocarcinoma. Note the contrast between tumor cells and the adjacent epithelium.

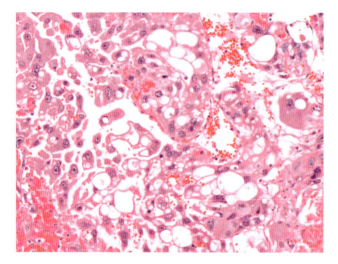

Figure 10.31 Choriocarcinoma. Cytoplasmic vacuolation is sometimes prominent in choriocarcinoma.

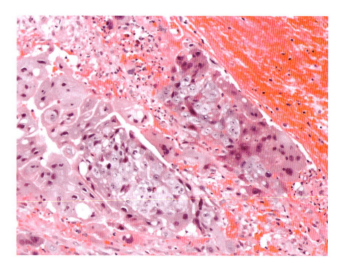

Figure 10.34 Choriocarcinoma. Tumor cells are usually present against a hemorrhagic background.

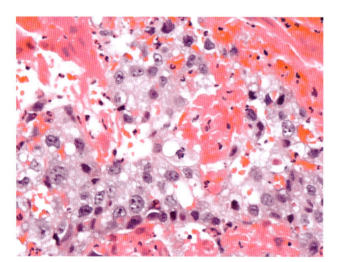

Figure 10.32 Choriocarcinoma. Note the malignant nuclear features of the mononucleate cells with mitotic activity.

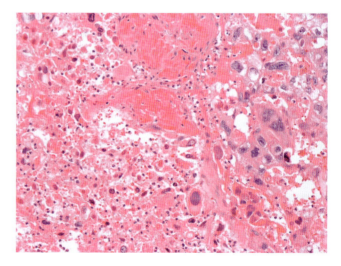

Figure 10.35 Choriocarcinoma. Hemorrhage and necrosis are important diagnostic clues.

morphologically indistinguishable from choriocarcinoma, that is separate from the molar villi.[48] It should be remembered that complete hydatidiform mole is commonly associated with quite significant atypia in the trophoblasts, which would not qualify as choriocarcinoma in the vast majority of cases.

Variant: Intraplacental choriocarcinoma

Intraplacental choriocarcinoma is a rare condition featuring cytologically malignant trophoblastic proliferation with classical morphology of choriocarcinoma, that arises directly from the chorionic villi of a placenta and extending into intervillous space.[59]

ANCILLARY STUDIES

The immunohistochemical profile of choriocarcinoma is as follows:

- Diffusely positive for cytokeratin[60]
- Generally positive for hCG (mainly in syncytiotrophoblasts and variable proportion of tumor cells)[61]
- Focally positive (usually in a minority of tumor cells) for hPL[61] and inhibin[60]
- Variably positive for p63[61]
- High Ki67 proliferation index, previously reported as 69% ± 20%[62]
- Generally positive for SALL4 (to variable extent)[61]
  - SALL4 has recently been proposed as a promising marker for distinguishing choriocarcinoma from other trophoblastic tumors, as it was found to be positive in all studied cases of choriocarcinoma, but negative for all cases of placental site trophoblastic tumor and epithelioid trophoblastic tumor tested.[61]

STR genotyping may be applied to delineate the genomic composition of choriocarcinoma.[58] The majority of gestational choriocarcinomas are androgenetic (paternal-only genome), which are associated with or presumably derived from CHM, usually found in the uterus but sometimes arising from a fallopian tube or ovary. A minority of cases are biparental, which may be intraplacental or preceded by normal pregnancy. In certain cases, this may also help to exclude the possibility of non-gestational choriocarcinoma, which would have identical allelic profiles as the patient but commonly with karyotypic abnormalities (Box 10.4).[58]

DIFFERENTIAL DIAGNOSIS

The differential diagnosis of gestational choriocarcinoma includes the following (with the key distinguishing features for each):

- Trophoblastic proliferations in very early gestation or CHM

> **BOX 10.4: Application of short tandem repeat (STR) genotyping in trophoblastic tumors**
>
> - As in the context of molar pregnancy, STR genotyping is also a powerful adjunct to the diagnosis of trophoblastic tumors.
> - Scenarios of diagnostic challenges which might require STR genotyping include the following:[69]
>   1. *Determining the origin of choriocarcinoma with concurrent pregnancy*: When choriocarcinoma is diagnosed in the context of an ongoing pregnancy, the tumor may be associated with current gestation or previous pregnancy. Determining the allelic profile of the choriocarcinoma could differentiate between biparental (from current pregnancy) and androgenetic (from previous complete mole) types.
>   2. *Trophoblastic tumors presenting at metastatic sites*: These cases may be mistaken as somatic tumor types arising from the extrauterine sites. Choriocarcinoma involving the ovary or other extrauterine sites may also raise the possibility of non-gestational choriocarcinoma of germ cell origin.
>   3. *Somatic-type malignancy masquerading as trophoblastic tumors*: Carcinoma of cervix may be confused with epithelioid trophoblastic tumor. Poorly differentiated carcinoma with trophoblastic differentiation in various organs (such as lung and pancreas) could resemble choriocarcinoma.

  - These should be distinguished by the microscopic nature of trophoblastic proliferation, lack of overtly malignant nuclear morphology and absence of mass lesion
- Exaggerated placental site
  - Lack of overtly malignant nuclear morphology, absence of mass lesion and low Ki67 index
- Placental site trophoblastic tumor
  - Typical pattern of vascular invasion (with other characteristic features) and usually more extensive hPL staining
- Epithelioid trophoblastic tumor
  - Mostly mononucleate cells with extracellular eosinophilic material
- Non-gestational choriocarcinoma
  - Clinical context (generally originate from extrauterine sites)
- Carcinoma with trophoblastic differentiation
  - Background of poorly differentiated carcinoma with scattered syncytiotrophoblasts, lacking typical admixture of various trophoblastic cell types

PLACENTAL SITE TROPHOBLASTIC TUMOR

Placental site trophoblastic tumor (PSTT) is a neoplasm with tumor cells showing implantation site intermediate trophoblast differentiation. The histologic features are characterised by a striking resemblance to changes at the normal implantation site.

CLINICAL FEATURES

PSTT could present in a relatively broad age range, reported as 19–63 years in the literature.[63] The preceding pregnancy may include term pregnancy, abortion or molar pregnancy, with an interval from preceding gestation to tumor diagnosis ranging from 0 to 216 months. The standard treatment is hysterectomy. The recurrence rate is variable from different studies, but about 10%–15% of cases are clinically malignant and the overall mortality rate is approximately 15%–20%.[1,63]

MACROSCOPIC FEATURES

PSTT usually presents as a mass lesion involving endometrium and myometrium, possibly extending to the uterine serosa. The cut surface is typically soft and tan, with only focal hemorrhage or necrosis.[1]

DIAGNOSTIC FEATURES

PSTT is recognised by the following histologic features:

- Relatively monomorphic proliferation of polygonal cells with moderately abundant cytoplasm,[63] including mostly mononucleate cells and occasional multinucleate cells[1] (Figures 10.36 through 10.40)

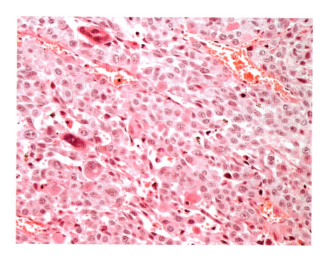

Figure 10.37 Placental site trophoblastic tumor. Mononucleate cells with moderate amount of eosinophilic cytoplasm usually predominate, with scattered multinucleate cells.

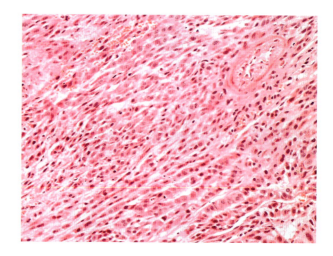

Figure 10.38 Placental site trophoblastic tumor. Arrangement of tumor cells in cords is sometimes observed.

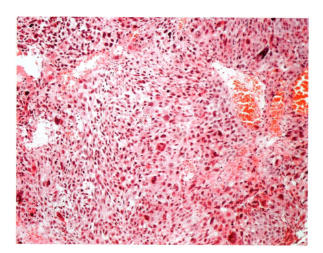

Figure 10.36 Placental site trophoblastic tumor. The low power impression is relatively monomorphic comprising sheets of polygonal cells.

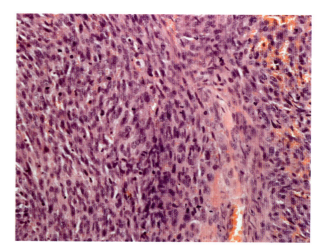

Figure 10.39 Placental site trophoblastic tumor. Spindle-shaped tumor cells may be predominantly found mimicking leiomyosarcoma.

Placental site trophoblastic tumor / Ancillary studies

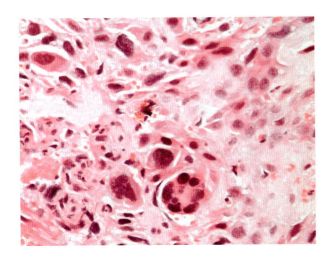

Figure 10.40 Placental site trophoblastic tumor. High-power view of the multinucleate tumor cells.

- Cytoplasm may be eosinophilic, amphophilic or clear[63]
- Nuclear atypia is generally prominent, with convoluted nuclei and occasional prominent nucleoli (Figure 10.41)[10]
- Mitotic rate is variable, with atypical mitosis common[63]
- Infiltrative border with isolated or sheets of tumor cells separating smooth-muscle fibers (resembling normal placental site) (Figure 10.42)[63]
- Extracellular eosinophilic fibrinoid material within vessel wall and surrounding groups of cells (resembling normal placental site)[1,63]
- Characteristic pattern of vascular invasion by replacing the vessel wall with tumor cells (resembling normal placental site and also a helpful clue) (Figure 10.43)[1]

Chorionic villi are usually absent.[1,63] Rare cases may show combination of choriocarcinoma with PSTT,[1,63] or ETT with PSTT.[1,61]

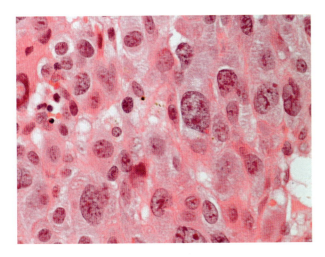

Figure 10.41 Placental site trophoblastic tumor. The degree of nuclear pleomorphism may be marked, but there could be much variation within a tumor.

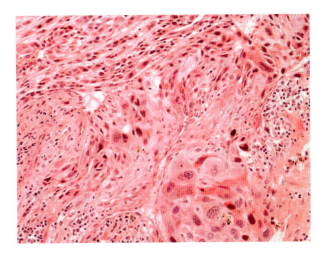

Figure 10.42 Placental site trophoblastic tumor. Infiltrative growth pattern is a typical feature.

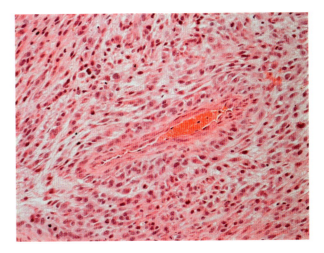

Figure 10.43 Placental site trophoblastic tumor. The pattern of vascular invasion by replacing the vessel wall with tumor cells is an important diagnostic clue.

ANCILLARY STUDIES

The immunohistochemical profile of PSTT is as follows:

- Diffusely positive for cytokeratin[1,60]
- Generally positive for hPL, often strong and extensive (Figure 10.44)[61,63-65]
- Generally positive for hCG (Figure 10.45), but usually focal, often limited to multinucleated cells[61,63]
- Commonly positive for inhibin, usually focal[5,60]
- Negative for p63[60,64,65]
- Ki67 proliferation index 8%–20%[55]
- Generally negative for SALL4, based on recent study[61]

Although genetic studies are seldom required for diagnosis of PSTT, an interesting observation from genotyping analysis is the consistent absence of Y chromosome in all cases that has been tested,[66] which might signify the role of a paternal X chromosome in the pathogenesis.

166 Gestational trophoblastic disease

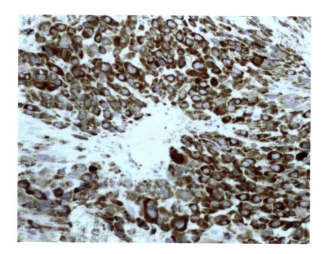

Figure 10.44 Placental site trophoblastic tumor. Immunoreactivity for human placental lactogen (hPL) is typically extensive in PSTT.

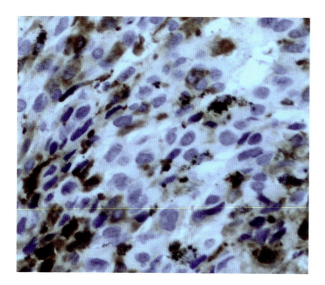

Figure 10.45 Placental site trophoblastic tumor. Focal immunoreactivity for hCG may be found.

DIFFERENTIAL DIAGNOSIS

The differential diagnosis of PSTT may include the following (with the key distinguishing features for each):

- Choriocarcinoma
  - Typical admixture of three types of trophoblastic cells and usually more extensive hCG staining, less extensive hPL and positive for SALL4
- Epithelioid trophoblastic tumor
  - Location in cervix or lower segment, pushing border, eosinophilic keratin-like material, positive staining for p63
- Exaggerated placental site
  - Lack of significant nuclear pleomorphism, absence of mass lesion and low Ki67 index
- Non-trophoblastic tumors (such as uterine sarcoma, PEComa, etc.)

EPITHELIOID TROPHOBLASTIC TUMOR

Epithelioid trophoblastic tumor (ETT) is a neoplasm demonstrating chorionic-type intermediate trophoblast differentiation, which could closely mimic non-trophoblastic tumors.

CLINICAL FEATURES

ETT generally presents in reproductive age (range 15–48 years), with most patients presenting with vaginal bleeding.[67,68] The preceding gestation may be term pregnancy, abortion or molar pregnancy, with a variable interval of 1 to 18 years from the pregnancy to tumor diagnosis.[67,68] Similar to PSTT, ETT is primarily treated by hysterectomy.[1] Approximately 25% of cases would develop metastasis, with about 10% dying of disease.[1]

MACROSCOPIC FEATURES

ETT has a predilection for the lower uterine segment and endocervix.[67,68] The usual finding is a discrete nodular mass invading the myometrium or cervix, with solid or cystic cut surface displaying a tan appearance.[1,67]

DIAGNOSTIC FEATURES

ETT has the following distinctive morphologic features:

- Islands of polygonal mononucleate cells with moderately abundant eosinophilic cytoplasm, arranged in nests, cords and sheets (Figures 10.46 through 10.48)[67]
  - The cells are usually larger than cytotrophoblasts but smaller than implantation site intermediate trophoblasts[1,67]
  - Scattered multinucleated cells possible (Figure 10.49)[68]

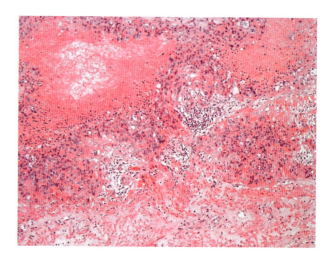

Figure 10.46 Epithelioid trophoblastic tumor. The tumor cells usually show a pushing or slightly infiltrative border with the underlying myometrium.

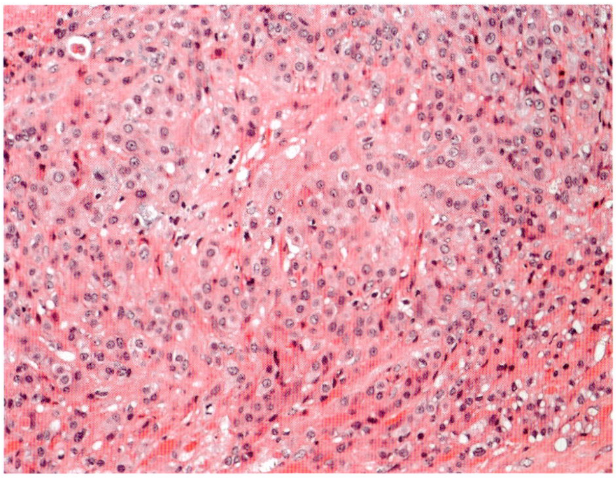

Epithelioid trophoblastic tumor / Ancillary studies 167

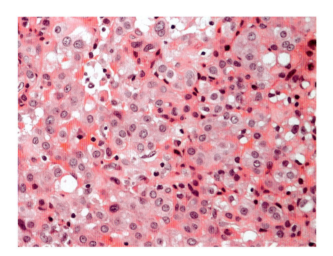

Figure 10.47 Epithelioid trophoblastic tumor. Mononucleate polygonal tumor cells are arranged in sheets, nests and cords.

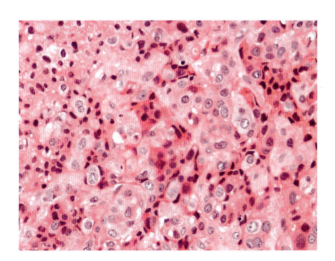

Figure 10.48 Epithelioid trophoblastic tumor. The tumor cells commonly exhibit round nuclei, reminiscent of chorionic-type intermediate trophoblasts.

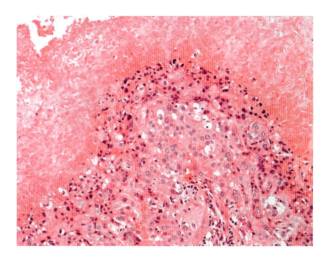

Figure 10.49 Epithelioid trophoblastic tumor. Occasional multinucleate cells are sometimes encountered.

Figure 10.50 Epithelioid trophoblastic tumor. Eosinophilic material with keratin-like appearance and necrotic debris are typically present, surrounded by tumor cells.

- Nuclei typically uniform and round with fine chromatin and occasional distinct nucleoli, but larger cells with irregular hyperchromatic nuclei (resembling implantation site intermediate trophoblasts) may be present[1,67]
- Mitotic count in the range of 0–9 per 10 high-power field[67]
- Surrounded by zones of hyaline material and necrotic debris producing geographic pattern (Figure 10.50)[1,67]
  - The hyaline material may resemble keratin,[68] thus mimicking keratinizing squamous cell carcinoma of cervix
- Usually nodular expansile growth, but foci of infiltrative pattern possible
- Replacement of endocervical glandular epithelium by tumor cells may be seen
  - Potentially mistaken as squamous intraepithelial lesion of cervix

Rare cases of ETT may coexist with choriocarcinoma or PSTT component.[67] Some cases may show placental site nodules intimately associated with ETT.[67]

ANCILLARY STUDIES

The immunohistochemical profile of ETT is as follows:

- Diffusely positive for cytokeratin[60]
- Variable for hCG and hPL, occasionally focally positive in scattered[67]
- Commonly positive for inhibin, usually focal[5,60]
- Positive for p63, usually diffuse and strong (Figure 10.51)[60,61,68]
- Ki67 proliferation index 10%–25%[67]
- Generally negative for SALL4, based on recent study on three cases only[61]

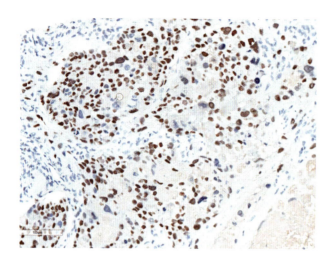

Figure 10.51 Epithelioid trophoblastic tumor. Positive p63 expression by immunohistochemistry.

In case of diagnostic difficulty, STR genotyping could help to confirm the gestational nature of the tumor and exclude non-gestational malignancy.

DIFFERENTIAL DIAGNOSIS

The differential diagnosis of ETT may include the following (with the key distinguishing features for each):

- Squamous cell carcinoma of cervix
  - Positive staining for p16, usually diffuse staining for CK5/6 (compared with occasional focal staining in ETT),[60] and negative staining for inhibin
  - STR genotyping (Box 10.4) and/or HPV testing may be employed in difficult cases
- Epithelioid smooth muscle tumor
  - Center of mass in myometrium, areas of smooth muscle morphology, immunoreactivity for h-caldesmon and desmin, with negative staining for inhibin

- Placental site trophoblastic tumor
  - Typical pattern of vascular invasion and infiltrative growth, with negative p63 and more extensive hPL staining
- Placental site nodule
  - Microscopic finding, absence of necrosis and Ki67 index <10%[1] (Summary Box 10.1)

EXAGGERATED PLACENTAL SITE

Exaggerated placental site (EPS) is a physiologic process characterised by exuberant infiltration of endomyometrium by implantation-site intermediate trophoblasts.[70] This is regarded as the upper end of the spectrum of histomorphologic changes at a normal implantation site, rather than a pathological process.[1,70] Genotyping studies were not supportive of any genetic association with PSTT.[70]

CLINICAL FEATURES

EPS may be observed in curettage specimens or suction evacuate after abortion or normal pregnancy.[70] There is no gross abnormality or evidence of mass lesion.[1] No treatment or follow-up is required.[1]

DIAGNOSTIC FEATURES AND ANCILLARY STUDIES

Histologically, EPS is characterised by abundant implantation-site intermediate trophoblasts involving the endometrium and superficial myometrium, with the trophoblastic cells having relatively pleomorphic and large nuclei, commonly including multinucleated forms (Figures 10.52 and 10.53).[1,70] As normally observed in the implantation site, infiltration among smooth-muscle fibers and replacement of vessel walls by trophoblasts are possible.[1,70] Mitotic figure is absent.[1] The Ki67 proliferation index is 0%–1%.[7,62,71] The

SUMMARY BOX 10.1: Summary of immunohistochemical profiles for differential diagnosis of trophoblastic tumors

Antibody	Choriocarcinoma	PSTT	ETT
Cytokeratin	Positive	Positive	Positive
hCG	Generally positive (mainly in syncytiotrophoblasts)	Generally positive (focal and mainly in multinucleated cells)	Variable (focal or negative)
hPL	Focally positive	Generally positive (often strong and extensive)	Variable (focal or negative)
α-inhibin	Focally positive	Commonly positive (focal)	Commonly positive (focal)
p63	Variable	Negative	Positive
Ki67[a]	>50%	>10%	>10%
SALL4[b]	Generally positive[b]	Generally negative[b]	Generally negative[b]

[a] The cutoffs for Ki67 proliferation index are adopted from Shih IM, Kurman RJ. Am J Surg Pathol 2004;28:1177–83.[7]
[b] Data on SALL4 are limited and based on a recent study only;[61] further studies may be required to confirm the validity.

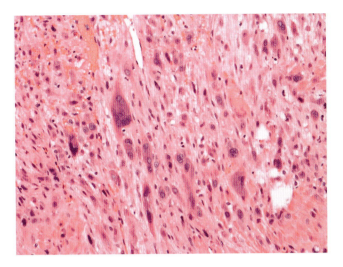

Figure 10.52 Exaggerated placental site. Proliferation of implantation site intermediate trophoblasts with prominent multinucleate forms and variable nuclear enlargement.

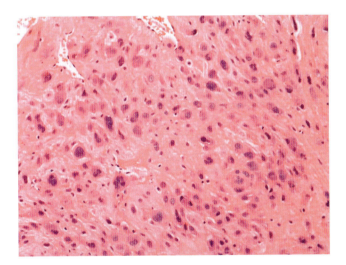

Figure 10.53 Exaggerated placental site.

immunohistochemical profile of trophoblasts in EPS is similar to normal implantation-site intermediate trophoblasts (hPL+, hCG+/−, p63−).[7]

Morphologic changes similar to EPS may be observed in the context of complete hydatidiform mole,[1] but those cases generally display greater nuclear atypia in the trophoblasts with slightly higher Ki67 index in the range of 5.2% ± 4.0%.[62]

DIFFERENTIAL DIAGNOSIS

The major differential diagnosis for EPS is placental site trophoblastic tumor, which is a true neoplasm of implantation-site intermediate trophoblasts. PSTT can be distinguished by the presence of macroscopic mass lesion, mitotic activity and Ki67 index >10%.[1,7]

PLACENTAL SITE NODULE

Placental site nodules (PSN; also known as 'placental site nodule and plaque') are non-neoplastic lesions of chorionic-type intermediate trophoblasts.

CLINICAL FEATURES

Placental site nodules are usually incidental findings in curettage or hysterectomy specimens.[1,2] Patients are generally of reproductive age with history of pregnancy or abortion, where the interval from latest pregnancy may be up to 108 months in reported cases.[1] The size of the lesion is usually microscopic and in the range of 1–14 mm,[1,72] but occasionally they may be grossly identified as yellow excrescences in the endometrium or cervix.[72] No treatment or follow-up is needed for placental site nodules without atypical features.[1]

DIAGNOSTIC FEATURES AND ANCILLARY STUDIES

Placental site nodules are diagnosed by the following histologic features:

- Circumscribed nodules or plaques of hyalinized extracellular matrix containing trophoblasts, surrounded by a rim of chronic inflammatory cells (Figure 10.54 and 10.55)[1,72]
- Trophoblasts arranged in single cells, small nests or cords (Figure 10.56)[1]
  - Nuclei are mostly uniform and small but some may be larger and irregular[72]
  - Multinucleated cells may be present (Figure 10.57)[1]

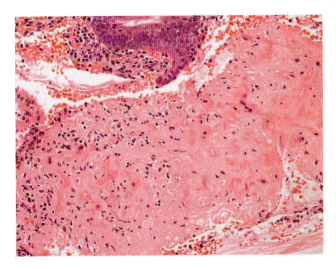

Figure 10.54 Placental site nodule. The typical setting is an incidental finding of hyalinized nodular lesion in curettage specimen, commonly accompanied by inflammatory cells at the periphery.

170 Gestational trophoblastic disease

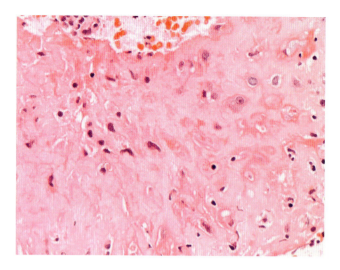

Figure 10.55 Placental site nodule. Isolated trophoblastic cells are present in a hyaline fibrinoid matrix.

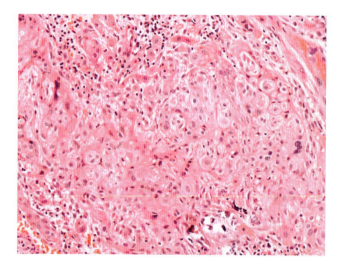

Figure 10.56 Placental site nodule. Some cases may display more closely packed trophoblasts in small nests.

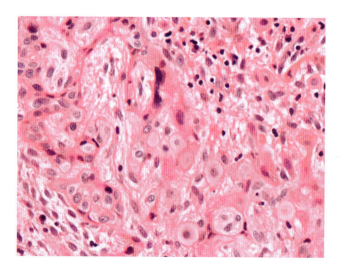

Figure 10.57 Placental site nodule. Scattered multinucleate cells with enlarged nuclei may be observed.

- Cytoplasm usually clear for smaller cells and eosinophilic or amphophilic for larger cells[72]
- Mitotic figures are rare or absent[1,72]

Immunohistochemically, the trophoblasts in placental site nodules display the usual immunophenotype of chorionic-type intermediate trophoblasts (hCG+/−, hPL+/−, p63+).[7] The Ki67 proliferation index is in the range of 3%–10%.[7]

Variant: Atypical placental site nodule

Atypical placental site nodules (APSN) have been increasingly recognised in recent years.[1,73] As mentioned in the WHO Classification,[10] APSN is characterised by the presence of cytologic atypia and proliferative activity that is intermediate between typical PSN and ETT. These lesions were reported to be generally larger than typical PSN, of higher cellularity, with more cohesive nests and cords, and higher Ki67 index than typical PSN.[1,73] The exact criteria for cytologic atypia and cutoffs for proliferation index have not been clearly established.[73] In a recent case series of APSN,[73] 3 out of 21 cases were diagnosed to have trophoblastic tumor (concurrently or upon follow-up), including two cases of PSTT and one case of ETT. This finding may indicate that patients with APSN warrant clinical and radiological investigations as well as follow-up,[73] but the actual clinical implications and optimal management are yet to be determined.

DIFFERENTIAL DIAGNOSIS

The differential diagnosis of PSN may include the following conditions (with the key distinguishing features for each):

- Epithelioid trophoblastic tumor
  - Presence of mass lesion, necrosis and Ki67 >10%
- Placental site trophoblastic tumor
  - Presence of mass lesion, infiltrative pattern, high cellularity, mitotic activity, Ki67 >10% and p63 negative
- Squamous cell carcinoma of cervix
  - Usually mitotically active with higher Ki67 index, positive staining for p16 and negative staining for inhibin

OTHER UNCLASSIFIED TROPHOBLASTIC LESIONS

Although most trophoblastic lesions could fit into the aforementioned entities, there undoubtedly are rare trophoblastic proliferations that may be difficult to classify. Apart from trophoblastic tumors with intermediate features between recognised entities, there are also some presumably non-neoplastic trophoblastic lesions reported in the literature that display unusual histologic or clinical features. Intriguingly, a number of peculiar trophoblastic lesions associated with cyst and fistula formation occurring after cesarean section have been reported under a variety of names,[72,74,75] such as 'uterine diffuse intermediate trophoblastic lesion resembling placental site plaque'[74] or 'atypical epithelioid trophoblastic lesions with cyst and fistula formation after cesarean section'.[75] The exact biological nature of these lesions requires further clarification with systematic analysis.

REFERENCES

1. Shih IM, Kurman RJ. The pathology of intermediate trophoblastic tumors and tumor-like lesions. *Int J Gynecol Pathol* 2001;20:31–47.
2. Shih IM, Seidman JD, Kurman RJ. Placental site nodule and characterization of distinctive types of intermediate trophoblast. *Hum Pathol* 1999;30:687–94.
3. Daya D, Sabet L. The use of cytokeratin as a sensitive and reliable marker for trophoblastic tissue. *Am J Clin Pathol* 1991;95:137–41.
4. Kurman RJ, Young RH, Norris HJ, Main CS, Lawrence WD, Scully RE. Immunocytochemical localization of placental lactogen and chorionic gonadotropin in the normal placenta and trophoblastic tumors, with emphasis on intermediate trophoblast and the placental site trophoblastic tumor. *Int J Gynecol Pathol* 1984;3:101–21.
5. Shih IM, Kurman RJ. Immunohistochemical localization of inhibin-alpha in the placenta and gestational trophoblastic lesions. *Int J Gynecol Pathol* 1999;18:144–50.
6. McCluggage WG. Value of inhibin staining in gynecological pathology. *Int J Gynecol Pathol* 2001;20:79–85.
7. Shih IM, Kurman RJ. p63 expression is useful in the distinction of epithelioid trophoblastic and placental site tumors by profiling trophoblastic subpopulations. *Am J Surg Pathol* 2004;28:1177–83.
8. Shih IM, Kurman RJ. Expression of melanoma cell adhesion molecule in intermediate trophoblast. *Lab Invest* 1996;75:377–88.
9. Singer G, Kurman RJ, McMaster MT, Shih IeM. HLA-G immunoreactivity is specific for intermediate trophoblast in gestational trophoblastic disease and can serve as a useful marker in differential diagnosis. *Am J Surg Pathol* 2002;26:914–20.
10. Kurman RJ, Carcangiu ML, Herrington CS, Young RH, eds. *WHO Classification of Tumours of Female Reproductive Organs*. International Agency for Research on Cancer. Lyon, 2014.
11. Hui P, Buza N, Murphy KM, Ronnett BM. Hydatidiform moles: Genetic basis and precision diagnosis. *Annu Rev Pathol* 2017;12:449–85.
12. Buza N, Hui P. Ancillary studies for precision diagnosis of hydatidiform moles. *Diagn Histopathology* 2017;23:292–302.
13. Niemann I, Hansen ES, Sunde L. The risk of persistent trophoblastic disease after hydatidiform mole classified by morphology and ploidy. *Gynecol Oncol* 2007;104:411–5.
14. Scholz NB, Bolund L, Nyegaard M, Faaborg L, Jørgensen MW, Lund H, Niemann I, Sunde L. Triploidy – Observations in 154 diandric cases. *PLOS ONE* 2015;10:e0142545.
15. Seckl MJ, Sebire NJ, Berkowitz RS. Gestational trophoblastic disease. *Lancet* 2010;376:717–29.
16. Fisher RA, Paradinas FJ, Soteriou BA, Foskett M, Newlands ES. Diploid hydatidiform moles with fetal red blood cells in molar villi. 2--Genetics. *J Pathol* 1997;181:189–95.
17. Ronnett BM, DeScipio C, Murphy KM. Hydatidiform moles: Ancillary techniques to refine diagnosis. *Int J Gynecol Pathol* 2011;30:101–16.
18. McConnell TG, Murphy KM, Hafez M, Vang R, Ronnett BM. Diagnosis and subclassification of hydatidiform moles using p57 immunohistochemistry and molecular genotyping: Validation and prospective analysis in routine and consultation practice settings with development of an algorithmic approach. *Am J Surg Pathol* 2009;33:805–17.
19. McConnell TG, Norris-Kirby A, Hagenkord JM, Ronnett BM, Murphy KM. Complete hydatidiform mole with retained maternal chromosomes 6 and 11. *Am J Surg Pathol* 2009;33:1409–15.
20. Fisher RA, Nucci MR, Thaker HM, Weremowicz S, Genest DR, Castrillon DH. Complete hydatidiform mole retaining a chromosome 11 of maternal origin: Molecular genetic analysis of a case. *Mod Pathol* 2004;17:1155–60.
21. DeScipio C, Haley L, Beierl K, Pandit AP, Murphy KM, Ronnett BM. Diandric triploid hydatidiform mole with loss of maternal chromosome 11. *Am J Surg Pathol* 2011;35:1586–91.
22. Lewis GH, DeScipio C, Murphy KM et al. Characterization of androgenetic/biparental mosaic/chimeric conceptions, including those with a molar component: Morphology, p57 immunohistochemistry, molecular genotyping, and risk of persistent gestational trophoblastic disease. *Int J Gynecol Pathol* 2013;32:199–214.
23. Lai CY, Chan KY, Khoo US, Ngan HY, Xue WC, Chiu PM, Tsao SW, Cheung AN. Analysis of gestational trophoblastic disease by genotyping and chromosome *in situ* hybridization. *Mod Pathol* 2004;17:40–8.
24. Vang R, Gupta M, Wu LS, Yemelyanova AV, Kurman RJ, Murphy KM, Descipio C, Ronnett BM. Diagnostic reproducibility of hydatidiform moles: Ancillary techniques (p57 immunohistochemistry and molecular genotyping) improve morphologic diagnosis. *Am J Surg Pathol* 2012;36:443–53.

25. Murphy KM, McConnell TG, Hafez MJ, Vang R, Ronnett BM. Molecular genotyping of hydatidiform moles: Analytic validation of a multiplex short tandem repeat assay. *J Mol Diagn* 2009;11:598–605.
26. Fukunaga M, Endo Y, Ushigome S. Clinicopathologic study of tetraploid hydropic villous tissues. *Arch Pathol Lab Med* 1996;120:569–72.
27. Sundvall L, Lund H, Niemann I, Jensen UB, Bolund L, Sunde L. Tetraploidy in hydatidiform moles. *Hum Reprod* 2013;28:2010–20.
28. Fukunaga M. Immunohistochemical characterization of p57Kip2 expression in tetraploid hydropic placentas. *Arch Pathol Lab Med* 2004;128:897–900.
29. Murphy KM, Descipio C, Wagenfuehr J, Tandy S, Mabray J, Beierl K, Micetich K, Libby AL, Ronnett BM. Tetraploid partial hydatidiform mole: A case report and review of the literature. *Int J Gynecol Pathol* 2012;31:73–9.
30. Niemann I, Bolund L, Sunde L. Twin pregnancies with diploid hydatidiform mole and co-existing normal fetus may originate from one oocyte. *Hum Reprod* 2008;23:2031–5.
31. Makrydimas G, Sebire NJ, Thornton SE, Zagorianakou N, Lolis D, Fisher RA. Complete hydatidiform mole and normal live birth: A novel case of confined placental mosaicism: Case report. *Hum Reprod* 2002;17:2459–63.
32. Surti U, Hill LM, Dunn J, Prosen T, Hoffner L. Twin pregnancy with a chimeric androgenetic and biparental placenta in one twin displaying placental mesenchymal dysplasia phenotype. *Prenat Diagn* 2005;25:1048–56.
33. Ariel I, Goldman-Wohl D, Yagel S, Gazit E, Loewenthal R. Triple paternal contribution to a normal/complete molar chimeric singleton placenta. *Hum Reprod* 2017;32:993–8.
34. Hoffner L, Dunn J, Esposito N, Macpherson T, Surti U. P57KIP2 immunostaining and molecular cytogenetics: Combined approach aids in diagnosis of morphologically challenging cases with molar phenotype and in detecting androgenetic cell lines in mosaic/chimeric conceptions. *Hum Pathol* 2008;39:63–72.
35. Kawasaki K, Kondoh E, Minamiguchi S, Matsuda F, Higasa K, Fujita K, Mogami H, Chigusa Y, Konishi I. Live-born diploid fetus complicated with partial molar pregnancy presenting with pre-eclampsia, maternal anemia, and seemingly huge placenta: A rare case of confined placental mosaicism and literature review. *J Obstet Gynaecol Res* 2016;42:911–7.
36. Sarno AP Jr, Moorman AJ, Kalousek DK. Partial molar pregnancy with fetal survival: An unusual example of confined placental mosaicism. *Obstet Gynecol* 1993;82(4 Pt 2 Suppl):716–9.
37. Fisher RA, Hodges MD, Newlands ES. Familial recurrent hydatidiform mole: A review. *J Reprod Med* 2004;49:595–601.
38. Zhao J, Moss J, Sebire NJ, Cui QC, Seckl MJ, Xiang Y, Fisher RA. Analysis of the chromosomal region 19q13.4 in two Chinese families with recurrent hydatidiform mole. *Hum Reprod* 2006;21:536–41.
39. Andreasen L, Christiansen OB, Niemann I, Bolund L, Sunde L. NLRP7 or KHDC3L genes and the etiology of molar pregnancies and recurrent miscarriage. *Mol Hum Reprod* 2013;19:773–81.
40. van der Smagt JJ, Scheenjes E, Kremer JA, Hennekam FA, Fisher RA. Heterogeneity in the origin of recurrent complete hydatidiform moles: Not all women with multiple molar pregnancies have biparental moles. *BJOG*. 2006;113:725–8.
41. Dixon PH, Trongwongsa P, Abu-Hayyah S, Ng SH, Akbar SA, Khawaja NP, Seckl MJ, Savage PM, Fisher RA. Mutations in NLRP7 are associated with diploid biparental hydatidiform moles, but not androgenetic complete moles. *J Med Genet* 2012;49:206–11.
42. Murdoch S, Djuric U, Mazhar B et al. Mutations in NALP7 cause recurrent hydatidiform moles and reproductive wastage in humans. *Nat Genet* 2006;38:300–2.
43. Reddy R, Akoury E, Phuong Nguyen NM et al. Report of four new patients with protein-truncating mutations in C6orf221/KHDC3L and colocalization with NLRP7. *Eur J Hum Genet* 2013;21:957–64.
44. Sebire NJ, Savage PM, Seckl MJ, Fisher RA. Histopathological features of biparental complete hydatidiform moles in women with NLRP7 mutations. *Placenta* 2013;34:50–6.
45. Sunde L, Niemann I, Hansen ES, Hindkjaer J, Degn B, Jensen UB, Bolund L. Mosaics and moles. *Eur J Hum Genet* 2011;19:1026–31.
46. El-Maarri O, Seoud M, Coullin P, Herbiniaux U, Oldenburg J, Rouleau G, Slim R. Maternal alleles acquiring paternal methylation patterns in biparental complete hydatidiform moles. *Hum Mol Genet* 2003;12:1405–13.
47. Sanchez-Delgado M, Martin-Trujillo A, Tayama C et al. Absence of maternal methylation in biparental hydatidiform moles from women with NLRP7 maternal-effect mutations reveals widespread placenta-specific imprinting. *PLoS Genet* 2015;11:e1005644.
48. Bynum J, Murphy KM, DeScipio C, Beierl K, Adams E, Anderson D, Vang R, Ronnett BM. Invasive complete hydatidiform moles: Analysis of a case series with Genotyping. *Int J Gynecol Pathol* 2016;35:134–41.
49. Robinson WP, Lauzon JL, Innes AM, Lim K, Arsovska S, McFadden DE. Origin and outcome of pregnancies affected by androgenetic/biparental chimerism. *Hum Reprod* 2007;22:1114–22.
50. Armes JE, McGown I, Williams M, Broomfield A, Gough K, Lehane F, Lourie R. The placenta in Beckwith-Wiedemann syndrome: Genotype-phenotype associations, excessive extravillous

trophoblast and placental mesenchymal dysplasia. *Pathology* 2012;44:519–27.
51. Kaiser-Rogers KA, McFadden DE, Livasy CA, Dansereau J, Jiang R, Knops JF, Lefebvre L, Rao KW, Robinson WP. Androgenetic/biparental mosaicism causes placental mesenchymal dysplasia. *J Med Genet* 2006;43:187–92.
52. Redline RW, Hassold T, Zaragoza M. Determinants of villous trophoblastic hyperplasia in spontaneous abortions. *Mod Pathol* 1998;11:762–8.
53. Sebire NJ, May PC, Kaur B, Seckl MJ, Fisher RA. Abnormal villous morphology mimicking a hydatidiform mole associated with paternal trisomy of chromosomes 3,7,8 and unipaternal disomy of chromosome 11. *Diagn Pathol* 2016;11:20.
54. Lipata F, Parkash V, Talmor M, Bell S, Chen S, Maric V, Hui P. Precise DNA genotyping diagnosis of hydatidiform mole. *Obstet Gynecol* 2010;115:784–94.
55. Zaragoza MV, Surti U, Redline RW, Millie E, Chakravarti A, Hassold TJ. Parental origin and phenotype of triploidy in spontaneous abortions: Predominance of diandry and association with the partial hydatidiform mole. *Am J Hum Genet* 2000 Jun;66:1807–20.
56. Redline RW, Hassold T, Zaragoza MV. Prevalence of the partial molar phenotype in triploidy of maternal and paternal origin. *Hum Pathol* 1998;29:505–11.
57. Mao TL, Kurman RJ, Huang CC, Lin MC, Shih IeM. Immunohistochemistry of choriocarcinoma: An aid in differential diagnosis and in elucidating pathogenesis. *Am J Surg Pathol* 2007;31:1726–32.
58. Savage J, Adams E, Veras E, Murphy KM, Ronnett BM. Choriocarcinoma in women: Analysis of a case series with genotyping. *Am J Surg Pathol* 2017;41:1593–606.
59. Black JO, Rufforny-Doudenko I, Shehata BM. Pathologic quiz case: Third trimester placenta exhibiting infarction. Intraplacental choriocarcinoma. *Arch Pathol Lab Med* 2003;127:e340–2.
60. Kalhor N, Ramirez PT, Deavers MT, Malpica A, Silva EG. Immunohistochemical studies of trophoblastic tumors. *Am J Surg Pathol* 2009;33:633–8.
61. Stichelbout M, Devisme L, Franquet-Ansart H, Massardier J, Vinatier D, Renaud F, Kerdraon O. SALL4 expression in gestational trophoblastic tumors: A useful tool to distinguish choriocarcinoma from placental site trophoblastic tumor and epithelioid trophoblastic tumor. *Hum Pathol* 2016;54:121–6.
62. Shih IM, Kurman RJ. Ki-67 labeling index in the differential diagnosis of exaggerated placental site, placental site trophoblastic tumor, and choriocarcinoma: A double immunohistochemical staining technique using Ki-67 and Mel-CAM antibodies. *Hum Pathol* 1998;29:27–33.
63. Baergen RN, Rutgers JL, Young RH, Osann K, Scully RE. Placental site trophoblastic tumor: A study of 55 cases and review of the literature emphasizing factors of prognostic significance. *Gynecol Oncol* 2006;100:511–20.
64. Luiza JW, Taylor SE, Gao FF, Edwards RP. Placental site trophoblastic tumor: Immunohistochemistry algorithm key to diagnosis and review of literature. *Gynecol Oncol Case Rep* 2013;7:13–5.
65. Shih IeM. Trophogram, an immunohistochemistry-based algorithmic approach, in the differential diagnosis of trophoblastic tumors and tumorlike lesions. *Ann Diagn Pathol* 2007;11:228–34.
66. Hui P, Wang HL, Chu P, Yang B, Huang J, Baergen RN, Sklar J, Yang XJ, Soslow RA. Absence of Y chromosome in human placental site trophoblastic tumor. *Mod Pathol* 2007;20:1055–60.
67. Shih IM, Kurman RJ. Epithelioid trophoblastic tumor: A neoplasm distinct from choriocarcinoma and placental site trophoblastic tumor simulating carcinoma. *Am J Surg Pathol* 1998;22:1393–403.
68. Fadare O, Parkash V, Carcangiu ML, Hui P. Epithelioid trophoblastic tumor: Clinicopathological features with an emphasis on uterine cervical involvement. *Mod Pathol* 2006;19:75–82.
69. Aranake-Chrisinger J, Huettner PC, Hagemann AR, Pfeifer JD. Use of short tandem repeat analysis in unusual presentations of trophoblastic tumors and their mimics. *Hum Pathol* 2016;52:92–100.
70. Dotto J, Hui P. Lack of genetic association between exaggerated placental site reaction and placental site trophoblastic tumor. *Int J Gynecol Pathol* 2008;27:562–7.
71. Yeasmin S, Nakayama K, Katagiri A, Ishikawa M, Iida K, Nakayama N, Miyazaki K. Exaggerated placental site mimicking placental site trophoblastic tumor: Case report and literature review. *Eur J Gynaecol Oncol* 2010;31:586–9.
72. Ismail SM, Lewis CG, Shaw RW. Postcaesarean section uterovesical fistula lined by persistent intermediate trophoblast. *Am J Surg Pathol* 1995;19:1440–3.
73. Kaur B, Short D, Fisher RA, Savage PM, Seckl MJ, Sebire NJ. Atypical placental site nodule (APSN) and association with malignant gestational trophoblastic disease; a clinicopathologic study of 21 cases. *Int J Gynecol Pathol* 2015;34:152–8.
74. O'Neill CJ, Cook I, McCluggage WG. Postcesarean delivery uterine diffuse intermediate trophoblastic lesion resembling placental site plaque. *Hum Pathol.* 2009;40:1358–60.
75. Liang Y, Zhou F, Chen X, Zhang X, Lü B. Atypical epithelioid trophoblastic lesion with cyst and fistula formation after a cesarean section: A rare form of gestational trophoblastic disease. *Int J Gynecol Pathol* 2012;31:458–62.

Index

A-S, *see* Arias-Stella
Abnormal (non-molar) villous lesion, 150, 160
   chromosomal trisomy syndromes, 161
   digynic triploid conceptions, 161
   hydropic abortions, 160
Abnormal cell divisions, 157
Abnormal endometrial development, 19
Abnormal placentation, 30
Abnormal pregnancy, 27
   absence of physiological changes with retention, 27
   absence of vascular changes in intradecidual spiral artery, 27
   acute atherosis, 29
   blood supply to placenta in intrauterine growth restriction, 28
   placenta accreta, 30
Abnormal uterine bleeding, 1, 43
Abortion, 24
   induced, tissue from, 24–25
   pregnancies of unknown location and ectopic pregnancy, tissue from, 26–27
   spontaneous, tissue from, 25–26
Acute atherosis, 29
Acute inflammatory cells, 16
Adenocarcinoma with myometrial invasion, 70; *see also* Choriocarcinoma
Adenofibroma, 73–74
Adenoma malignum-like infiltration, 120
Adenomyomatous polyp, 68–70
Adenomyosis, 60, 117–118
Adenosarcoma, 68–69, 74
Adhesion molecules, 18
Adipose
   metaplasia, 85
   tissue, 2
Adjuvant therapy, 115
AH, *see* Atypical hyperplasia
α-inhibin, 148, 168
AMCAR stain, clear cell carcinoma with, 141
AMGP, *see* Atypical mucinous glandular proliferation

Ancillary studies, 70, 163, 165–170
Androgenetic/biparental mosaic/chimeric conceptions, 157
   clinical significance, 160
   immunohistochemical and genotyping studies, 158–160
   morphologic features, 157–158
Androgenetic genome, 157, 163
Anovulatory cycles, 44
Anti-human placental lactogen, 25
Anti-keratin antibodies, 25
Apoptosis, 16, 44
Arias-Stella (A-S), 26–27
   effect, 99
   endometrium with, 141
   reaction, 139
Arterioles, 71
Artifactual crowding of glands, 4
Atypical endometrial hyperplasia, 98
Atypical hyperplasia (AH), 91
   endometrial polyp with, 67
'Atypical hyperplasia superimposed by secretory changes', *see* Secretory-type EIN/AH
Atypical mucinous glandular proliferation (AMGP), 82
Atypical placental site nodule (APSN), 170
Atypical polypoid adenomyoma (APA), 69–70, 97

Basal endometrium, 10, 18
Basalis layer of endometrium, 68
Basal layer, 8, 11, 15
Benign cystic polyps, 18
Benign endometrial changes, *see* Endometrial metaplasia
Benign endometrium, reactive reparative changes of, 106
Benign hyperplasia, 91; *see also* Endometrial intraepithelial neoplasia atypical hyperplasia (EIN/AH)
   differential diagnosis, 93
   DPE, 93

   etiology and genetic profile, 91
   histopathology, 92–93
   prognosis and predictive factors, 92
   secretory endometrium, 93–94
Benign mucinous metaplasia, 81
Benign tumors and tumor-like conditions
   adenofibroma, 73–74
   adenomyomatous polyp, 68–69
   APA, 69–70
   endometrial metaplasia and related changes, 76–86
   endometrial polyp, 65–68
   ESN, 70–73
   tumor-like lesions, 74–76
β-human chorionic gonadotropin (β-hCG), 148
BiCHM, *see* Biparental complete hydatidiform moles
Biopsy, 1, 18
   endometrial, 1–2, 18, 26, 45, 98–99
   material, 99
   out-of-phase, 44
   specimens, 8, 132
Biparental complete hydatidiform moles (BiCHM), 157
Bizarre stromal cells, 65–66
Blood
   supply, 10–11
   vessels, 22
B lymphocytes, 25, 35

Carcinoma with trophoblastic differentiation, 163
Cartilaginous metaplasia, 85
CD10, 75, 85, 118
   immunohistochemistry, 72
   positive for, 116
CD56+ granulated lymphocytes, 35–36, 48
CD56+ natural killer cells, 10
CD68, 85
   immunohistochemistry in nodular histiocytic hyperplasia, 75
   immunostaining, 36
Central necrosis, 77, 79

175

Cervical invasion assessment, 121
Chemokines, 18
Chemotherapy, 32
Chlamydia trachomatis, 39
CHM, *see* Complete hydatidiform mole
Choriocarcinoma, 147, 161; *see also* Endometrial adenocarcinoma
    ancillary studies, 163
    clinical features, 161
    diagnostic features, 161–163
    differential diagnosis, 163
    macroscopic features, 161
    variant, 163
Chorionic villi, 26, 147, 161, 165
Chromosomes
    HM with gain or loss of, 156
    trisomy syndromes, 161
Chronic endometritis, 10, 38–39; *see also* Endometritis
    acute on, 59
    nonspecific, 37, 39
    postpartum, 37
    with prominent lymphoid infiltrate, 74
Chronic inflammatory cells, 39, 51, 169
Ciliated-cell carcinoma, 126
Ciliated-cell metaplasia, *see* Tubal metaplasia
CK, *see* Cytokeratin
Clear-cell carcinoma (CCC), 138; *see also* Endometrial serous carcinoma (ESC); Endometrioid carcinoma
    clear cell carcinoma with AMCAR stain, 141
    clinical features, 138
    with cystic tubular growth pattern, 139
    differential diagnosis, 138
    endometrioid carcinoma, 140–141
    immunohistochemistry, 138
    intraluminal papillae, 140
    markers, 143
    molecular features, 138
    with Napsin A stain, 141
    with p53 staining, 140
    pathologic findings, 138
    prognostic and predictive factors, 138
Clear-cell EmGD
    future direction, 108–109
    morphologic features, 107–108
Clear-cell metaplasia, 77, 83
Clomiphene (clomifene), 56
Combined hormone-therapy regimes, 54–56
    narrow secretory-pattern glands, 55
    secretory glands and inactive stroma, 55
    sequential hormone therapy, 56
Combined oral contraceptive pill (COP), 47
Complete hydatidiform mole (CHM), 149, 151–152, 154
Contraception, 47
    COP, 47
    progestins, 47–49
Corpus luteum, 7–8, 12–13, 21, 26, 44–45
Cowden syndrome, 94, 114
CTNNB1 (β-catenin gene), 70
Curettage, 1–3, 31, 70, 84, 98
    findings and material, 26
    specimens, 25, 70, 99
Cyproterone acetate with ethinylestradiol, 60–61
Cystic tubular growth pattern, CCC with, 139
Cytokeratin (CK), 72, 85, 148, 168
    CK7, 143
Cytokines, 18
Cytologic
    atypia, 91
    demarcation, 93, 95
Cytoplasm, 9, 165
Cytotrophoblasts, 147, 161
    cells, 21
    shell, 21

Danazol, 61
Decidua basalis, 23, 25
Decidualization, 21
Decidua myometrium, 28
Decidua vera, 21, 23–25
Dedifferentiated carcinoma, 142–143
Deep myometrial invasion, endometrial cancer with, 117
Defective decidualization, 30
Depomedroxyprogesterone acetate, 48
Depth of myometrial invasion (DMI), 118
Desmin, 72
Desmoplastic reaction, 119
Dianette®, *see* Cyproterone acetate with ethinylestradiol
'Diffusely infiltrative endometrial adenocarcinoma', *see* Adenoma malignum-like infiltration
Digynic triploid conceptions, 160–161
Dilatation, 1–3, 12, 95
    aneurismal, 160
    of blood vessels, 22
    cystic dilatation of glands, 57
Disordered proliferative endometrium (DPE), 44, 92–94, 114
Dispermic fertilization, 157
Distended spiral arteries, 22
DMI, *see* Depth of myometrial invasion
Dysfunctional uterine bleeding, 43–44

Early proliferative-phase endometrium, 13, 35–36
ECCC, *see* Endometrial clear-cell carcinoma
Ectopic pregnancy, 26–27, 161
EIN, *see* Endometrial intraepithelial neoplasia
EIN/AH, *see* Endometrial intraepithelial neoplasia/atypical hyperplasia
Emergency contraceptive pill (ECP), 48
EmGD, *see* Endometrial glandular dysplasia
Endocervical-type adenomyoma, 69, 74
Endocervical adenocarcinoma, 124, 128
Endocrine manipulation strategies, 44
Endogenous estrogenic stimulation, 114
Endometrial-myometrial junction, 116–117
Endometrial ablation, 32, 59–60
Endometrial adenocarcinoma, 39, 98
    anecdotal reports, 114
    development, 113
    endometrial polyp with, 67
    high-grade glandular, 135
Endometrial aspirate, outpatient sampling by, 2–3
Endometrial biopsy, 19, 26, 45, 72, 98, 115, 130; *see also* Biopsy
    dating, 18
    EIN/AH diagnosis in, 99
    histological evaluation, 1
    Pipelle, 2
Endometrial cancer(s), 91, 113–114
    adenomyosis, 117–118
    assessment, 122
    cervical invasion assessment, 121
    with deep myometrial invasion, 117
    endometrial-myometrial junction, 116–117
    endometrial carcinoma grading, 115–116
    myometrial invasion measurement, 116
    myometrial invasive patterns, 118–120
    pathologic characteristics of, 115
Endometrial cavity, 3, 7, 39, 41, 60, 123, 130–131
Endometrial clear-cell carcinoma (ECCC), 107, 138
    future direction of clear-cell EmGD, 108–109
    immunophenotypes, 135

morphologic features of, 107
putative precursor for, 107
Endometrial cytomegalovirus infection, 40
Endometrial effects
    dense spindly stroma with granulated lymphocytes, 50
    hysterectomy specimen, 48
    of medroxyprogesterone acetate, 50–51
    of progestin treatment, 48
    pseudodecidualized stroma, 49
    pseudodecidualized stroma with focal necrosis, 50
    scanty narrow glands, 48
    of tamoxifen treatment, 57
Endometrial epithelial metaplasias, 76–77
    clear-cell metaplasia, 83
    eosinophilic metaplasia, 79–80
    hobnail metaplasia, 82–83
    mucinous metaplasia, 80–81
    papillary proliferation, 83–84
    papillary syncytial metaplasia, 81–82
    squamous metaplasia and morules, 76–78
    tubal metaplasia, 78–79
Endometrial epithelium, 35, 78–79, 81, 97, 102
Endometrial glands, 9, 27, 44
Endometrial glandular dysplasia (EmGD), 91, 101–102, 114
    comparison among lesions of SEIC and, 103
    differential diagnosis, 106
    etiology and genetic profile, 102
    histopathology, 102
    immunohistochemistry in diagnosis, 103–105
    with p53 stain, 104
    with papillary architecture, 105
    prognosis and predictive factors, 102
Endometrial granulated lymphocytes, 15–16, 35
Endometrial granulocytes, 10
Endometrial histology, 18
Endometrial hyperplasia, 66, 100
    without atypia, 92
    and cancer, 1
Endometrial inflammation
    endometritis, 37
    morphological subtypes of endometritis, 39–41
    nonspecific endometritis, 37–39
    normal endometrium, 35–37
Endometrial intraepithelial neoplasia (EIN), 91

Endometrial intraepithelial neoplasia/atypical hyperplasia (EIN/AH), 94, 96, 126; see also Benign hyperplasia
    atypical polypoid adenomyoma, 97
    diagnostic criteria for, 95
    differential diagnosis, 96
    endometrial metaplasia, 97
    endometrial polyps, 96
    endometrioid carcinoma, 98–99
    ESC, 99
    etiology and genetic profile, 94
    histopathology, 95–96
    immunohistochemistry in diagnosis, 101
    loss of PAX2 expression in, 101
    oversized, 97
    progestin-treated, 99–100
    prognosis and predictive factors, 94
    secretory-type, 98
    subdiagnostic lesions, 99
    tissue fragmentation and sampling artifact, 96–97
Endometrial ischemia, 32
Endometrial malignant lesions
    clear-cell carcinoma, 138–142
    clinical presentation and management, 114–115
    endometrial serous carcinoma, 131–138
    endometrioid carcinoma, 123–130
    etiology and risk factors, 113–114
    mucinous carcinoma, 130–131
    pathogenesis, 114
    pathologic characteristics of endometrial cancer, 115–123
    undifferentiated and dedifferentiated carcinoma, 142–143
Endometrial metaplasia, 97, 106
    endometrial epithelial metaplasias, 76–84
    endometrial stromal metaplasias and changes, 84–86
    and related changes, 76
Endometrial mucinous carcinoma, 129–130
Endometrial ossification, 32
Endometrial polyp(s), 55–56, 65–66, 69, 74, 96, 106
    ancillary studies, 68
    association with hyperplasia and malignancy, 66–67
    with atypical hyperplasia, 67
    diagnostic features, 65
    differential diagnosis, 68
    with endometrial adenocarcinoma, 67

gastric metaplasia in, 81
    morphologic variation, 65–66
    with serous EIC, 67
Endometrial precancerous lesions, 91
Endometrial premalignant lesions, 91
    precursors of endometrial serous carcinoma, 101–106
    precursors of endometrioid carcinoma, 91–101
    putative precursor for endometrial clear-cell carcinoma, 107–109
Endometrial serous carcinoma (ESC), 99, 113–114, 128, 131–132, 139; see also Clear-cell carcinoma (CCC)
    clinical features, 131
    differential diagnosis, 135
    EmGD, 101–106
    histopathology, 131–134
    immunohistochemistry, 134
    immunophenotypes, 135
    macroscopy, 131
    molecular features, 134–135
    precursors, 101
    prognostic and predictive factors, 135–138
Endometrial spiral arteries, 11
Endometrial stromal metaplasia, 78
    adipose metaplasia, 85
    cartilaginous metaplasia, 85
    extramedullary hematopoiesis, 85–86
    glial tissue in endometrium, 85
    osseous metaplasia, 84
    and other stromal changes, 84
    pseudorosette-like proliferation, 85
    smooth-muscle metaplasia, 85
    synovial-like metaplasia, 85
Endometrial stromal nodule (ESN), 70–71; see also Placental site nodule (PSN)
    Approach to diagnosis of, 72–73
    CD10 immunohistochemistry in, 72
    clinical and macroscopic features, 70
    diagnostic features, 70–71
    differential diagnosis, 71–72
    endometrial stromal tumor with limited infiltration, 71
    immunohistochemistry, 72
    molecular findings, 72
Endometrial tumors, 2
Endometrial undifferentiated carcinoma, 142
Endometrioid adenocarcinoma, 66–67, 94
    in tamoxifen-associated polyp, 58
Endometrioid carcinoma
    benign hyperplasia, 91–94
    EIN/AH, 94–101
    precursors, 91

Endometrioid carcinoma, 98–99, 123–130, 140–141; *see also* Clear-cell carcinoma (CCC)
  clinical features, 123
  corded and hyalinized variant, 127
  differential diagnosis, 126
  differential diagnosis between endocervical adenocarcinoma and, 124
  endometrioid carcinoma mimicking ovarian sex-cord tumor, 127
  histopathology, 123–124
  immunohistochemistry and molecular features, 124
  immunophenotypes, 135
  intra-luminal papillae in, 128
  macroscopy, 123
  prognosis and predictive factors, 130
  with squamous differentiation, 125
  variants, 125–126
  vimentin positive, 129
Endometritis, 1, 31, 37, 41
  classification, 37
  morphological subtypes, 39–41
Endometrium, 16, 21, 168–169
  blood supply, 10–11
  composition, 9
  dilatation and curettage, 1–2
  endometrial glands, 9
  endometrial tissue, 3
  extramedullary hematopoiesis in, 85–86
  forms, 7
  glial tissue in, 85
  indications for sampling endometrium, 1
  inflammatory cells, 10
  late secretory-phase, 36
  lymphoma-like lesion, 74–75
  nodular histiocytic hyperplasia, 75
  outpatient sampling by endometrial aspirate, 2–3
  plexiform tumorlet of uterus, 75–76
  sampling, 1–2
  stroma, 9–10
  tissue artifacts, 3–4
  tumor-like lesions of, 74
Endomyometrium, 168
Endoreduplications, 157
Endovascular trophoblast, 21–22
  cells, 22
  intraluminal, 28, 31
  migration and conversion, 27
Eosinophilic metaplasia, 77, 79–80
Eosinophilic syncytial change, *see* Papillary syncytial metaplasia

Eosinophils, 10, 36–38
Epithelial
  cells, 139
  cytokeratins, 39
  nucleus, 12
Epithelioid smooth muscle tumor, 168
Epithelioid trophoblastic tumor (ETT), 147, 163, 166, 170; *see also* Placental site trophoblastic tumor (PSTT)
  ancillary studies, 167–168
  clinical features, 166
  diagnostic features, 166–167
  differential diagnosis, 168
  macroscopic features, 166
ESC, *see* Endometrial serous carcinoma
ESN, *see* Endometrial stromal nodule
Estrogen, 47, 54, 91
  deficiency, 43, 45, 53
  estrogen-associated endometrial malignancies, 114
  estrogen-only hormone therapy, 54
Estrogen receptor (ER), 72, 75
European Society for Medical Oncology (ESMO), 101, 124
Exaggerated placental site (EPS), 163, 168
  clinical features, 168
  diagnostic features and ancillary studies, 168–169
  differential diagnosis, 169
Excessive blood loss, 30
Extracellular eosinophilic fibrinoid material, 165
Extramedullary hematopoiesis in endometrium, 78, 85–86
Extrauterine
  lesion, 157
  pregnancy, 26
Extravillous trophoblast, 21–23, 25, 27–28, 30–31

Fallopian tube, 7, 10, 21, 122, 163
Familial biparental hydatidiform mole (FBHM), 157
Fertilization of ovum, 21
Fetal somatic tissue, 25
Fetus, 24–26, 32
FFPE, *see* Formalin-fixed paraffin-embedded
Fibrillary tissues, 25, 27
Fibrin, 17, 41, 72
Fibroblastic metaplasia of stromal cells, 117
FIGO, *see* International Federation of Gynecology and Obstetrics
Fluorescence in-situ hybridization (FISH), 72

Foamy cells, 123–124, 128
Focal necrotising endometritis, 37, 41
Follicle-stimulating hormone (FSH), 7–8
Follicular phase, 7–8, 18
Formalin-fixed paraffin-embedded (FFPE), 153–154
Functional abnormal uterine bleeding
  anovulatory cycles, 44
  dysfunctional uterine bleeding, 43–44
  estrogen deficiency, 45
  irregular shedding, 45
  luteal phase defect, 44–45

Gastric metaplasia, 77, 81
Genetic factors of endometrial carcinoma risk, 114
Genome-wide methods, 113
Genomic aberrations, 147
Genomic constitutions, 147, 149
Genotyping
  analysis, 84
  interpretation of STR genotyping data, 154–155, 156
  principles and technical aspects of STR genotyping, 153–154
  problems with STR genotyping, 155
  by STR polymorphism analysis, 152
  studies, 158–160
Germ cell origin, 161
Gestational choriocarcinoma, 161, 163
Gestational endometrium, 21, 26
Gestational trophoblastic disease (GTD), 147
  abnormal (non-molar) villous lesion, 160–161
  androgenetic/biparental mosaic/chimeric conceptions, 157–160
  choriocarcinoma, 161–163
  EPS, 168–169
  ETT, 166–168
  HM, 149–157
  normal histology and immunohistochemistry of trophoblasts, 147–149
  placental site trophoblastic tumor, 164–166
  PSN, 169–170
  unclassified trophoblastic lesions, 170–171
Gestational trophoblastic neoplasia (GTN), 149
Gestations, 147, 160–161
Gestrinone, 60–61
Gland-in-gland structure, 96–97
Gland-to-stroma ratio, 3, 93, 95
Gland-within-gland artifact, 4

Gland crowding, 95–96, 99
Glandular epithelium, 3, 9, 16, 36, 39, 96, 99
Glandular growth pattern, 132–133
Glandular lumina, 11, 37–38, 77
Glial tissue in endometrium, 78, 85
Gonadotrophin-releasing hormone agonists (GnRH agonists), 60
　endometrial effects of, 61
Granulated lymphocytes, 15–16, 35
Granulomatous endometritis, 39–40
Growth factors, 18
GTD, see Gestational trophoblastic disease
GTN, see Gestational trophoblastic neoplasia
Gynecologic Oncology Group (GOG), 115

H-caldesmon, 70, 72, 75, 85, 143, 168
hCG assay, see Human chorionic gonadotropin assay
Hematologic diseases, 86
Hematoxylin-and-eosin staining, 11
Hemorrhage, 2, 93, 161
　focal, 164
　postpartum, 30
Hemostasis, 17
Hereditary nonpolyposis colorectal cancer syndrome (HNPCC), 94, 114
Herpes simplex cervicitis, 40–41
Histiocytic endometritis, see Xanthogranulomatous endometritis
Histiocytic nodules, 41
Histologic features of HM, 150
　CHM, 151, 154
　differential diagnostic difficulties in, 153
　PHM, 151–152, 154
Histopathology of early pregnancy, 27
HM, see Hydatidiform mole
HNF-1β biomarker, 135, 138
Hobnail metaplasia, 77, 82–83, 97, 106
Hormone replacement therapy (HRT), see Hormone therapy
Hormone therapy, 53, 60–61
　combined hormone-therapy regimes, 54–56
　estrogen-only, 54
　progestin-only, 56
　SERMs, 56–59
　TSEC, 59
　WHI trial, 53–54
hPL, see Human placental lactogen
Human chorionic gonadotropin assay (hCG assay), 25, 148

Human placental lactogen (hPL), 148, 165–166
Hydatidiform mole (HM), 147, 149
　clinical significance, 149
　genotyping by STR polymorphism analysis, 152–155
　histologic features, 150, 151–154
　immunohistochemistry for P57, 150, 152, 154–155
　invasive, 157
　molecular pathology, 149
　unusual genotypic findings or presentations in, 155–157
Hydropic abortions, 160
Hyperemesis, 149
Hyperplasia, 1, 91; see also Metaplasia
Hyperplasia without atypia, see Benign hyperplasia
Hyperprolactinemia, 45
Hypoplastic endometrium, 45
Hypothalamic dysfunction, 45
Hypothalamic–pituitary–ovarian axis, 43, 45
Hysterectomy specimen(s), 3, 48, 75, 107, 169
　of postmenopausal endometrium, 17
　radical, 123
　from tamoxifen-treated women, 57
Hysteroscopic-directed sampling, 2
Hysteroscopy, 1–3

Iatrogenic disease
　contraception, 47–49
　endometrial ablation, 59–60
　hormone therapy, 53–59
　hormone treatment, 60–61
　intrauterine contraceptive devices, 49–51
　SPRM, 51–53
Ichthyosis uteri, 76–77
Immunohistochemical
　and genotyping studies, 158–160
　markers for types of trophoblasts, 147–149
　profiles for differential diagnosis of trophoblastic tumors, 168
Immunohistochemistry, 72, 147
　and CCC, 138
　in diagnosis of EIN/AH, 101
　in EmGD diagnosis, 103–105
　and endometrioid carcinoma, 124
　interpretation of, 155
　for P57, 150, 152
　of trophoblasts, 147–149
　typical results and interpretation, 154
　and undifferentiated carcinomas, 142
Inconspicuous

　cytoplasm, 9
　spiral arteries, 114
Induced abortion, tissue from, 24–25
Infertility, 1, 18–19, 40, 44–45, 84
Infiltrative border, 71–72, 165
Inflammation, 25, 31, 38; see also Endometrial inflammation
　acute, 31, 119
　ligneous, 41
　neutrophilic, 99
Inflammatory cells, 7, 10, 16, 35, 130
　chronic, 59
　stromal, 49
Intermediate trophoblasts (IT), 148, 161
International Federation of Gynecology and Obstetrics (FIGO), 43, 115
　grade 3 endometrioid carcinoma, 142–143
　grading system, 115–116
　group of ovulatory disorders, 43
　staging system, 121
Interstitial trophoblast, 21–22, 28
Intestinal metaplasia, 77, 80
Intra-luminal papillae, 133, 140
　in endometrioid carcinoma, 128
Intracytoplasmic
　mucin, 80, 130
　organisms, 39
Intraepithelial lymphocytes, 36
Intraluminal endovascular trophoblast, 28, 31
Intraluminal mucin, 130
Intramyometrial segments, 27
Intraplacental choriocarcinoma, 163
Intrauterine contraceptive devices (IUCD), 48–51
　endometrial effects of non-medicated intrauterine devices, 52–53
Intrauterine pregnancy, 1, 24–26
Invasive HM, 157
Invasive mole, 157
Involuted placental beds, 30
Irregular endomyometrial junction, 116
Irregular shedding, 26, 45
Isolated tumor cells (ITCs), 115
Isthmic endometrium, 18, 68
Isthmus, 8

JAZF1-SUZ12 gene fusion, 72

Ki67 proliferation index, 168–169
Killer immunoglobulin-like receptors (KIR), 22–23
KRAS mutation analysis, 70, 81–82, 130

Lacunae, 21–22
Langhans giant cells, 40

Laser ablation
   endometrial cavity, 60
   endometrium following, 59
Leucocytes, 10, 16
   endometrial stromal, 35
   in postmenopausal endometrium, 37
Levonorgestrel-releasing intrauterine contraceptive devices, 48
   endometrial atrophy, 51
   pseudodecidualized surface stroma, 51
   surface epithelial cells, 51
Ligneous
   endometritis, 41
   inflammation, 41
Lipids, 13, 18
   lipid-laden macrophages, 28
Low grade endometrial stromal sarcoma (LG-ESS), 71
Luteal phase, 7–8
   defect, 18, 44–45
Luteinizing hormone (LH), 7–8
Lymphoid aggregates, 10, 30, 35, 37
Lymphoma-like lesion, 74–75
Lymphovascular invasion, 157
   endometrioid carcinoma with, 122
Lymphovascular space invasion (LVSI), 121
Lynch syndrome (LS), 1, 94, 114, 124

Macroscopy, 123, 131
Malakoplakia, 37, 39, 75
Mast cells, 10, 36–37
Maternal allele(s), 150, 153–155
Medroxy-progesterone acetate (MPA), 48, 115
   endometrial effects, 50
   scanty mitoses in glands and stroma, 51
MELF myometrial invasive pattern, *see* Microcystic elongated and fragmented myometrial invasive pattern
Menometrorrhagia, 43
Menopausal hormone therapy (MHT), *see* Hormone therapy
Menorrhagia, 43, 61
Menstrual cycle(s), 7–9, 11, 44
   histological features of endometrium through, 12
   menstrual phase, 16–17
   proliferative, 11, 13–14
   secretory, 11–16
Menstrual phase, 10, 16–17
Menstruation, 7–8, 11, 17, 30, 35–36, 43–45, 139
Mesenchymal malignancies, 143

Metaplasia, 76
   changes, 76–86
   endometrial, 76–86, 106
   endometrial epithelial, 76–84
Metastatic mole, 157
Metrorrhagia, 43
Microabscesses, 51
Microcystic elongated and fragmented myometrial invasive pattern (MELF myometrial invasive pattern), 118–120, 122
Micrometastasis (MM), 115
Microsatellite instability (MSI), 142
Mid proliferative-phase endometrium, 13
Mifepristone, 53
Minipill, *see* Progestin-only contraceptive pill (POP)
Miscarriage, 18, 24–26, 28, 31–32, 40
Mismatch repair genes (MMR genes), 124
Mitotic activity, 8–9, 11–13, 38, 47, 55, 57, 69, 73–74, 80, 83, 97, 126, 130, 169–170
   in A-S reaction, 139
   brisk, 84, 106
   variable, 93
Mixed endometrial carcinoma, 143
Mixed ESC and endometrioid carcinoma, 134
Molar pregnancy, 24–25, 31, 160–161, 163–164, 166
Molecular mediators, 18
Molecular pathology of HM, 149
Mononuclear cytotrophoblast cells, 21
Mononucleate cells, 161–164, 166
Monospermic fertilization, 157
Morphological subtypes of endometritis, 39
   granulomatous endometritis, 39–40
   malakoplakia, 39
   miscellaneous, 41
   viral endometritis, 40–41
   xanthogranulomatous endometritis, 39
Morular metaplasia, *see* Morules
Morules, 69, 76–78
   central necrosis, 79
   in endometrial hyperplasia, 79
MPA, *see* Medroxy-progesterone acetate
MSI, *see* Microsatellite instability
Mucinous
   adenocarcinoma, 81
   carcinoma, 130–131
   metaplasia, 80–82
Müllerian adenosarcoma, *see* Adenosarcoma
Multinuclear syncytiotrophoblast cells, 21
Myelomonocytic cells, 21
Myomatous stroma, 69–70

Myometrial invasion, 73, 91, 98, 115–116, 135
   adenocarcinoma with, 70
   measurement, 116, 118
   patterns, 118–120
Myometrium, 7–8, 10, 15, 27, 60, 68–70, 73, 75, 85, 117, 120, 164, 166; *see also* Endometrium
   interface, 116
   without intervening decidua, 29
   penetration, 30
   superficial, 28, 117, 168

Napsin A stain, CCC with, 141
Narrow secretory-pattern glands, 55
Natural killer cells (NK cells), 10, 35
Necrosis, 25, 31, 161
Neisseria gonorrhoea, 39
Neutrophils, 38
Nitabuch's layer, 23
NLRP7/KHDC3L gene mutations, 157
Nodular histiocytic hyperplasia, 41, 75
Non-gestational choriocarcinoma, 163
Non-molar
   conceptions, 152
   gestation, 154, 156
Non-necrotising granulomas, 40
Non-neoplastic trophoblastic lesions, 147
Noninvolution, *see* Subinvolution
Nonmedicated intrauterine contraceptive devices, 49, 51
   endometrial effects, 52–53
Nonspecific chronic endometritis, 37, 39
Nonspecific endometritis, 37
   etiology, 38–39
   pathological features, 37–38
Nonvillous migratory trophoblast, 21
Normal blood supply to placenta, 24
Normal endometrial inflammatory cells, 35
Normal endometrium, 35–37; *see also* Endometrium; Myometrium
   composition, 9–11
   cuboidal epithelium with clefts dipping into spindly stroma, 7
   dating endometrium, 18–19
   endometrium in body of uterus, 8
   functional layer, 9
   menstrual cycle, 11–17
   postmenopausal endometrium, 17–18
Normal placentation, 23
Normal pregnancy, 161, 163, 168
Nuclear atypia, 80, 95, 130, 165

Occasional hemosiderin-laden macrophages, 30
Occasional multinucleate giant cells, 39

Osseous metaplasia, 78, 84–85
Oval hyperchromatic nuclei, 9
Ovarian dysfunction, 43
Ovulatory phase, 7–8

p16 immunohistochemistry in endometrial polyp, 68
p53 marker
    CCC with, 140
    EmGD with, 104
    expression in clear-cell EmGD, 108
    gene, 124
    stain, 103
p57 marker
    immunohistochemistry for, 150, 152
    immunostaining, 152–153
    interpretation, 155
    results and interpretation, 154
p63 marker, 78, 125, 148
PAEC, see Progesterone receptor modulator-associated endometrial changes
Palisaded histiocytes, 60
PALM-COEIN, see Polyp, adenomyosis, leiomyoma, malignancy and hyperplasia, coagulopathy, ovulatory disorders, endometrium, iatrogenic and not otherwise classified
Papillary
    growth pattern, 132
    proliferation, 83–84
    syncytial metaplasia, 81–83, 97
Parametrial invasion, 122–123
Parietalis, 25
Partial hydatidiform mole (PHM), 149, 151, 154, 160
PAS stain, see Periodic acid–Schiff stain
PAX2 biomarker, 94, 97, 101, 124, 134–135
Pelvic artery embolization, 32
Periodic acid–Schiff stain (PAS stain), 41, 80
Perivascular lymphocytic infiltrate, 28
Phloxine-tartrazine stain, 10
PHM, see Partial hydatidiform mole
'Physiological vascular changes', 23
Phytoestrogens, 59
Pill, see Combined oral contraceptive pill (COP)
Pipelle device, 2–3
Placenta accreta, 30, 32
Placenta increta, 29
Placental alkaline phosphatase (PLAP), 148
Placental mesenchymal dysplasia (PMD), 156, 160; see also Endometrial glandular dysplasia (EmGD)

Placental site nodule (PSN), 168–169
    atypical, 170
    clinical features, 169
    diagnostic features and ancillary studies, 169–170
    differential diagnosis, 170
Placental site nodule and plaque, see Placental site nodule (PSN)
Placental site trophoblastic tumor (PSTT), 147, 163–164, 168–170; see also Epithelioid trophoblastic tumor (ETT)
    ancillary studies, 165–166
    clinical features, 164
    diagnostic features, 164–165
    macroscopic features, 164
Placenta percreta, 29
Placentation, 21
    decidua vera, 24
    implantation site and nine weeks gestation, 22
    interstitial trophoblast infiltrating interstitium, 22
    normal blood supply to placenta, 24
    normal placentation, 23
Plasma cells, 10, 36, 38–39, 41
Plasma progesterone levels, 7–8, 12, 21
Platelet plugs, 17
Plexiform tumorlet of uterus, 75–76
Polar trophoblastic proliferation, 160
Polymenorrhea, 43
Polymorphic fetal human leukocyte antigen-C molecules, 22–23
Polyp, adenomyosis, leiomyoma, malignancy and hyperplasia, coagulopathy, ovulatory disorders, endometrium, iatrogenic and not otherwise classified (PALM-COEIN), 43
POP, see Progestin-only contraceptive pill
Post-laser ablation, 59
Postmenopausal endometrium, 17–18, 37
Postpartum hemorrhage, 30
PR, see Progesterone receptor
Pre-pregnancy, 21
Precursors
    of endometrial serous carcinoma, 101–106
    of endometrioid carcinoma, 91–101
Pregnancy
    abnormal, 27–30
    abortion, 24–27
    chemotherapy, 32
    endometrial ablation, 32
    pelvic artery embolization, 32
    placentation, 21–24

    postpartum hemorrhage, 30–32
    radiotherapy, 32
    therapy, 32
Primary ovarian disease, 45
Primary postpartum hemorrhage, 30
Progesterone receptor (PR), 72
Progesterone receptor modulator-associated endometrial changes (PAEC), 53
Progestin-only contraceptive pill (POP), 48
Progestin(s), 47–49
    levonorgestrel-releasing intrauterine devices, endometrial effects of, 51–52
    medroxyprogesterone acetate, endometrial effects of, 50–51
    progestin-only hormone therapy, 56
    progestin-releasing intrauterine devices, 49
    progestin treatment, endometrial effects of, 48–50
    treatment effect, 100
Progestogens, 47
Proliferative endometrium, 44
Proliferative phase, 11
    early proliferative-phase endometrium, 13
    inconspicuous spiral arteries, 114
    late proliferative-phase endometrium, 13
    mid proliferative-phase endometrium, 13
Pseudodecidua, 21
Pseudolipomatosis, 4
Pseudorosette-like proliferation, 85
Pseudostratification, 11
PSN, see Placental site nodule
PSTT, see Placental site trophoblastic tumor
PTEN gene, 70, 94, 101, 114, 124
Putative precursor for ECCC, 107–109

Quantitative fluorescent polymerase chain reaction (QF-PCR), 159

Radiation, 114
Radiotherapy, 32
Raloxifene, 56
Reactive reparative changes of benign endometrium, 106
Recurrent HM, 156–157
Retained placental fragment, 30–31
Retraction of stroma around glands, 4
Reverse transcriptase-polymerase chain reaction (RT-PCR), 72
Rohr's striae, 23

Sampling artifacts, 96–97; *see also* Tissue artifacts
Scattered multinucleated cells, 166
Secondary postpartum hemorrhage, 30
Secretory-type EIN/AH, 98
Secretory carcinoma, 125–126
Secretory endometrium, 16, 26, 37, 93–94, 138
Secretory exhaustion, 16
Secretory phase, 11
　granulated lymphocytes, 16
　plasma progesterone levels, 12
　prominent spiral arteries, 15
　secretory-phase endometrium, 14–15, 44
　stratum compactum adjacent, 15
　stromal cells, 13
Selective estrogen receptor modulators (SERMs), 56
　endometrial cancer, 57, 59
　endometrial effects of tamoxifen treatment, 57
　endometrioid adenocarcinoma in tamoxifen-associated polyp, 58
　hysterectomy specimen from tamoxifen-treated woman, 57
　macroscopic features of tamoxifen-associated diffuse endometrial hyperplasia, 58
　tamoxifen-associated endometrial hyperplasia, 58
Selective progesterone receptor modulator (SPRM), 51–53
　endometrial effects, 53–54
Sequential hormone therapy, 54, 56
Serous carcinoma markers, 143
Serous endometrial intraepithelial carcinoma (SEIC), 67, 101, 106, 114, 131–132, 135
Sex hormones, 17–18
Short tandem repeat (STR), 153, 163
　interpretation of STR genotyping data, 154–155, 156
　principles and technical aspects of STR genotyping, 153–154
SIL, *see* Squamous intraepithelial lesion
Single nucleotide polymorphism (SNP), 159
Smooth-muscle
　markers, 72, 75, 143
　metaplasia, 78, 85, 117
Solid growth pattern, 132, 134
　CCC with, 139
Somatic-type malignancy, 163
Spindle-cell variant, 126
Spindly fibroblast-like stroma, 45
Spiral arteries, 16, 22–23, 26
　and arterioles, 11
　lumen, 29
Spontaneous abortion, tissue from, 24–26
SPRM, *see* Selective progesterone receptor modulator
Squamous
　epithelial, 125
　metaplasia, 76, 78
　morule, 125
Squamous cell carcinoma of cervix, 168, 170
Squamous intraepithelial lesion (SIL), 128
STR, *see* Short tandem repeat
Stroma(l), 8–10, 16
　cells, 9
　edema, 9, 12–13
　granulocytes, 35
　invasion, 126
　lymphocytes, 39
　mitosis, 9
Subinvolution, 30–31
Submucosal cellular leiomyoma, 71
Subnuclear vacuolation, 11–12
Superficial myometrium, 28, 117, 168–169
Supra-nuclear vacuolation, 12
Surface papillary syncytial change, *see* Papillary syncytial metaplasia
Syncytiotrophoblasts, 147, 152, 161
Synovial-like metaplasia, 85

Tamoxifen, 56
　tamoxifen-associated endometrial hyperplasia, 58
　tamoxifen-associated polyps, 57
　therapy, 65
T cells, 21, 23, 35, 37, 74
Telescope' glands, *see* Gland-in-gland structure
Telescoping effect of glands, 4
Tetraploid hydatidiform mole, 155–156
The Cancer Genome Atlas (TCGA), 113, 124, 134, 138
Tibolone, 60–61
Tissue
　fragmentation, 96–97
　from induced abortions, 24–25
　from pregnancies of unknown location and ectopic pregnancy, 26–27
　from spontaneous abortions, 25–26
Tissue-selective estrogen complex (TSEC), 59
Tissue artifacts, 3
　artifactual crowding of glands, 4
　gland-within-gland artifact, 4
　pseudolipomatosis, 4
　retraction of stroma around glands, 4
　telescoping effect of glands, 4
T lymphocytes, 10, 35
Toxemia, 149
TP53 mutations, 124, 131, 138
Trans-tubal metastasis, 122
Transcervical resection of endometrium, 60
Transvaginal ultrasonography and hysteroscopy, 1
Trauma, 2
Trophoblastic/trophoblasts, 147–148, 161
　atypia, 160
　cells, 161
　hyperplasia, 158
　immunohistochemical markers for types, 147–149
　normal histology and immunohistochemistry, 147
　pseudoinclusion, 160
　syncytium, 21–22
　tumors, 147, 163, 168
　unclassified trophoblastic lesions, 170–171
TSEC, *see* Tissue-selective estrogen complex
Tubal metaplasia, 77–79
Tuberculous endometritis, 19, 40
Tumor-like lesions of endometrium, 74–76
Twin gestation with HM coexisting with non-molar gestation, 156–157

Ulipristal acetate, 53
Ultrasound, 115
　assay, 25
　scan, 149
Undifferentiated carcinoma, 142–143
Unopposed estrogen, 1, 54, 92, 114
Unusual genotypic findings or presentations in HM, 155
　HM with gain or loss of chromosomes, 156
　recurrent HM, 156–157
　tetraploid hydatidiform mole, 155–156
　twin gestation with HM coexisting with non-molar gestation, 156
Uterine
　artery, 10
　bleeding, 43
　lumen, 16
　natural killer cells, 21–23
'Uterine adenomyoma', *see* Adenomyomatous polyp
Uterine tumor resembling ovarian sex cord tumor (UTROSCT), 72, 75

Uteroplacental
  artery, 23
  circulation, 22
Uterus, 8, 10, 17–18, 56, 94
  blood supply to, 11
  plexiform tumorlet of, 75–76

Vabra aspirator, 2
Vacuolar stromal edema, 49
Vascular endothelial growth factor (VEGF), 11

Very early CHM (VECHM), 150
Villi, 23–26, 29, 147, 150, 156, 158, 160
Villoglandular
  carcinoma, 125
  endometrioid carcinoma with lymphovascular invasion, 121
  ESC with villoglandular architecture, 133
Villous tissue, 154–155
Vimentin positive, 85, 129
Vira

  endometritis, 37, 40–41
  infection, 40

'Window of implantation or receptivity', 18
Women's Health Initiative (WHI), 53–54

Xanthogranulomatous endometritis, 37, 39

Zygote, 21, 157

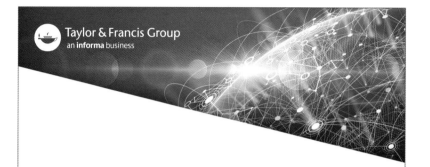